DRUGS FOR HEART DISEASE

DRUGS FOR HEART DISEASE

SECOND EDITION

Edited by

John Hamer MD. Ph.D F.R.C.P.

Formerly Consultant Cardiologist
St Bartholomew's Hospital
London

SPRINGER-SCIENCE+BUSINESS MEDIA, B.V.

© 1987 Springer Science+Business Media Dordrecht
Originally published by Chapman and Hall Ltd in 1987
Softcover reprint of the hardcover 2nd edition 1987

ISBN 978-0-412-26540-2

British Library Cataloguing in Publication Data

Drugs for heart disease.—2nd ed.
  1. Cardiovascular system—Diseases—
Chemotherapy
  I. Hamer, John, *1927–*
616.1'061   RC669

ISBN 978-0-412-26540-2   ISBN 978-1-4899-3294-5 (eBook)
DOI 10.1007/978-1-4899-3294-5

Contents

Contents

Contents

Contents

Contents

Preface to the second edition

This book is the outcome of a cardiologist switching to clinical pharmacology in mid-career and may be seen as representing the interface between the two disciplines. In this second edition I have not tried to be encyclopaedic, but have asked the contributors to give a brief account of current practice, so that it represents the present state of cardiac therapeutics.

Although some contributors are from Bart's, I have tried to spread my net widely and produce a general view from the English speaking world. I hope this will be enough to draw the teeth of my colleagues who will react at once to say that 'this is not what we do at Bart's.'

Some chapters, mostly the early ones, are drug orientated and describe the use and properties of individual groups of drugs. Other later chapters are disease orientated and describe the use of various groups of drugs in different conditions, such as angina or hypertension. This necessarily leads to some overlap, but I have not tried to produce a uniformity of view, but have been content with Chairman Mao 'to let a hundred flowers bloom'. I am grateful to my cardiological colleague, Professor A. John Camm for his help and advice on current cardiological practice.

To improve the flow of the text I have limited the references to key publications, rather than trying to quote all the papers published on each topic. Obsessional collectors of bibliography will find their needs met by collecting the references in the references.

Surrey   John Hamer
1986

Preface to the first edition

This book reviews the clinical pharmacology of cardiovascular drugs. I have started from the premise that 'clinical pharmacology' is the scientific study of the use of drugs in man. It is inevitably necessary to refer to much basic work in animals as it is not technically feasible to investigate drug actions on the myocardium at a cellular level in man, or ethically acceptable to use invasive methods to study drug action in patients unless opportunities arise during diagnostic investigation. I have sought to avoid the detailed consideration of mechanisms derived from animal pharmacology, but to draw on animal work for features helpful in the understanding of the response of human disease to treatment.

The apparent remoteness of animal pharmacology from clinical practice is in part responsible for the emergence of Clinical Pharmacology as a new independent discipline with immediate relevance to the treatment of patients, and it is this aspect of pharmacology I am seeking to emphasize in relation to my experience as a clinical cardiologist. In numerical terms, cardiovascular disease forms half of medicine and it is hoped that the book will be of interest to general physicians as well as to specialist cardiologists and trainees.

The early activity of clinical pharmacology has been connected with the development of techniques to measure drug concentrations in blood and other biological fluids. This development has led to a close concern with 'pharmacokinetics', i.e. the way drugs are handled in the body, and is dealt with in the final chapter (13) which outlines the advantages of measuring drug blood levels and the techniques in current use; it is hoped that this section will be helpful to physicians planning to set up such a service. Blood level measurements lend themselves to the study of pharmacokinetics, including the comparison of different formulations of a drug (bioavailability), and to the study of drug interactions. Although a knowledge of how drugs are handled in the body is fundamental to their sensible use in treatment, I hope to avoid the impression that blood level measurement is the essential basis of the discipline.

Clinical pharmacology is primarily concerned with the selection of appropriate therapy, and adjustment of dose and administration of drugs to the needs of the patient. I have attempted to consider the mechanisms

xiii

Preface to the first edition

of drug action, the absorption, metabolism excretion of drugs (pharmaco-kinetics); the effects of the drugs in man (pharmacodynamics), and the rational use of the drugs in disease, including interactions with other drugs and toxic effects.

I have attempted to marshall and synthesize the often contradictory reports from the continuously growing medical literature to give a picture of the current state of therapeutics in the light of my experience as a clinical cardiologist in academic, hospital and private practice, and as an undergraduate and postgraduate teacher both in England and in the United States. My early experience as a registrar to both William Evans and Clifford Hoyle, who showed the way with a sound study of drugs for angina, gave me a healthy scepticism about the effects of drugs in heart disease, which susbequent contact with the pharmaceutical industry has failed to eradicate, although it has helped me to appreciate the problems of the development of new drugs and their introduction into thera-peutics. I was personally fortunate to be early in the field when beta-blockers appeared and comparative studies have led to a continued interest in antiarrhythmic drugs.

This is something of a Bart's book and I am particularly grateful for outside help with the prostaglandin chapter from my friends of the Wellcome Foundation. I seek understanding from authors who will feel that insufficient prominence is given to their research and from phar-maceutical companies who may consider the advantages of their drugs inadequately described. If many doctors handle drugs badly the fault must lie in part with their training. It is my aim to correct such faults in my own field and to expiate my previous sins in this respect!

London   John Hamer
November, 1977

xiv

Contributors

Ann Errichetti, MD
Fellow in Clinical Pharmacology
University of Massachusetts Medical School
Department of Medicine
Worcester
Massachusetts 01605
USA

Dr D.J. Galton, MSc, MD, FRCP
Consultant Physician
St Bartholomew's Hospital
London EC1A 7BE

Dr John Hamer, MD, PhD, FRCP
Consultant Cardiologist, now retired
Department of Clinical Pharmacology
St Bartholomew's Hospital
London EC1A 7BE

Dr Roger Hayward, MD, MRCP
Senior Registrar
Department of Cardiology
Middlesex Hospital
Mortimer Street
London W1N 8AA

Professor Brian F. Johnson, MB, FRCP
Professor of Medicine and Pharmacology
University of Massachusetts Medical School
Department of Medicine
Worcester
Massachusetts 01605
USA

Contributors

Mr Atholl Johnston
Head of Analytical Unit
Department of Clinical Pharmacology
St Bartholomew's Hospital
London EC1A 7BE

Dr N.I. Jowett
Honorary Senior Registrar
Department of Diabetes and Lipids
St Bartholomew's Hospital
London EC1A 7BE

Dr Cyrus R. Kumana, B.Sc, MB, FRCP (London & Canada)
Reader in Clinical Pharmacology
University of Hong Kong
Department of Medicine
Queen Mary Hospital
Hong Kong

Professor Ariel Lant
Department of Therapeutics
Charing Cross and Westminster Medical School
Page St Wing
Westminster Hospital
London SW1P 2AP

Professor J.R.A. Mitchell, BSc, MD, DPhil, MA, FRCP
Foundation Professor of Medicine
Department of Medicine
University Hospital
Queen's Medical Centre
Nottingham NG7 2UH

Mr S.G. Moody
Department of Clinical Therapeutics
Wellcome Research Laboratories
Langley Court
Beckenham
Kent BR3 3BS

Dr J. O'Grady, MD, MRCP
Clinical Research Manager
May & Baker Limited
Rainham Road South
Dagenham
Essex RM10 7XS

Professor Lionel H. Opie, MD, PhD, FRCP
Professor of Medicine
University of Cape Town
Department of Medicine
Medical School
Observatory 7925
Cape Town
South Africa

Professor Leon Resnekov, MD, FRCP
Frederick H. Rawson Professor of Medicine
University of Chicago
Department of Medicine/Cardiology
950 East 59th Street
Chicago
Illinois 60637, USA

Professor U. Thadani, MBBS, MRCP, FRCP (c)
Professor of Medicine and Director of Clinical Cardiology
Department of Medicine
University of Oklahoma
Oklahoma City
Oklahoma 73190
USA

1 Antiarrhythmic drugs

JOHN HAMER

1.1 Introduction – pharmacokinetics

The classification of antiarrhythmic drugs proposed by Vaughan Williams in 1970 [1, 2] has stood the test of time and is widely used as a shorthand expression of drug effect. The four classes, conventionally described by Roman numerals (I–IV) on the basis of effect on action potential (Fig. 1.1), have remained unchanged and although criticized as not clinically relevant seem to describe fundamental ways in which abnormal rhythms can be controlled. Class I has been subdivided (Ia, Ib, Ic) on the perhaps naive basis of the effect of those drugs on action potential duration (APD) [2]. Class V was initiated for a new group of drugs which seemed to slow the rate by an effect on Cl ion currents in the pacemaker [3]. These drugs have not been developed because of toxicity problems. They might have found a place in control of angina but are not truly antiarrhythmic and were described cynically as antiarrhythmic drugs searching for an arrhythmia to treat.

Overlap between the classes is seen with several drugs and has caused some confusion among pharmacologists. For instance the beta-blocker, propranolol (Class II), has membrane-stabilizing actions (Class I) in high concentration, but these are a pharmacological curiosity not achieved in ordinary antiarrhythmic treatment [4]. The concept of a drug having actions of several classes has seemed useful at times. For instance amiodarone is Class II acutely after an intravenous dose and Class III in long-term oral therapy. I was shocked to hear a well-known pharmacologist say that one should not do that as 'a drug does what a drug does', but I am unrepentant as the concept of overlapping classes seems to aid understanding.

The effect of Class I drugs on cell membrane Na current, seen as reduced rate of rise of the depolarization of the negative intracellular resting potential (Fig 1.1), suggests an action on the cell membrane which might be closely related to the plasma level of drug bathing the cell

1

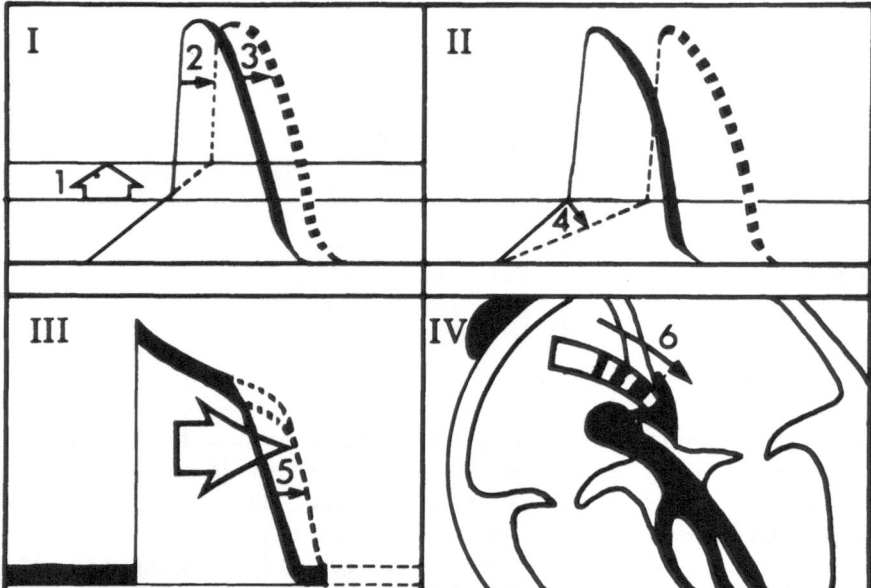

Fig. 1.1 Modified with permission from Krikler.[5] Diagrammatic representation of the effect of the four Vaughan Williams classes (Roman numerals) of anti-arrhythmic drugs on the action potential. Control action potential is shown as a solid line, action potential after the drug by a dotted line. The arabic numerals show the major drug effects. *Class I* Membrane stabilizing drugs such as quinidine and lignocaine act mainly by block of passive depolarizing Na ion entry evident as: 1. Elevation of threshold potential of pacemaker cells. Rising diastolic (pacemaker) potential must continue longer before depolarization is triggered, so that pacemaker rate is slowed. 2. Reduced rate of rise of action potential due to interference with Na ion influx. This sensitive index of Class I effect is not usually obvious without electrical differentiation of the rate of rise, but has the secondary effect of reducing conduction of activation from cell to cell which may be the major antiarrhythmic effect of the Class I drugs, and gives rise to QRS prolongation which may be a useful index of drug effect. 3. Prolongation of the action potential is seen with subclass Ia drugs (quinidine) probably as a secondary effect on K efflux during repolarization. It produces a long QT interval in the electrocardiogram and is generally regarded as an indication of toxicity of these drugs. *Class II* Sympathetic antagonism is seen with beta-adrenergic blocking drugs as: 4. Slowing of the rate of rise of the diastolic (pacemaker) potential which is under autonomic control, so that the pacemaker rate is slowed. The action potential when triggered is normal. This mechanism blocks any tachycardia due to sympathetic stimulation and may play a part in reducing the activity of ectopic pacemakers produced by sympathetic stimulation. Conduction in the atrioventricular (AV) node is also slowed by block of sympathetic tone. *Class III* Drugs acting specifically to prolong the action potential, such as amiodarone, by: 5. Delay of repolarization by selective interference with K efflux currents, without change in the activation process of Na ion entry shown by the rate of rise of the action potential. The prolonged action potential delays resetting of resting poten-

surface, giving support to the concept of plasma level monitoring [6, 7] and stresses the importance of understanding the pharmacokinetics of a drug in interpreting its clinical action. Half the time lignocaine does not work it is because of a misunderstanding of its pharmacokinetics [8]. Simple correlation of effect with plasma levels is complicated by secondary factors such as plasma-binding or the presence of active metabolites [2, 7]. It is the free (unbound) fraction which is important in producing a pharmacodynamic effect. Sophisticated plasma measurements may be needed to separate these effects by measuring free levels [10] or by separate measurement of drug and metabolites. One of the properties sought for an ideal antiarrhythmic drug [2] is prolonged duration of effect, allowing once a day treatment. This is often achieved by active metabolites, but has the disadvantage that the intravenous effect of the drug itself in an acute state may differ from the action in long-term oral therapy where the metabolites play a part [7]. The problem of effective plasma levels in ischaemic tissue where arrhythmias may be generated has been little explored [9].

The philosophy of antiarrhythmic therapy must remain as described previously [9], correct diagnosis leading to consideration of possible alternative lines of treatment such as electroversion or pacing. Application of drug therapy in the light of full knowledge of pharmacokinetics is tempered by the knowledge that all drugs are toxic and may worsen arrthymias [2, 11]. This is particularly evident in the case of 'torsade de pointes' [12] which is characteristically a drug-induced arrhythmia (Fig. 1.2) likely to terminate in ventricular fibrillation and needing a change of approach rather than additional treatment with a possibly provocative drug. Any underlying hypokalaemia should be corrected and over-drive pacing may control the situation temporarily until the effect of the provocative drug has subsided or can be eliminated.

---

tial for further elevation, so that effective refractory period is prolonged, preventing re-entry and terminating arrhythmias. *Class IV* Drugs blocking Ca ion entry such as verapamil, act specifically on the specialized cells of the AV node which rely on slow Ca ion currents, rather than fast Na currents for depolarization. The rate of rise of the slow (calcium current) action potential is probably reduced (not shown). 6. Conduction in the AV node is slowed (barred arrow) and the major action is production of AV nodal block to prevent re-entry or slow the ventricular response to an atrial arrhythmia such as fibrillation. Arrhythmias due to abnormal Ca ion action potentials in other cardiac cells may also be directly inhibited by these drugs. Analogous effects on AV node conduction are produced through modulation of autonomic control such as beta-adrenergic blockade (Class II), the vagal stimulation of digitalis, or the direct effect of adenosine.

3

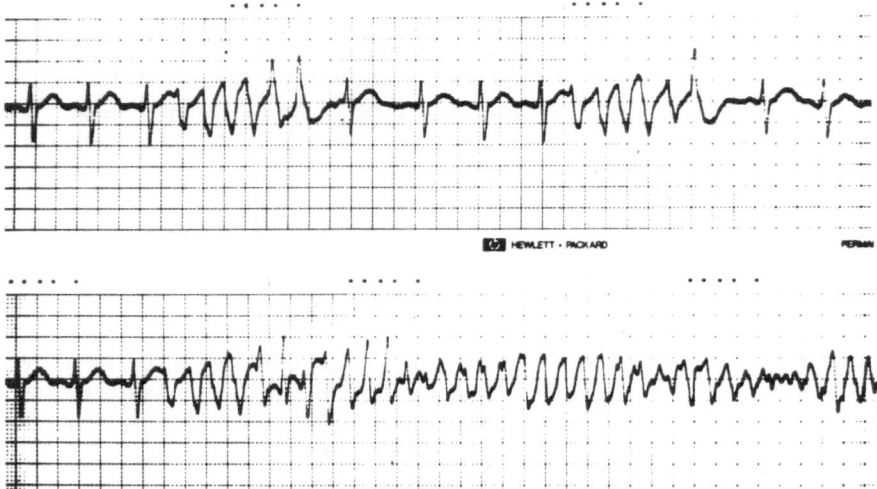

Fig. 1.2 Torsade de pointes without QT prolongation. Two consecutive strips from the coronary care unit ECG monitor. A normal ECG without QT prolongation or T wave changes is interrupted by two bursts (upper row) of torsade de pointes, a polymorphous ventricular tachycardia with changing QRS axis, terminating spontaneously. In the lower row a third burst degenerates into ventricular fibrillation.

1.2 Need for treatment

The major problem is sudden cardiac death, usually due to ventricular fibrillation (VF), either early in cardiac infarction or as a manifestation of extensive coronary artery disease without infarction, as shown by the lack of infarction in some survivors, or in other chronic myocardial disease. Very early in myocardial infarction, at the time of pain, increased sympathetic activity may be a major factor in producing VF [13] suggesting the use of beta-blockers. Later local metabolic changes in the infarct become more important [9] and membrane-stabilizing drugs (Class I) seem more appropriate. The concept of warning arrhythmias allowing the appropriate prophylactic use of antiarrhythmic drugs to prevent VF has proved unreliable [14] leading to the suggestion that routine prophylactic treatment might be employed. The high incidence of adverse effects in the majority not benefiting from treatment does not justify this policy and has led to a probably unrewarding search for alternative new non-toxic drugs. The alternative policy of no treatment while awaiting events in a coronary care unit is countered by the finding that good apparent immediate results of resuscitation may not be maintained in the long term [15]. Most physicians adopt some compromise of prophylactic therapy in patients apparently at high risk in a general setting of a coronary care unit with prompt resuscitation.

The suggestion of risk of sudden death from VF in patients with frequent or bizarre (complex) ventricular ectopic beats in association with acute myocardial infarction or with chronic myocardial disease, justified by the beneficial effect of antiarrhythmic treatment [16] has led to the extension of the concept to healthy subjects in conformity with ideas that go back to Wenckebach that ectopic beats should be sought and stamped out wherever they occur.

These ventricular ectopic beats are very frequent in the normal population [17], although rarely noticed in the absence of anxiety. This approach has given rise to much unnecessary stress to patients told they must take drugs for a 'life-threatening arrhythmia'. Many physicians prefer to follow the teaching of William Evans, formerly on the London Hospital, who held reassuringly that not only were they harmless in a normal heart; but a sign of health! A good long-term study with ambulatory Holter monitoring has confirmed this commonsense idea [18]. Even Dr Lown is converted and has written of ectopic beats in a normal heart 'They no more augur sudden death than a sneeze portends pneumonia' [19]. Clearly some patients with occult disease may be included as apparently healthy in population surveys but in general there seems no need to give potentially toxic drugs to these healthy subjects [20].

The induction of ventricular ectopic beats after exercise during recovery from infarction has proved unreliable as an indication for treatment [21]. The control of spontaneous ectopic beats on Holter monitor may not protect against VF, making the application of effective drug treatment difficult [22]. Similar considerations apply to the situation of ventricular ectopic beats in mitral valve prolapse. The mild cases with a benign course [23] clearly not needing treatment which can be reserved for patients with malignant arrhythmias who may have an associated cardiomyopathy.

1.3 Alternative treatment

The difficulties of antiarrhythmic drug treatment have led to the assessment of alternative approaches. Surgical treatment has attractions where feasible. Resection of ventricular aneurysm has long been known to relieve accompanying arrhythmias which seem to arise in the surrounding intact marginal tissue, so that simple resection of the scar may be ineffective. A large series [24] operated for recurrent ventricular tachycardia with additional endocardial resection also improved left ventricular function. Patients with arrythmias related to local cardiomyopathy, often found in the right ventricle, may similarly be relieved by subendocardial resection, guided by intra-operative mapping [25]. The ability to ablate the His bundle by high energy endocardial shocks suggests a similar approach to arrhythmic foci if they can be located accurately [26].

Paroxysmal junctional tachycardias can be dealt with by scanning pacemakers which interrupt the re-entry process. The implantable defibrillator [27] will provide an alternative to drug treatment for recurrent VF and should provide an ideal group of patients for risk-free drug testing.

1.4 Electrophysiological testing

A new dimension to the study of antiarrhythmic drugs is provided by the possibility of studying the effect of drugs on ventricular arrhythmias induced by programmed electrical stimulation. Although this has theoretical appeal it is difficult to be sure that suppression of evoked responses will be followed by abolition of dangerous arrhythmias, such as recurrent VF, during long-term therapy [28, 29]. It is difficult to compare the results of different studies as investigators vary in the aggression of their programme to produce an evoked response and in their criteria of a positive result [30]. Response may vary with the site of pacing in relation to the origin of the arrhythmia. New drug studies are often confined to patients not responding to conventional drugs, but these may differ from one centre to another. Although an undoubted trial for the patient these studies appear to be acceptably safe in expert hands [29], and there is a general correlation of suppression of ventricular tachycardia or VF with clinical response. Studies may allow the detection of drugs with adverse effects, tending to exacerbate a tachycardia [31].

The assumption that suppression means effective treatment is not always justified [30]. Drugs may effect spread rather than initiation of the arrhythmia. A study of a small number of patients for one year after arrest from cardiac infarction showed no advantage for drug selection by electrophysiological study [32]. A comparative study of various regimens in sustained ventricular tachycardia showed that procainamide predicted the response to other drugs and tests did not aid selection of treatment [33]. It is concluded that after infarction either any known effective drug may suppress or the arrhythmias are self-limiting [32]. Attempts to show synergism with drug combinations have been unsuccessful [34], the more potent drug tending to dominate the response, confirming the traditional view that it is better to learn to use one drug properly.

1.5   Class I drugs: membrane-stabilizing agents

The action of this group of antiarrhythmic drugs in blocking Na ion entry into the cell is evident at higher concentration as a local anaesthetic effect in nerve [1, 2]. It is evident as a reduction in the rate of rise of the intracellular potential on depolarization (Fig. 1.1). The antiarrhythmic effect mainly relates to a consequent reduction in the rate of conduction of the activation process from cell to cell which will terminate re-entry. The effect depends in part on the rate of recovery of the Na channel. Side effects are often related to entry into the brain, producing giddiness, ataxia, tremor, nausea, and eventually convulsions or confusional states [2]. Three subgroups of Class I (a,b,c) are recognized on the perhaps naive basis of effect on action potential duration (APD) Group Ia, including the type drug quinidine, tends to prolong the action potential duration (APD) presumably through a secondary effect on reactivation and may prolong effective refractory period (ERP). This action is evident clinically in the electrocardiogram (ECG) as prolongation of the QT interval and is associated with toxic effects and production of arrhythmias such as torsade de pointes and VF. Group Ib, typified by lignocaine, tends to shorten APD, perhaps on the basis of rapid recovery of the Na channel. Group Ic contains a number of new drugs (such as encainide and flecainide) with little effect on APD. They produce prolonged block of the Na channel and have a major effect on Purkinje fibre conduction and the abolition of ventricular ectopic beats which presumably originate in Purkinje system re-entry; although QT is not prolonged these drugs have a strong tendency to produce arrhythmias such as torsade de pointes (Fig. 1.2).

1.5.1   CLASS IA

(a)   Quinidine

Quinidine, the first of the antiarrhythmic drugs, introduced in 1912 [9], is often, because of its great potency, regarded as the standard for comparison for newer agents. Quinidine is notorious for its high incidence of toxic effects which relate in part to attempts at the rapid production of effective plasma levels for the reversion of atrial fibrillation, though even moderate doses may provoke dangerous ventricular arrhythmias with long QT [35], even in the absence of digitalis. Coincident digitalis therapy may account for some of the reported problems with quinidine, as the pharmacological advice to have the patient digitalized before reversion to prevent a rapid ventricular response if atrial flutter developed was given before the effect of quinidine on digoxin excretion with raising of plasma levels and increased effect [2] was fully understood (Chapter 5).

Unexpected high plasma levels and associated quinidine syncope or sudden death due to ventricular flutter or fibrillation often in torsade de pointes [2] are avoided in long-term therapy by the use of slow-release preparations, though problems may arise from active metabolites not measured in the plasma levels of unchanged quinidine. In addition, long-term maintenance therapy with quinidine is often disturbed by gastrointestinal side effects. The use of Aludrox to prevent diarrhoea without impairing absorption [36], does not seem to have become popular.

Electrophysiological testing in ventricular tachycardia showed a response in about 40% of patients which in general predicted long-term effect over two months [37]. Problems of combination therapy are shown by the slight rise in serum level of both quinidine and disopyramide when given together [38]. Phenytoin on the other hand reduced plasma quinidine levels through enzyme induction [39]. Adding a second Class I drug did not seem to increase protection and sometimes made induction of ventricular tachycardia easier, suggesting the possibility of a worse clinical effect [40].

(b) Procainamide

A product of the local anaesthetic series [9] procaine amide is similar to quinidine (Class Ia), but less potent. The short half-life, partly prolonged by the active metabolite' N-acetyl procaine amide (NAPA) [41] is easily overcome pharmaceutically by slow-release preparations, allowing satisfactory oral treatment with few side effects, but with the possibility of high toxic plasma levels in slow acetylators [9]. The major draw-back in long-term therapy is the development of drug-induced disseminated lupus erythematosus particularly in slow acetylators [2, 42]. Virtually all patients have antinuclear antibodies after one year.

NAPA has been introduced into treatment as a primary agent on the grounds that it may be less likely to produce drug-induced lupus. It is similar in action to procainamide, though there are some electrophysiological differences [43]. The suggestion that torsade de pointes after QT prolongation is related to increased dispersion of effective refractory period (ERP) was not confirmed in a clinical study using procainamide [44].

Both ranitidine and cimetidine increase plasma levels of procainamide and NAPA, probably by competition for the renal tubular cationic secretory pathway [45]. Procainamide crosses the placental barrier and has been used to treat a fetal tachycardia [46].

The Rauwolfia alkaloid, ajmaline, which has a consistent Class I effect which can be used intravenously to block accessory pathway conduction in the Wolff–Parkinson–White (WPW) syndrome, abolishing the delta wave, can conveniently be replaced by procainamide [47].

(c) Disopyramide

Disopyramide is relatively new to the English-speaking world, although well-known in France for several years. Its relatively simple pharmacokinetics and moderate Class Ia effect with relatively little toxicity led to its rapid acceptance and approval by the FDA, as the first acceptable new antiarrhythmic since procainamide.

Although capable of the usual Class I toxic effects, its use was at first limited by an atropine-like action, producing dry mouth, urinary retention and precipitation of glaucoma, although quinidine has similar effects [48]. A striking vagolytic effect on the atrioventricular (AV) node will improve block at the nodal level, while the Class I action paradoxically increases atrioventricular block in the His–Purkinje system [9]. This vagolytic action may increase the ventricular rate in atrial fibrillation or flutter [2]. Studies in transplanted hearts suggest that the vagal block counteracts some of the direct depressant effect [49]. After extensive use, disopyramide acquired a reputation for an adverse effect on myocardial activity and tendency to precipitate congestive heart failure although most of the reports are related to acute high doses and chronic treatment in less severely affected patients seems well-tolerated [50].

There has been difficulty in the rapid establishment of effective plasma levels on acute myocardial infarction [51]. Complex but impractical dose schedules have been suggested to give an adequate loading dose intravenously without toxicity [52]. Similar oral treatment is too slowly effective to be of use [53]. A further problem is the complex protein-binding which involves the acute phase reactant, alpha-1-acid-glycoprotein (AAG) which is increased after infarction [10] reducing further the effective free plasma level.

The major metabolite is mono-N-dealkyl-disopyramide (MND) which is similarly protein bound but to a lesser extent and has reduced activity exposing treatment to the hazards of enzyme induction [54]. In contrast to quinidine, disopyramide does not interact with warfarin [55].

Studies in re-entry atrioventricular nodal tachycardia show that these were stopped by block of the fast retrograde limb [56]. The effect in ten cases of WPW syndrome was similarly mainly in the retrograde accessory pathway [57]. An electrophysiological evaluation in severe, sustained ventricular tachycardia or fibrillation showed more clinical effectiveness than expected from the prevention of induction by stimulation [58].

(d) Pirmenol

This new Class Ia agent seems effective for 24 hours, suggesting daily oral treatment [59]. A short intravenous half-life suggests that it could also be useful for intravenous control of ventricular arrhythmias [60].

Antiarrhythmic drugs

(e) Amino-steroids

ORG 6001 should be classed as Ia rather than Ib as it prolongs APD and ERP [1]. It shows promise as a non-toxic antiarrhythmic [9].

1.5.2 CLASS IB

(a) Lignocaine (=Lidocaine US)

This potent product of the local anaesthetic series [8] is the type drug of Class Ib. Although not suitable for oral use, because of extensive first pass metabolism it has proved moderately safe and effective and has become established as the standard intravenous antiarrhythmic. The shortening of APD characteristic of Class Ib is well seen in Purkinje fibres where a long APD may contribute to the gate effect at the termination of the Purkinje system; abolition of this effect may contribute to the antiarrhythmic action [1]. Free entry to the central nervous system produces the usual toxic effects which generally appear before serious cardiac toxicity [9].

Half the time lignocaine does not work there is misunderstanding of the pharmacokinetics [9]. A loading dose is needed to fill body stores, the volume of distribution, and produce an adequate plasma level. It is followed by a maintenance infusion at a rate to replace the loss due to hepatic metabolism. A usual dose is 100 mg by slow initial injection followed by a 2 mg per min infusion. A sag of plasma levels before the infusion can build up its effect may lead to loss of arrhythmia control at 30–60 min, and can be countered by a secondary bolus of 50 mg [9]. Complex infusion regimens have not in general improved the situation and are liable to dangerous errors. Blood level monitoring has in the past been only of retrospective help, but the situation has been transformed by the rapid EMIT assay [61]. Reduced liver blood flow in congestive heart failure or shock, or from the effect of drugs such as propranolol, may lead to accumulation of lignocaine [9] and require a reduced infusion rate (1 mg per min or less).

In general the rapid metabolism quickly relieves overdose and lignocaine has proved a relatively safe and effective drug even in inexperienced hands in coronary care units [62].

(b) Lignocaine in myocardial infarction

Lignocaine is widely used as suggested by Lown and Vassaux [62] to suppress ventricular ectopic beats after myocardial infarction on the hypothesis that this approach will prevent cardiac arrest from VF and reduce the mortality of infarction [62]. This suggestion is supported by the somewhat dubious process of adding the results of all known trials [63]. In the only convincing trial [14], an infusion of 4 mg per min was needed and there was consequently a greater than usual incidence of side effects. Doubts about the free use of lignocaine in coronary care arose from the realization that the so-called 'warning' arrhythmias may be misleading and patients may be exposed to an undue risk of side effects [64]. The more widespread use of prophylactic lignocaine may expose more patients to the risk of toxic effects [65].

Beta-blockade may be a more useful approach early in infarction when sympathetic tone is increased [4, 13]. If we had a perfect drug there might be a case for routine treatment of all patients with infarction [66]. This suggestion has led to intensive search for more potent and less toxic lignocaine analogues and has led to the more potent Class Ic drugs, which might find a use in this way. As usual life is not like this and greater potency is often associated with more toxicity!

(c) Phenytoin (epanutin, dilantin)

This well-known anticonvulsant has good Class Ib antiarrhythmic properties with a favourable effect on AV node conduction, probably by central sympathetic stimulation which makes it particularly suitable for treatment of digitalis toxicity where tachyarrhythmias are accompanied by vagal AV nodal block [9]. Nystagmus may give warning of toxicity which usually presents as giddiness and ataxia or nausea and vomiting.

Phenytoin suffers from several pharmacokinetic disadvantages, well understood from its widespread use in epilepsy, which make it difficult to handle as an antiarrhythmic. A large volume of distribution requires a large loading dose for acute intravenous work which cannot be given as a single bolus without producing toxic plasma levels. For intravenous loading, 50–100 mg every 5 min till arrhythmia control, toxicity, or a total of 1 g is recommended [9]. Even in digitalis toxicity the more familiar lignocaine which has little effect on AV conduction is generally preferred.

Although well-absorbed and effective orally, it is the classical example of saturable kinetics, so that small changes in maintenance dose can produce large changes in plasma level, making it difficult to handle as a long-term antiarrhythmic. Oral therapy can begin with 1 g on the first day, reducing to 100 mg two or three times daily. It is a potent inducer of liver enzymes and may change metabolism of other drugs given simultaneously [39].

(d) Mexiletine

Mexiletine was deliberately developed as an orally effective lignocaine analogue and has many similarities of action and effect [9]. It suffers, like phenytoin from a large volume of distribution, needing a large loading dose, about 1 g, and requiring complex loading schedules [9]. The absence of hepatic metabolism makes it less flexible for intravenous use than lignocaine. The lack of liver metabolism prevents any first pass effect, so that oral treatment is effective, but the flexible control of plasma levels seen with lignocaine intravenously is lost and elimination relies on renal excretion which varies with urinary pH [67], being practically shut off in an alkaline urine.

Although moderately effective in electrophysiological studies [63], long-term use is relatively ineffective [68] and is limited by side effects [69], though combination in a reduced dose with another drug may be helpful. There is a suggestion that the Class Ib effect of shortening APD may limit QT prolongation on quinidine, which is Class Ia and prolongs APD, reducing the risk of torsade [70]. There is no evidence of effectiveness on mortality in cardiac infarction [9].

(e) Aprindine

This lignocaine analogue is perhaps more potent and toxic than lignocaine itself [9]. It can be given orally and seemed promising for long-term therapy, but unfortunately seems to be disqualified by the frequent occurrence of agranulocytosis [71]. Although shortening APD as a Class Ib drug, torsade has been reported with preliminary QT prolongation [72].

(f) Tocainide

This orally effective lignocaine analogue avoids some of the problems of mexiletine as it is eliminated both by renal excretion, presumably pH dependent, and hepatic metabolism. It seemed promising both intravenously and in coronary care [73] and as an oral treatment in refractory ventricular arrhythmias [74] but has been effectively disqualified by producing a high incidence of agranulocytosis [75].

(g) Ethmozine

This Russian phenothiazine shortens APD in dog studies [76] and seems to prevent ventricular ectopic beats with few side effects [77].

1.5.3 CLASS IC

These new drugs, selected for potent effect against ventricular ectopic beats, have little effect on APD, ERP or QT interval [1]. They act mainly against the His–Purkinje system, prolonging the HV interval and lengthening QRS duration. They have prolonged effect, either pharmacokinetically by slow excretion (flecainide) or by having active metabolites (encainide and lorcainide) [7], allowing once daily treatment. Despite lack of prolongation of APD these drugs may produce ventricular tachycardia without long QT as seen with flecainide [2] suggesting that disordered conduction rather than a repolarization effect is responsible for this arrhythmia. Ventricular tachycardia (not torsade) with long QT is also reported on flecainide [78]. A similar effect is seen with encainide, sustaining induced ventricular tachycardia [31].

(a) Flecainide

Flecainide is a characteristic Class Ic drug, abolishing ventricular ectopics and prolonging QRS in the ECG; it effectively blocks the retrograde pathway of AV nodal re-entry [79], but produces only minor, transient negative inotropic effects [80]. Changes in free plasma levels due to the rise in AAG after infarction do not seem to be a problem [10].

Prolonged action is related to slow urinary excretion which may be accelerated by acidification in case of toxicity [2]. Flecainide is effective in eliminating ventricular ectopic beats [2, 81], but may increase inducibility of arrhythmias, usual polymorphic ventricular tachycardias, degenerating to VF [82]. Spontaneous ventricular arrhythmias may complicate treatment [2]. Caution is advised in sinus node disease [83]. In a comparison with quinidine [84], flecainide was more effective in suppressing chronic ventricular ectopic beats, with a similar incidence but different spectrum of side effects. QRS widening did not predict the antiarrhythmic effect. A lesser effect on the J-T interval (Q-T interval less the widened QRS) than with quinidine may indicate a lesser risk of torsade. Flecainide seems relatively free of unexpected adverse effects [85].

(b) Encainide

Encainide maintains prolonged activity through active metabolites, mainly O-desmethylencainide (ODE) [7], with a long half-life. This introduces problems in relation to genetic polymorphism of metabolism [86, 2]. ODE is formed extensively only in good metabolizers. Poor metabolizers (5–10% of the population) do not form so much ODE, but accumulate encainide itself with prolongation of effect [6]. Encainide metabolism can be predicted from debrisoquine [86]. The similar action of ODE and encainide allows intravenous electrophysiological testing to be used to predict the results of chronic oral therapy when ODE accumulates [87], though there is a suggestion that ODE may be responsible for QRS widening, which is not seen in poor metabolizers [86].

Oral encainide was effective in suppressing ventricular ectopic beats without impairment of left ventricular function [88]. Over half refractory ventricular tachycardias responded in an electrophysiological study [87]. A similar response was rated in a study of 80 patients with ventricular tachycardia or fibrillation [89], but there was a high incidence of worsening arrhythmia related to larger doses and higher plasma levels of encainide and ODE, but not evident as QRS or QT widening.

(c) Lorcainide

Lorcainide similarly maintains activity through an active metabolite, norlorcainide, which takes a week to wash out. Norlorcainide has a similar antiarrhythmic effect to lorcainide itself but seems not to affect the AH interval or ERP [7]. Long-term oral therapy was effective in suppressing ventricular ectopic beats [90]. Central side effects such as perspiration, vivid dreams and insomnia are major problems in long-term use [2]. There seems relatively little tendency to toxic arrhythmias such as torsade de pointes [2], but pre-existing conduction disturbances may be worsened. It has been suggested that QRS widening can be used to monitor the effects of the drug, as lorcainide and norlocainide have similar actions [91]. There was prolongation of PR, QRS and QT intervals, but no side effects on 100 mg twice daily [90]. In WPW syndrome, AV node conduction did not seem to be affected but conduction was slowed or blocked in the accessory pathway, terminating or slowing re-entry and slowing the ventricular rate in atrial fibrillation [92]. These findings suggest a useful effect in WPW syndrome. Sinus node function was unchanged but exit block sometimes caused a slow rate in patients with sinus node disease [92].

(d) Propaphenone

This new drug has been widely studied in Europe. In an animal preparation, guinea-pig atria, it showed Class I effect and also beta-blockade [93]. In clinical work it shows little evidence of beta-blockade in that heart rate is not slowed [94]. The finding of worsening arrhythmia without QT prolongation suggests classification with the Class Ic drugs. It does not have a long half-life and usually needs 8 hourly doses [94]. Plasma levels and half-life are very variable and there is some non-linearity of response [94] suggesting saturation of metabolism. A controlled trial showed effective suppression of ventricular ectopic beats with some prolongation of PR and QRS intervals [95]. There was a suggestion of exacerbation of heart failure and serum digoxin was increased by 83% [95], suggesting the possibility of a dangerous interaction.

1.6   Class II – sympathetic antagonism

This group is practically reduced to the beta-blockers (Chapter 2) as other agents with antisympathetic effects, for instance the Rauwolfia alkaloids, are now rarely used as antiarrhythmics or are found to have other actions as in the case of the Class III effect of bretylium. The main use of beta-blockers has been in the control of arrhythmias provoked by increased sympathetic tone, as in anxiety states with sinus tachycardia or ectopic beats or the early stages of myocardial infarction [4, 13].

An additional effect is the removal of normal sympathetic tone at the AV node to impair conduction and block re-entrant AV nodal tachycardias, or slow the ventricular rate in atrial fibrillation (AF). One of the complaints about the Vaughan Williams classification is that it leaves no place for other drugs acting by autonomic effects on the AV node. The vagal effect of digitalis is widely used to control the ventricular rate in AF (Chapter 5). Adenosine (below) has a vagomimetic effect that can be used similarly to block AV nodal re-entry. Beta-blockers may be useful to prevent exercise tachcyardias from sympathetically mediated improved conduction when the resting ventricular rate is well controlled by digitalis [4].

1.6.1 ADENOSINE

The vagomimetic effect of adenosine triphosphate (ATP) has recently been used to block the AV node to terminate AV nodal re-entrant tachycardia [96] in the same way as beta-blockers or digitalis or verapamil. Side effects are minor and transient, but there may be bradycardia from an effect on the sinus node. Asthma must be avoided. Adenosine which is rapidly formed from ATP *in vivo* is itself similarly effective [97]. The action is not truly vagal as it is unaffected by atropine, but probably involves a specific receptor as it is blocked by methylxanthines in animal work. It seems a safe and effective treatment without haemodynamic disturbance, but has no effect on the anomalous pathway (bypass tract) in WPW syndrome. The possible negative inotropic effects of the alternatives of beta-blockade or verapamil are avoided [98]. The very short half-life allows titration with increasing doses to avoid sinus node depression and bradycardia [98]. Adenosine may be first choice [98]. Most use for these drugs has been in infants where paroxysmal tachycardia may be troublesome and digitalis is unreliable in its effect [99]. Verapamil and ATP had a high success rate. Verapamil may produce arrest in adverse circumstances, such as hypocalcaemia or previous beta-blockade, and ATP can produce alarming sinus pauses [95] so dose titration [98] seems a good approach.

A new therapeutic approach is suggested by the hypothesis that the bradycardias and tachycardias of the sick sinus syndrome are due to sensitivity to adenosine [100]. The tachycardias may be AV nodal re-entry due to local slow conduction and both slow rate and impaired AV conduction are produced by adenosine. Suppression of adenosine effect here might be of therapeutic value.

15

1.7 Class III

Prolonged APD with little change in depolarization (Fig. 1.1), resembling the cardiac effects of hypothyroidism was the basis of the description of Class III to explain the effects of amiodarone [1]. An associated prolongation of refractory period (ERP) preventing re-entry may be the basis of the antiarrhythmic action. The effect of prolonged APD is seen in the electrocardiogram as QT prolongation and has been associated with toxic arrhythmias such as torsade de pointes. The success and relative toxicity of amiodarone has led to an intensive search for new Class III agents.

1.7.1 AMIODARONE

The long latent interval (10 years) due to fears of corneal damage following the observed micro-deposits, delayed general release of this drug, but allowed intensive work on its clearly excellent long-term antiarrhythmic effects.

A complication has been the apparent different acute effect of intravenous amiodarone, used in Europe for control of supraventricular tachycardias [101]. Animal work [102] shows a non-competitive sympathetic blockade of sinus and AV nodes (Class II effect) with superperfusion. It is only on long-term oral therapy for 4–6 weeks [98] that the Class III effects of prolonged APD and ERP are seen with reduction in serum T_3 (triiodothyronine). A clinical study [103] produced comparable results. Treatment was given for comparable prolongation of AV node ERP. Only intravenous treatment prolonged A-H interval and oral therapy was more active on ERP of atria and ventricles and the H-V interval.

Long-term oral therapy is complicated by the slow pharmacokinetics and slow onset of action of the drug [104]. Not surprisingly intravenous tests even after 4–7 day infusion failed to predict the long-term oral response [105]. As the side effects seem to be dose-related it is best to aim for the minimum effective dose.

Bioavailability is also variable and may relate to metabolism to *N*-desethylamiodarone in gut wall as well as high hepatic extraction [106] which give low and variable bioavailability (72–86%) [107]. High lipid solubility results in extensive storage in fat which forms a reservoir giving a long half-life of 35–40 days, or more in the obese.

These considerations suggest that pharmacodynamic or pharmacokinetic monitoring would be useful. The most striking change is the QT interval in the electrocardiogram, although interpretation may be made difficult by U waves or bifid T waves [104]. QT interval is closely related to plasma and myocardial levels on long-term treatment [108]. Monitoring

QT interval may detect failure of compliance and great prolongation may show risk of torsade de pointes [104].

An alternative approach is to look at the possible underlying effect on thyroid hormones which seems to be a diversion from T_3 to inactive reverse T_3 (rT_3) synthesis which may be fundamental to the mode of action in the heart [109], but rT_3 is subject to other influences and may be unreliable in itself [104].

Plasma levels may be useful and change slowly with the slow pharmacokinetics. It is best to measure the total amiodarone plus desethylamiodarone. The therapeutic level is not known [104], but bioavailability problems can be detected and overcome in this way, and values above 1.5 μg per ml are often toxic.

A loading dose of 0.6–2.0 g daily is needed for 1–8 weeks and the usual maintenance doses are 200 mg daily for paroxysmal AF or WPW, but recurrent ventricular tachycardia and fibrillation may need 300–800 mg daily [110]. A lower dose may be effective in a week and is generally used to avoid adverse effects [110].

More extensive use has revealed frequent side effects which are less troublesome when the drug is used in lower doses (200–400 mg daily) for minor problems, than when larger doses are needed to control malignant ventricular arrhythmia [111]. The corneal microdeposits do not interfere with vision and seem harmless and reversible. Other problems in chronic use include thyroid effects, both hypothyroidism from general systemic T_3 to rT_3 diversion or hyperthyroidism from the effect of iodine load. Also seen are pulmonary fibrosis, liver damage, myopathy, tremor, ataxia, neuropathy, anorexia and photosensitivity leading to skin pigmentation [111]. Both digoxin and warfarin effects are potentiated with increases in serum digoxin and prothrombin time [110], and the doses of these drugs should be reduced.

Good results are reported with tachycardias involving bypass tracts [112]. There is prolongation of AH and ERP and intravenous control seemed to predict therapy in this group [112]. Other drugs seem equally predictive and ajmaline or procainamide (Class Ia) were found to predict the response to amiodarone [47], so it may represent just a general ease of control in the responsive subjects. Good control of serious ventricular arrhythmias on oral therapy may be associated with persistent inducibility in electrophysiological study [113]. Anticoagulant therapy may be potentiated by amiodarone and a halving of warfarin dose is suggested [114]. Disappointment is expressed that amiodarone is less effective and more toxic than generally appreciated [115]: this must relate to excessive expectations of a panacea. It seems reasonable to reserve it for life-threatening arrhythmias [110].

1.7.2 THE LONG QT PROBLEM

The production of long QT in the ECG as a reflection of APD prolongation as part of the Class III effect gives rise to problems as long QT is associated with toxic arrhythmias such as torsade de pointes [116]. It is usually suggested that the arrhythmias result from increased dispersion of re-polarization which is evident as long QT, while the therapeutic Class III effect may result from uniform prolongation of APD and ERP.

Correction of measured QT for heart rate is difficult [117]; the simple Bazett square root of R-R' interval correction is inadequate. The best way to assess drug effect is to compare QT intervals at identical paced rates. An alternative approach to study of drug effects without rate problems is to look at the evoked response to a paced beat [118]: the evoked T wave was satisfactorily prolonged after amiodarone.

An investigation of the effect of procainamide [44] failed to show relation of induction of torsade to increased dispersion of refractoriness. QT was prolonged in relation to the increase in ERP, though dispersion was not increased. The occurrence of torsade with drugs such as flecainide which do not widen APD or QT (Fig. 1.2) suggests that the arrhythmia may be related to disturbances of activation (Class I effect) rather than changes in refractoriness (Class III) which may be just a marker of drug effect. An apparent additive effect between amiodarone (Class III) and quinidine (Class I) may be related to elevation of plasma quinidine levels on amiodarone [119]. With amiodarone it seems that some degree of QT prolongation is part of the therapeutic effect, related to plasma levels [108], but extreme changes may give rise to torsade. Other arrhythmias seem to be polymorphous ventricular tachycardias rather than true torsade de pointes, and may have a different basis.

1.7.3 BRETYLIUM

Well known as a sympathetic blocker in hypertension, this quarternary amine was found to have antiarrhythmic effects with prolongation of APD [120]. As a sympathetic blocker it was at first assumed to act by a Class II effect. It remains effective as an antiarrhythmic when sympathetic neurone uptake (uptake-1) is blocked by a tricyclic antidepressant uptake blocker, though this idea is hard to apply clinically, and it is presumably taken into the myocardium by the alternative uptake-2 system [121].

It has mainly been used in the intravenous treatment of postoperative ventricular arrhythmias when the patient is recumbent, minimizing the postural hypotensive effect [8]. Electrophysiological studies failed to show much effect on the inducibility of ventricular tachycardias [122].

Other quarternary amines, such as clofilium, may be similar [120, 123].

They seem to concentrate in the myocardium and prolong APD. Although quarternary amines present problems of bioavailability they seem to be absorbed from the gut in long-term oral therapy. Meobentine resembles bretylium but does not produce ganglion blockade.

Quarternary amine derivatives of lignocaine and propranolol have antiarrhythmic effects, but their chemical properties as highly ionized bases make it difficult to assess their pharmacodynamics. They are local anaesthetics in nerve but and are not beta-blockers, but may alter repolarization by blocking K channels [9].

Bethanidine is a antihypertensive related to bretylium, though not a quarternary amine. It prolongs APD and the QT of the paced evoked responses [124]. It is a useful antiarrhythmic [124] and postural hypotension can be prevented by uptake-1 block with protriptyline, allowing oral ambulant therapy, although this combined approach seems open to hazards of failure of compliance.

Melperone, an established neuroleptic with few side effects has Class III effect [125]. As it is also an alpha-adrenergic blocker and has a positive inotropic effect it may be useful in myocardial infarction or congestive heart failure. It is suggested that positive inotropic effect may be a feature of all Class III drugs as prolonged APD allows greater cellular Ca ion entry [126], but this view may be naive as many opposing factors contribute to the plateau of the action potential.

1.7.4 BETA-BLOCKERS

Some prolongation of QT interval and of APD has been reported with long-term treatment with a number of beta-blockers [4, 127]. A study in dogs of the paced evoked response suggests that it may be a universal feature of beta-blockade [128], although particularly associated with sotalol [127] which prolongs QT even in ordinary treatment of hypertension and probably carries an increased risk of torsade [129], especially in the case of renal failure, which reduces sotalol excretion [127]. Sotalol has been used as an antiarrhythmic agent for its Class III effect, but it is difficult to separate the clinical response from the effect of its beta-blocking (Class II) action. The effect of the isolated d-isomer is awaited with interest as it should be free of beta-blocking action which is practically confined to the l-isomer [4, 130].

1.8 Class IV

The Class IV drugs such as verapamil and diltiazem are Ca-current antagonists with predominant effects on the AV nodal tissues that are not overwhelmed by the sympathetic reflex response to vasodilatation (Chapter 3). They find their main role in the control of supraventricular arrhythmias by AV nodal block. An additive effect with digoxin allows their use in combination where either alone is unsuccessful in the control of atrial fibrillation [131]. They will come into their own in the control of atrial fibrillation in the denervated transplanted heart.

The suspicion [9] that some arrhythmias might have their basis in abnormal Ca currents [2] and may be responsive to Class IV drugs has not in general been sustained. However, the variant of ventricular tachycardia with the bifascicular block pattern of right bundle branch block and left axis deviation seems specifically to respond to verapamil [132]. It presumably arises by re-entry in the conducting system and a slow response (Ca current) origin is suspected.

Lidoflazine, sometime classed as a Ca-antagonist (Chapter 3) has many effects on the cell membrane, including Class 1a action with prolongation of QT [8]. However, its tendency to produce ventricular arrhythmias [133] disqualifies it from serious consideration.

1.9 Class V

The announcement of a new class of antiarrhythmic drugs for a group of specific bradycardic agents [3] had little impact as these drugs, although potentially useful in the management of angina, appear to have little relevance to the treatment of arrhythmias.

Alinidine (St567) is *N*-allyl clonidine [134] and is metabolized to clonidine with sedative and hypotensive side effects. The possibility of a new action on pacemaker current has attracted attention [3] and an effect on Cl currents is suspected [135]. *AQ-A39* has similar effects [136]

References

1. Vaughan Williams, E.M. (1984) A classification of antiarrhythmic actions reassessed after a decade of new drugs. *J. Clin. Pharm.*, **24**. 129–47.
2. Muhiddin, K.A. and Turner, P. (1985) Is there an ideal antiarrhythmic drug? A review – with particular reference to class I antiarrhythmic agents. *Postgrad. Med, J.*, **61**, 665–78.
3. Millar, J.S. and Vaughan Williams, E.M. (1981) Anion antagonism – a fifth class of antiarrhythmic action? *Lancet*, i, 1291–2.
4. Hamer, J. (1979) Beta-adrenergic blocking drugs. In *Drugs for Heart Disease* (ed. J. Hamer), Chapman and Hall, London.
5. Krikler, D.M. (1974) A fresh look at cardiac arrhythmias. Therapy. *Lancet*, i, 1034–7.

6. Kates, R.E. (1983) Plasma level monitoring of antiarrhythmic drugs. *Am. J.. Cardiol.*, **52**, 8–15C.
7. Kates, R.E., Woosley, R.L. and Harrison, D.C. (1984) Clinical importance of metabolites of antiarrhythmic drugs. *Am. J. Cardiol.*, **53**, 248–51.
8. Alderman, E.L., Kerber, R.E. and Harrison, D.C. (1974) Evaluation of lidocaine resistance in man using intermittent large-dose infusion techniques. *Am. J. Cardiol.*, **34**, 342–9.
9. Kumana, C. and Hamer, J. (1979) Anti-arrhythmic Drugs. In *Drugs for Heart Disease* (ed. J. Hamer), Chapman and Hall, London.
10. Caplin, J.L., Johnston, A., Hamer, J. and Camm, A.J. (1985) The acute changes in serum binding of disopyramide and flecainide after myocardial infarction. *Eur. J. Clin. Pharmacol.*, **28**, 253–5.
11. Ruskin, J.N., McGovern, B., Garan, H., DiMarco, J.P. & Kelly, E. (1983) Antiarrhythmic drugs: a possible cause of out-of-hospital cardiac arrest. *N. Eng. J. Med.*, **309**, 1302–6.
12. Krikler, D.M. and Curry, P.V.L. (1976) Torsade de pointes, an atypical ventricular tachycardia. *Br. Heart J.*, **38**, 117–20.
13. Pantridge, J.F., Webb, S.W., Odgees, A.A.J. and Geddes, T.S. (1974) The first hour after the onset of acute myocardial infarction. in *Progress in Cardiology – 3* (ed. Paul V. Yu & John F. Goodwin, Lea and Febiger), Philadelphia.
14. Lie, K.I., Wellens, H.J., van Capelle, F.J. and Durrer, D. (1974) Lidocaine in the prevention of primary ventricular fibrillation. A double-blind, randomized study of 212 consecutive patients. *N. Engl. J. Med.*, **291**, 1324–6.
15. Sloman, G. and Prineas, R.J. (1973) Major cardiac arrhythmias in acute myocardial infarction: implications for longterm survival. *Chest*, **63**, 513–16.
16. Hoffmann, A., Schütz, E., White, R., Follath, F. and Burckhardt, D. (1984) Suppression of high-grade ventricular ectopic activity by antiarrhythmic drug treatment as a marker for survival in patients with chronic coronary artery disease. *Am. Heart J.*, **107**, 1103–8.
17. Clarke, J.M., Hamer, J., Shelton, J.R., Taylor, S. and Venning, G.R. (1976) The rhythm of the normal human heart. *Lancet*, ii, 508–12.
18. Kennedy, H.L., Whitlock, J.A., Sprague, M.K., Kennedy, L.J., Buckingham, T.A. and Goldberg, R.J. (1985) Long-term follow-up of asymptomatic healthy subjects with frequent and complex ventricular ectopy. *N. Engl. J. Med.*, **312**, 193–7.
19. Graboys, T.B. and Lown, B. (1983) Coffee, arrhythmias and common sense. *N. Engl. J. Med.*, **308**, 835–6.
20. Ruskin, J.N. (1985) Ventricular extrasystoles in healthy subjects. *N. Engl. J. Med.*, **312**, 238–9.
21. Sami, M., Kraemer, H. and De Bush, R.F. (1979) Reproducibility of exercise-induced ventricular arrhythmia after myocardial infarction. *Am. J. Cardiol.*, **43**, 724–30.
22. Myerburg, R.J., Zaman, L., Kessler, K.M. and Castellanos, A. (1982) Evolving concepts of management of stable and potentially lethal arrhythmias. *Am. Heart J.*, **103**, 615–25.
23. Oakley, C.M. (1984) Mitral valve prolease: harbinger of death or variant of normal? *Br. Med. J.*, **288**, 1853–4.
24. Martin, J.L., Untereker, W.J., Harken, A.H., Horowitz, L.N. and Josephson,

21

Antiarrhythmic drugs

M.E. (1982) Aneurysmectomy and endocardial resection for ventricular tachycardia: favourable hemodynamic and antiarrhythmic results in patients with global left ventricular dysfunction. *Am. Heart J.*, **103**, 960–5.

25. Cox, J.L. (1983) Anatomic-electrophysiologic basis for the surgical treatment of refractory ischemic ventricular tachycardia. *Ann. Surg.*, **198**, 119–29.

26. Josephson, M.E. (1984) Catheter ablation of arrhythmias. *Ann. Intern. Med.*, **101**, 234–7.

27. Reid, P.R., Mirowski, M., Mower, M.M., Platia, E.V., Griffith, L.S.C., Watkins, L., Bach, S.M., Imran, M. and Thomas, A. (1983) Clinical evaluation of the internal automatic cardioventer-defribillator in survivors of sudden cardiac death. *Am. J. Cardiol.*, **51**, 1608–13.

28. Graboys, T.B. (1982) The stampede to stimulation – numerators and denominators revisited relative to electrophysiologic study of ventricular arrhythmias. *Am. Heart J.*, **103**, 1089–90.

29. Horowitz, L.N., Spielman, S.R., Greenspan, A.M. and Josephson, M.E. (1982) Role of programmed stimulation in assessing vulnerability to ventricular arrhythmias. *Am. Heart J.*, **103**, 604–10.

30. Rasmussen, K. (1983) Induction of ventricular tachyarrhythmias-rationality gained or ethics lost? *Acta Med. Scand.*, **214**, 177–9.

31. Rinkenberger, R.L., Prystowsky, E.N., Jackman, W.N., Naccarelli G.V., Heger, J.J. and Zipes, D.P. (1982) Drug conversion of nonsustained ventricular tachycardia to sustained ventricular tachycardia during serial electrophysiologic studies: identification of drugs that exacerbate tachycardia and potential mechanisms. *Am. Heart J.*, **103**, 177–84.

32. Hamer, A., Vohra, J., Sloman, G. and Hunt, D. (1983) Electrophysiologic studies in survivors of late cardiac arrest after myocardial infarction. *Am. Heart J.*, **105**, 921–7.

33. Waxman, H.L. Buxton, A.E., Sadowski, L.M. and Josephson, M.E. (1983) The response to procainamide during electrophysiologic study for sustained ventricular tachyarrhythmias predicts the response to other medications. *Circulation*, **67**, 30–7.

34. Ross, D.L., Sze, D.Y., Keefe, D.L., Swerdlow, C.D., Echt, D.S., Griffin, J.C., Winkle, R.A. and Maston, J.W. (1982) Antiarrhythmic drug combinations in the treatment of ventricular tachycardia. Efficacy and electrophysiologic effects. *Circulation*, **66**, 1205–10.

35. Koster, R.W. and Wellens, H.J.J. (1976) Quinidine-induced ventricular flutter and fibrillation without digitalis therapy. *Am. J. Cardiol.*, **38**, 519–23.

36. Romankiewicz, J.A., Reidenberg, M., Drayer, D. and Franklin, J.E. (1978) The noninterference of aluminium hydroxide gel with quinidine sulfate absorption: an approach to control of quinidine-induced diarrhea. *Am. Heart J.*, **96**, 518–20.

37. Dimarco, J.P., Garan, H. and Ruskin, J.N. (1983) Quinidine for ventricular arrhythmias: value of electrophysiologic testing. *Am. J. Cardiol.*, **51**, 90–5.

38. Baker, B.J., Gammill, J., Massengill, J., Schubert, E., Karin, A. and Doherty, J.E. (1983) Concurrent use of quinidine and disopyramide: evaluation of serum concentrations and electrocardiographic effects. *Am. Heart J.*, **105**, 12–15.

39. Urbano, A.M. (1983) Phenytoin-quinidine interaction in a patient with recurrent ventricular tachyarrhythmias. *N. Engl. J. Med.*, **308**, 225.

40. Duffy, C.E., Swiryn, S., Bauernfeind, R.A., Strasberg, B., Palileo, E. and Rosen, K.M. (1983) Inducible sustained ventricular tachycardia refractory to individual class I drugs: effect of adding a second class I drug. *Am. Heart J.*, **106**, 450–8.

41. Woosley, R.L. and Roden, D.M. (1983) Importance of metabolites in antiarrhythmic therapy. *Am. J. Cardiol.*, **52**, 3C–7C.

42. Woosley, R.L., Drayer, D.E., Reidenberg, M.M., Nies, A.S., Carr, K. and Oates, J.A. (1975) Effect of acetylator phenotype on the rate at which procainamide induces antinuclear antibodies and the lupus syndrome. *N. Engl. J. Med.*, **298**, 1157–59.

43. Sung, R.J., Juma, Z. and Saksena, S. (1983) Electrophysiologic properties and antiarrhythmic mechanisms of intravenous N-acetylprocainamide in patients with ventricular dysrhythmias. *Am. Heart J.*, **105**, 811–19.

44. Shechter, J.A., Caine, R., Friehling, T., Kowey, P.R. and Engel, T.R. (1983) Effect of procainamide on dispersion of ventricular refractoriness. *Am. J. Cardiol.*, **52**, 279–82.

45. Somogyi, A. and Bochner, F. (1984) Dose and concentration dependent effect of ranitidine on procainamide disposition and renal clearance in man. *Br. J. Clin. Pharmacol.*, **8**, 175–81.

46. Dumesic, D.A., Silverman, N.H., Tobias, S. and Golbus, M.S. (1982) Transplacental cardioversion of fetal supraventricular tachycardia with procainamide. *N. Engl. J. Med.*, **107**, 1128–31.

47. Brugada, P., Dassen, W.R., Braat, S., Gorgels, A.P. and Wellens, H.H.J. (1983) Value of the ajmaline-procainamide test to predict the effect of long-term oral amiodarone on the anterograde effective refractory period of the accessing pathway in the Wolff–Parkinson–White syndrome. *Am. J. Cardiol.*, **52**, 70–2.

48. Danilo, P. and Rosen, M.R. (1976) Cardiac effects of disopyramide. *Am. Heart. J.*, **92**, 532–6.

49. Bexton, R.S., Hellestrand, K.J., Cory-Pearce, R., Spurrell, R.A.J., English, T.A.H. and Camm, A.J. (1983) The direct electrophysiologic effects of disopyramide phosphate in the transplanted human heart. *Circulation*, **67**, 38–45.

50. Gottdiener, J.S., DiBianco, R., Bates, R., Sauerbrunn, B.J. and Fletcher, R.D. (1983) Effects of disopyramide on left ventricular function: assessment by radionuclide cineangiography. *Am. J. Cardiol.*, **51**, 1554–8.

51. Ilett, K.F., Madsen, B.W. Woods, J.D. (1979) Disopyramide kinetics in patients with acute myocardial infarction. *Clin. Pharm. Ther.*, **26**, 1–7.

52. Simpson, R.J., Foster, J.R., Berge, C., Baker, S. and Gettes, L.S. (1983) Safety of multiple bolus loading of intravenous disopyramide. *Am. Heart J.*, **106**, 505–8.

53. Kumana, C.R., Rambihar, V.S., Willis, K., Gupta, R.N., Tanser, P.H., Cairns J.A., Wilderman, R.A., Johnston, M., Johnson, A.L. and Gent, M. (1982) Absorption and antidysrhythmic activity of oral disopyramide phosphate after acute myocardial infarction. *Br. J. Clin. Pharm.*, **14**, 529–37.

54. Aitio, M.-L., Mansury, L, Tata, E., Haataja, M. and Aitio, A. (1981) The effect of enzyme induction on the metabolism of disopyramide in man. *Br. J. Clin. Pharm.*, **11**, 279–85.

55. Sylven, C. and Anderson, P. (1983) Evidence that disopyramide does not

interact with warfarin. *Br. Med. J.*, **286**, 1181.
56. Sethi, K.K., Jaishankar, S., Khalilullah, M. and Gupta, M.P. (1983) Selective blockade of retrograde fast pathway by intravenous disopyramide in paroxysmal supraventricular tachycardia mediated by dual atrioventricular nodal pathways. *Br. Heart J.*, **49**, 532–43.
57. Kerr, C.R., Prystowsky, E.N., Smith, W.M., Cook, L. and Gallagher J.J. (1982) Electrophysiologic effects of disopyramide phosphate in patients with Wolff-Parkinson-White syndrome. *Circulation*, **65**, 869–78.
58. Lerman, B.B., Waxman, H.L., Buxton, A.E. and Josephson, M.E. (1983) Disopyramide: evaluation of electrophysiologic effects and clinical efficacy in patients with sustained ventricular tachycardia or ventricular fibrillation. *Am. J. Cardiol.*, **51**, 759–64.
59. Lee, T.G., Goldberg, A.D., Chang, T., Serkland, M.T., Yakatan, G.J., Johnson, E.L., Toole, J.G. and Goldstein, S. (1983) Pharmacokinetics and efficacy of pirmenol hydrochloride in the treatment of ventricular dysrhythmia. *J. Cardiovasc. Pharmacol.*, **5**, 632–7.
60. Anderson, J.L., Lutz, J.R., Sanders, S.W. and Nappi, J.M. (1983) Efficacy of intravenous pirmenol hydrochloride for treatment of ventricular arrhythmias. A controlled comparison with lidocaine. *J. Cardiovasc. Pharmacol.*, **5**, 213–20.
61. Deglin, S.M., Deglin, J.M., Wurtzbacher, J., Litton, M., Rolfe, C. & McIntire, C. (1980) Rapid serum lidocaine determination in the coronary care unit. *J. Am. Med. Assoc.*, **244**, 571–3.
62. Lown, B. and Vassaux, C. (1968) Lidocaine in acute myocardial infarction. *Am. Heart J.*, **76**, 586–7.
63. DeSilva, R.A., Hennekens, C.H., Lown, B. and Casscells, W. (1981) Lignocaine prophylaxis in acute myocardial infarction: an evaluation of randomized trials. *Lancet*, **ii**, 855–58.
64. Kertes, P. and Hunt, D. (1984) Prophylaxis of primary ventricular fibrillation in acute myocardial infarction. The case against lignocaine. *Br. Heart J.*, **52**, 241–7.
65. Lown, B. (1985) Lidocaine to prevent ventricular fibrillation. Easy does it. *N. Engl. J. Med.*, **313**, 1154–6.
66. Harrison, D.C. (1978) Should lidocaine be administered routinely to all patients after acute myocardial infarction? *Circulation*, **58**, 581–4.
67. Kiddie, M.A., Kaye, C.M., Turner, P. and Shaw, T.R.D. (1974) The influence of urinary pH on the elimination of mexiletine. *Br. J. Clin. Pharm.*, **1**, 229–32.
68. Palileo, E.V., Welch, W., Hoff, J., Strasberg, B., Bauernfeind, R.A., Swiryn, S., Coelho, A. and Rosen, K.M. (1982) Lack of effectiveness of oral mexiletine in patients with drug-refractory paroxysmal sustained ventricular tachycardia. A study utilising programmed stimulation. *Am. J. Cardiol.*, **50**, 1075–81.
69. Waspe, L.E., Waxman, H.L., Buxton, A.E. and Josephson, M.E. (1983) Mexiletine for control of drug-resistant ventricular tachycardia: clinical and electrophysiologic results in 44 patients. *Am. J. Cardiol.*, **51**, 1175–81.
70. Duff, H.J., Roden, D., Primm, R.K., Oates, J.A. and Woosley, R.L. (1983) Mexiletine in the treatment of resistant ventricular arrhythmias: enhance-

ment of efficacy and reduction of dose-related side effects by combination with quinidine. *Circulation*, **67**, 1124–8.

71. van Leeuwen, R. and Meyboom, R.H.B. (1976) Agranulocytosis and aprindine. *Lancet*, **ii**, 1137.

72. Scagliotti, D., Strasberg, B., Hai, H.A., Kehoe, R. and Rosen, K. (1982) Aprindine-induced polymorphous ventricular tachycardia. *Am. J. Cardiol.*, **49**, 1297–300.

73. Allen-Narker, R.A.C., Roberts, C.J.C., Marshall, A.J., Jordan, S.C., Barritt, D.W. and Goodfellow, R.M. (1984) Prophylaxis against ventricular arrhythmias in suspected acute myocardial infarction: a comparison of tocainide and disopyramide. *Br. J. Clin. Pharmacol.*, **18**, 725–32.

74. Podrid, P.J. and Lown, B. (1982) Tocainide for refractory symptomatic ventricular arrhythmias. *Am. J. Cardiol.*, **49**, 1279–86.

75. Volosin, K., Greenberg, R.M. and Greenspon, A.J. (1985) Tocainide associated agranulocytosis. *Am. Heart J.*, **109**, 1392–93.

76. Tsuji, Y., Nishimura, M., Osada, M. and Watanabe, Y. (1983) Membrane action of ethmozin on normoxic and hypoxic canine Purkinje fibers. *J. Cardiovasc. Pharmacol.*, **5**, 961–7.

77. Pratt, C.M., Yepsen, S.C., Taylor, A.A., Mason, D.T., Miller, R.R., Quinones, M.A. and Lewis, R.A. (1983) Ethmozine suppression of single and repetitive ventricular premature depolarizations during therapy: documentation of efficacy and long-term safety. *Am. Heart J.*, **106**, 85–91.

78. Lui, H.K., Lee, G., Dietrich, P., Low, R.I. and Mason, D.T. (1982) Flecainide-induced QT prolongation and ventricular tachycardia. *Am. Heart J.*, **103**, 567–9.

79. Hellestrand, K.J., Nathan, A.W., Bexton, R.S., Spurrell, R.A. and Camm, A.J. (1983) Cardiac electrophysiologic effects of flecainide acetate for paroxysmal reentrant junctional tachycardia. *Am. J. Cardiol.*, **51**, 770–6.

80. Legrand, V., Vardormael, M. Collignon, P. and Kulbertus, H.E. (1983) Hemodynamic effects of a new antiarrhythmic agent, flecainide (R-818), in coronary heart disease. *Am. J. Cardiol.*, **51**, 422–6.

81. Meinertz, T., Zehender, M.K., Geibel, A., Treese, N., Hoffmann, T., Kasper, W. and Pop, T. (1984) Long-term antiarrhythmic therapy with flecainide. *Am. J. Cardiol.*, **54**, 91–6.

82. Oetgen, W.J., Tibbits, P.A., Abt, M.E.O. and Goldstein, R.E. (1983) Clinical and electrophysiologic assessment of oral flecainide acetate for recurrent ventricular tachycardia: evidence for exacerbation of electrical instability. *Am. J. Cardiol.*, **52**, 7–50.

83. Vik-Mo, H., Ohm, O.-J. and Lund-Johansen, P. (1982) Electrophysiologic effects of flecanide acetate in patients with sinus nodal dysfunction. *Am. J. Cardiol.*, **50**, 1090–4.

84. The Flecainide–Quinidine Research Group (1983) Flecainide versus quinidine for treatment of chronic ventricular arrhythmias. A multicenter clinical trial. *Circulation*, **67**, 1117–23.

85. CSM Update. Recurrent ventricular tachycardia: adverse drug reactions (1986) *Brit. Med. J.*, **292**, 50.

86. Wang, T, Roden, D.M., Wolfenden, H.T., Woosley, R.L., Wood, A.J.J. and Wilkinson, G.R. (1984) Influence of genetic polymorphism on the metabolism and disposition of encainide in man. *J. Pharm. Exp. Ther.*, **228**, 605–11.

Antiarrhythmic drugs

87. Anderson, J.L., Stewart, J.R., Johnson, T.A., Lutz, J.R. and Pitt, B. (1982) Response to encainide of refractory ventricular tachycardia: clinical application of assays for parent drug and metabolites. *J. Cardiovasc. Pharmacol.*, **4**, 812–19.

88. Sami, M.H., Derbekyan, V.A. and Lisbona, R. (1983) Hemodynamic effects of encainide in patients with ventricular arrhythmia and poor ventricular function. *Am. J. Cardiol.*, **52**, 507–11.

89. Chesnie, B., Podrid, P., Lown, B. and Raeder, E. (1983) Encainide for refractory ventricular tachyarrhythmia. *Am. J. Cardiol.*, **52**, 495–500.

90. Keefe, D.L. Peters, F. and Winkle, R.A. (1982) Randomized double-blind placebo controlled crossover trial documenting oral lorcainide efficacy in suppression of symptomatic ventricular tachyarrhythmias. *Am. Heart J.*, **103**, 511–18.

91. Meinertz, T., Kasper, W., Kersting, F., Just, H., Bechtold, H. and Janchen, E. (1979) Lorcainide II. Plasma concentration-effect relationship. *Clin. Pharm. Ther.*, **26**, 198–204.

92. Manz, M., Steinbeck, G. and Luderitz B. (1982) Electrophysiological effects of lorcainide in sinoatrial disease and in Wolff-Parkinson-White syndrome. *Eur. Heart J.*, **3**, 56–66.

93. Ledda, F., Mantelli, L., Manzini, S., Amerini, S. and Mugelli, A. (1981) Electrophysiological and antiarrhythmic properties of propafenon in isolated cardiac preparations. *J. Cardiovasc. Pharmacol.*, **3**, 1162–73.

94. Connolly, S.J., Kates, R.E., Lebsack, C.S., Harrison, D.C. and Winkle, R.A. (1983) Clinical pharmacology of propafenone. *Circulation*, **68**, 589–96.

95. Salerno, D.M., Granrud, G., Sharkey, P., Asinger, R. and Hodges, M. (1984) A controlled trial of propafenone for treatment of frequent and repetitive ventricular premature complexes. *Am. J. Cardiol.*, **53**, 77–83.

96. Behlhassen, B., Pelleg, A., Shoshani, D., Geva, B. and Laniado, S. (1983) Electrophysiologic effects of adenosine-5-triphosphate on atrioventricular reentrant tachycardia. *Circulation*, **68**, 827–33.

97. DiMarco, J.P., Sellers, T.D., Berne, R.M., West, G.A. and Belardinelli, L. (1983) Adenosine: electrophysiolgic effects and therapeutic use for terminating paroxysmal supraventricular tachycardia. *Circulation*, **68**, 1256–63.

98. Belhassen, B. and Pelleg, A. (1984) Acute management of paroxysmal supraventricular tachycardia: verapamil, adenosine triphosphate or adenosine? *Am. J. Cardiol.*, **54**, 225–7.

99. Greco, R., Musto, B., Arienzo, V., Alborino, A., Garofalo, S. and Marsico, F. (1982) Treatment of paroxysmal supraventricular tachycardia in infancy with digitalis, adenosine-5'-triphosphate, and verapamil: a comparative study. *Circulation*, **66**, 504–8.

100. Watt, A.H. (1985) Hypothesis. Sick sinus syndrome: an adenosine-mediated disease. *Lancet*, **i**, 786–8.

101. Faniel, R. and Schoenfeld, P.H. (1983) Efficacy of i.v. amiodarone in converting rapid atrial fibrillation and flutter to sinus rhythm in intensive care patients. *Eur. Heart J.*, **4**, 180–5.

102. Kadoya, M., Konishi, T., Tamamura, T., Ikeguchi, S., Hashimoto, S. and Kawai, C. (1985) Electrophysiological effects of amiodarone on isolated rabbit heart muscles. *J. Cardiovasc. Pharmacol.*, **7**, 643–8.

103. Wellens, H.J.J., Brugada, P., Abdollah, H. and Dassen, W.R. (1984) A

comparison of the electrophysiologic effects of intravenous and oral amiodarone in the same patient. *Circulation*, **69**, 120–4.

104. McKenna, W.J. and Krikler, D.M. (1984) Clinical evaluation of the efficacy of oral amiodarone. *Br. Heart J.*, **51**, 241–2.

105. Saksena, S., Rothbart, S.T., Shah, Y. and Cappello, G. (1984) Clinical efficacy and electropharmacology of continuous intravenous amiodarone infusion and chronic oral amiodarone in refractory ventricular tachycardia. *Am. J. Cardiol.*, **54**, 347–52.

106. Berdeaux, A., Roche, A., Labaille, T., Giroux, B., Edouard, A. and Giudicelli, J.F. (1984) Tissue extraction of amiodarone and N-desethylamiodarone in man after a single oral dose. *Br. J. Clin. Pharm.*, **18**, 759–63.

107. Riva, E., Gerna, M., Latini, R., Giani, P., Volpi, A. and Maggioni, A. (1982) Pharmacokinetics of amiodarone in man. *J. Cardiovasc. Pharmacol.*, **4**, 264–9.

108. Debbas, N.M.G., du Cailar, C., Bexton, R.S., DeMaille, J.G., Camm, A.J. and Puech, P. (1984) The QT interval: a predictor of the plasma and myocardial concentration of amiodarone. *Br. Heart J.*, **51**, 316–20.

109. Nademanee, K., Singh, B.N., Hendrickson, J.A., Reed, A.W., Melmed, S. and Hershman, J. (1982) Pharmacokinetic significance of serum reverse T_3 levels during amiodarone treatment: a potential method for monitoring chronic drug therapy. *Circulation*, **16**, 202–11.

110. McKenna, W.J., Rowland, E. and Krikler, D.M. (1983) Amiodarone: the experiences of the past decade. *Br. Med. J.*, **287**, 1654–6.

111. Rotmensch, H.H., Belhassen, B. and Ferguson, R.K. (1982) Amiodarone – benefits and risks in perspective. *Am. Heart J.*, **104**, 1117–19.

112. Alboni, D., Shanthe, N., Pirani, R., Beggioni, F., Scarfo, S., Tomasi, A.M. and Masoni, A. (1984) Effects of amiodarone on supraventricular tachycardia involving bypass tracts. *Am. J. Cardiol.*, **53**, 93–8.

113. Waxman, H.L., Groh, W.C., Marchlinski, F.E. Buxton, A.E., Sadowski, L.M., Horowitz, L.N., Josephson, M.E. and Kastor, J.A. (1982) Amiodarone for control of sustained ventricular tachyarrhythmia: clinical and electrophysiologic effects in 51 patients. *Am J. Cardiol.*, **50**, 1066–74.

114. Hamer, A., Peter, T., Mandel, W.J., Scheinman, M.M. and Weiss, D. (1982) The potentiation of warfarin anticoagulation by amiodarone. *Circulation*, **65**, 1025–9.

115. Fogoros, R.N., Anderson, K.P., Winkle, R.A., Swerdlow, C.D. and Mason, J.W. (1983) Amiodarone: clinical efficacy and toxicity in 96 patients with recurrent, drug-refractory arrhythmias. *Circulation*, **68**, 88–94.

116. Surawicz, B. and Knoebel, S.B. (1984) Long QT: good, bad or indifferent? *J. Am. Coll. Cardiol.*, **4**, 398–413.

117. Staniforth, D.H. (1983) The QT interval and cycle length: the influence of atropine hyoscine and exercise. *Br. J. Clin. Pharm.*, **16**, 615–21.

118. Donaldson, R.M. and Rickards, A.F. (1982) Evaluation of drug-induced changes in myocardial repolarisation using the paced evoked response. *Br. Heart J.*, **48**, 381–7.

119. Tartini, R., Kappenberger, L., Steinbrun, W. and Meyer, U.A. (1982) Dangerous interaction between amiodarone and quinidine. *Lancet*, **i**, 1327–9.

120. Patterson, E. and Lucchesi, B.R. (1983) Bretylium: a prototype for future development of antidysrhythmic agents. *Am. Heart J.*, **106**, 426–31.

Antiarrhythmic drugs

121. Iversen, L.L. (1973) Catecholamine uptake processes. *Brit. Med. Bull.*, **29**, 130–5.
122. Bauernfeind, R.A., Hoff, J.V., Swiryn, S., Palileo, E., Strasberg, B., Scagliotti, D. and Rosen, K.M. (1983) Electrophysiologic testing of bretylium tosylate in sustained ventricular tachycardia. *Am. Heart J.*, **105**, 973–80.
123. Bexton, R.S. and Camm, A.J. (1982) Drugs with a class III antiarrhythmic action. *Pharmacol. Ther.*, **17**, 315–55.
124. Bacaner, M.B. and Benditt, D.G. (1982) Antiarrhythmic, antifibrillatory and hemodynamic actions of bethanidine sulfate: an orally effective analog of bretylium for suppression of ventricular tachyarrhytmias. *Am. J. Cardiol.*, **50**, 728–34.
125. Smiseth, O.A., Platou, E.S., Refsum, H. and Mjos, O.D. (1981) Haemodynamic and metabolic effects of the antiarrhythmic drug melperone during acute left ventricular failure in dogs. *Cardiovasc. Res.*, **15**, 724–30.
126. Platou, E.S., Myhre, E.S.P., Smiseth, O.A. and Refsum, H. (1983) Melperone: alpha-adrenoceptor blocker with class III antiarrhythmic action. In *Alpha-Adrenoceptor Blockers in Cardiovascular Disease* (ed. Helge Referum & Ole D. Mios), Churchill Livingstone, Edinburgh, pp. 311–22.
127. Neuvonen, P.J., Elonen E., Tanskanen, A. and Tuomilehto, J. (1982) Sotalol prolongation of the QTc interval in hypertensive patients. *Clin. Pharm. Ther.*, **32**, 25–32.
128. Taggart, P., Donaldson, R., Abed, J. and Nashat, F. (1984) Class III action of β-blocking agents. *Cardiovasc. Res.*, **18**, 683–9.
129. Krapf, R. and Gertsch, M. (1985) Torsades de pointes induced by sotalol despite therapeutic plasma sotalol concentration, *Br. Med. J.*, **290**, 1784–5.
130. Taggart, P., Sutton, P. and Donaldson, R. (1985) d-Sotalol: a new potent class III anti-arrhythmic agent. *Clin. Sci.*, **69**, 631–6.
131. Schwartz, J.B., Keefe, D., Kates, R.E., Kirsten, E. and Harrison, D.C. (1982) Acute and chronic pharmacodynamic interaction of verapamil and digoxin in atrial fibrillation. *Circulation*, **65**, 1163–70.
132. Lin, F–C., Finley, C.D., Rahimtoola, S.H. and Wu, D. (1983) Idiopathic paroxysmal ventricular tachycardia with a QRS pattern of right bundle branch block and left axis deviation: a unique clinical entity with specific properties. *Am. J. Cardiol.*, **52**, 95–100.
133. Kennelly, B.M. (1977) Comparison of lidoflazine and quinidine in prophylactic treatment of arrhythmias. *Br. Heart J.*, **39**, 540–6.
134. Kobinger, W., Lillie, C. and Pichler, L. (1979) N-allyl-derivative of clonidine, a substance with specific bradycardic action at a cardiac site. *Arch. Pharmacol.*, **306**, 255–62.
135. Brutsaert, D.L., de Clerck, N.M. and Sys, S.U. (1982) Activation stabilization – further support for a new class of cardioactive substances *J. Cardiovasc. Pharmacol.*, **4**, 808–11.
136. Hilaire, J., Broustet, J.P., Colle, J.P. and Theron, M. (1983) Cardiovascular effects of AQ–A 39 in healthy volunteers. *Br. J. Clin. Pharm.*, **16**, 627–31.

2 Beta-adrenergic blocking drugs

CYRUS R. KUMANA

2.1 Introduction

The following account deals with the practical aspects of treatment with beta-adrenoceptor blocking drugs (popularly referred to as beta-blockers). Of the very many well-established, as well as tentative indications for treating patients with these drugs, some (angina, hypertension, secondary prevention of myocardial infarction) involve very large numbers of patients and long-term treatment. Hence, apart from clinical need, powerful commercial considerations have had an unduly important role in prompting the pharmaceutical industry into developing and marketing a myriad of alternative agents. The latter often differ from each other with respect to one or other of their minor ancillary properties, and frequently these form the basis on which individual agents are promoted. From the ensuing publications about different drugs and their respective differences from each other, an enormous quantity of medical literature has accumulated. Much of this was reviewed in the previous edition of this book [1]. More recent reviews, as well as detailed proceedings from symposia or workshops devoted to particular applications or particular drugs possessing specific ancillary properties, have appeared in profusion. A limited selection of these publications [2–5] can provide a useful update on most aspects of beta-blocking therapy.

This chapter discusses many of the most current clinicopharmacological topics referred to in these sources, as well as several other topics which are nevertheless important in the author's view. On the other hand, there has been no attempt whatsoever, nor would it be feasible in a chapter of this size, to review all the recent literature dealing with beta-blocking drugs. Rather, there has been a concerted effort to evaluate critically a number of important or controversial clinical issues which could influence the treatment of individual patients. Fundamental aspects of cardiac pharmacology pertinent to using beta-blockers in patients with heart disease have been discussed in the corresponding

29

chapter of the previous edition of this book [1] and elsewhere, and have not been covered here. Particular emphasis has been given to clinical pharmacology, with special reference to the impact of beta-blockade on blood pressure.

In practical terms it is both convenient and expedient to compare and contrast the pharmacological properties of different beta-adrenoceptor antagonists in relation to those of propranolol. Propranolol, the longest established and most widely used drug in this category, is endowed with (1) membrane stabilizing activity, (2) high lipid solubility and the absence of (3) selectivity, (4) partial agonist activity and (5) alpha-receptor antagonist activity.

It is unrealistic to expect clinicians to contemplate, let alone try to remember how the multitude of different beta-blocking agents differ from propranolol with respect to each of these various properties. A more useful exercise is to consider each ancillary property in turn, and evaluate the data pertaining to one or two antagonists which are outstandingly different from propranolol with respect to the particular property under consideration. It is also undoubtedly an over simplification to attribute all differences between individual beta-blocking drugs to one or more of the properties listed above, since there may very well be alternative explanations involving a complex series of metabolic, pharmacokinetic, and other factors.

2.2 Membrane stabilizing activity (MSA)/local anaesthetic activity

This property of propranolol, which is also possessed to a lesser extent by several other beta-blockers, is readily demonstrable *in vitro*, but requires the drug to be present in very high concentrations. Furthermore, unlike beta-blocking activity, which is confined to the l-isomer, MSA is possessed by both d- and l-forms. In the case of propranolol, MSA becomes evident at concentrations around 1000-fold those of free (unbound) plasma propranolol encountered during routine systemic therapy. Since these concentrations could only be achieved by local application, hitherto, the clinical importance of MSA has been largely discounted. Indeed, the only reason for considering this property was so that it could be avoided in agents selected for the topical treatment of glaucoma, lest they caused local anaesthesia. Not surprisingly beta-blockers lacking MSA such as timolol, have been exploited for such topical treatment in preference to propranolol.

An exciting development is the realization that, probably because of its MSA, propranolol was a potent inhibitor of sperm motility. This led to preliminary studies of its use as a vaginally applied contraceptive [6]. By this route however, a substantial amount is absorbed systemically and produces cardiovascular effects [7]. To avoid such effects, consideration is now being given to utilizing the MSA of d-propranolol for this purpose, as the latter is devoid of beta-blocking activity.

2.3 Selectivity (cardioselectivity, beta 1-selectivity)

A beta-adrenoceptor antagonist can be described as selective if it can be shown to exert less bronchial and/or vascular beta-receptor blockade than doses of propranolol which have equipotent cardiac beta-blocking activity. This aspect of beta-blockade has been the subject of intense discussion and debate [8–11], both with respect to theories to account for selectivity as well as the means of measuring it. Currently, though, the importance of selectivity appears to be in doubt. This is probably because the so-called selective antagonists (mainly atenolol and metoprolol) display only marginally less pronounced effects on clinically relevant tests of airway function and vascular tone than equipotent cardiac beta-blocking doses of propranolol. Nor has it been possible to demonstrate clinically significant differences in outcome when patients are treated with selective as opposed to non-selective drugs. The possible clinical significance of selectivity with respect to bronchial and vascular beta-blocking is discussed briefly in the following section. Even more contentious aspects, namely the effects of various selective and non-selective beta-blocking drugs on metabolism and muscle tremor will not be considered here.

2.3.1 SELECTIVITY AND BRONCHIAL BETA-RECEPTOR BLOCKADE

Selectivity may be readily revealed in pharmacological studies using isolated bronchial and cardiac tissues. However, in intact humans (patients or volunteers) it is surprisingly difficult to demonstrate clinically significant differences between so-called selective and non-selective drugs. Indeed, studies purporting to show very clear-cut differences have usually suffered from one or more important methodological flaws [11]. The variety of different approaches attempting to demonstrate clinically relevant selectivity (viz. inhalation of beta-agonists, performance of airway function tests during exercise, histamine challenge testing in asthmatics) as well as the disagreements amongst researchers using the same and different techniques [12–15], attest to the currently available 'selective' antagonists having clinically insignificant differences from propranolol. This being so, the following generalizations are probably valid with respect to the use of beta-blockers in patients with obstructive airway disease.

31

Beta-adrenergic blocking drugs

(1) All beta-blockers affect tests of airway function adversely, even in non-asthmatics. By definition, selective antagonists do so only whilst exerting relatively greater degrees of cardiac beta-blocking activity.

(2) Symptomatic exacerbation of obstructive airway disorder by beta-blockers [11] is an infrequent complication, usually, but not invariably affecting patients with an asthmatic history. Prolonged treatment over years results in <5% of those exposed being affected; though admittedly, patients with asthmatic histories would usually have been excluded from such series. The willingness of respiratory physicians and hospital ethics committees to approve research involving treatment with beta-blockers for asthmatics having bronchial provocation tests also attests to the risks being small.

(3) Thus, despite asthma being a relative contraindication to beta-blockers, in the presence of overriding indications it is prudent to (a) give a selective antagonist, (b) use small doses (with larger doses selectivity may not be retained), (c) give additional selectivity (beta$_2$) agonist treatment, preferably by inhalation.

(4) In patients with chronic obstructive lung disease (bronchitis and emphysema) the same precautions are warranted as in asthma. This is because many such patients have a true asthmatic component, most have diminished airway functional reserve, and many appear to be physically and/or psychologically dependent on inhaled bronchodilators.

2.3.2 SELECTIVITY AND VASCULAR BETA-BLOCKADE

Symptomatic peripheral vascular insufficiency due to treatment with non-selective and selective beta-blockers was reviewed by McDevitt [16]. Cold extremities, Raynaud's phenomenon (affecting about 6% of North American patients exposed to propranolol), exacerbation of intermittent claudication, and even digital gangrene have all been described. They are presumed to result from (a) antagonism of beta$_2$-receptor-mediated vasodilatation, which is theoretically spared (in relative terms) by selective beta-blockade, and (b) cardiac beta$_1$-receptor blockade (not influenced by selectivity) diminishing perfusion pressure. It has been very difficult to determine the relative risks of developing symptoms of peripheral vascular insufficiency in patients receiving equipotent cardiac beta-blocking doses of selective and non-selective antagonists. Retrospective surveys of adverse effects in large series of patients treated with selective and non-selective drugs have not revealed important differences in their incidence. However, in some patients, such symptoms may already have been the basis for pre-selection to one or other treatment, possibly accounting for the failure to note any advantage with selective drugs.

32

Selectivity (cardioselectivity, beta 1-selectivity)

Using indirect means of assessing tissue blood flow (skin temperature, xenon uptake, plethysmography), at least two double-blind studies have attempted to compare the influence of selective and non-selective beta-blockers on the peripheral circulation in man. One of these studies [17], entailed oral metoprolol and propranolol in 10 healthy males and four hypertensives (given as single equipotent cardiac beta-blocking doses), and inferred greater reductions in skin and muscle blood flow after propranolol than metoprolol. Their account was unclear as to whether a within-subject comparison was used. Furthermore, the statistically significant differences they found were between subjects on propranolol and on placebo, and not between individuals taking the two active drugs. Also, such differences as did occur were not substantially greater after exercise than at rest, implying that clinically significant amounts of circulating adrenaline were unlikely to have been released during exercise. Using the same drugs, another study [18] was conducted in 12 healthy male volunteers and employed a crossover design with sequential testing and regular treatment for 4 weeks with equipotent cardiac beta-blocking doses increasing at weekly intervals. In the doses used, metoprolol had slightly greater effect lowering blood pressure (at rest and post-exercise) than propranolol. The most striking and statistically significant difference they encountered on the two treatments, was the very much larger dose of isoprenaline required to decrease vascular resistance (and increase heart rate) in subjects taking propranolol. Thus, the greatest benefit from using selective beta-blockade may occur whenever an abundance of circulating adrenaline or like substance is responsible for vascular instability. Under these circumstances non-selective beta-blockade may be more liable to antagonize $beta_2$-receptor mediated vasodilatation and unmask alpha-receptor mediated peripheral vasoconstriction.

It remains a matter of speculation as to how and if these differences between pharmacological effects of selective and non-selective antagonists translate into clinically significant differences in symptomatology. It might nevertheless be prudent to prefer treatment with selective beta-blockade whenever patients have peripheral vascular insufficiency. These issues concerning selectivity and blood vessel calibre are equally relevant to peripheral vascular resistance and to the influence of selective and non-selective beta-blocking drugs on hypertensive surges.

2.4 Partial agonist activity

Paradoxically, competitive agonists with weak agonistic activity may behave predominantly as antagonist drugs, by competing with more potent agonists and displacing them from their respective receptors. Such is the case with the drugs referred to as beta-blockers with partial agonist activity (PAA); previously known as intrinsic sympathomimetic activity (ISA). By analogy, drugs which competitively bind to beta-adrenoceptors yet manifest no agonism, constitute the so-called pure antagonists (without PAA). Par excellence, the drug pindolol exhibits a most pronounced degree of PAA, but other drugs (practolol, alprenolol, and oxprenolol) also exhibit this property to a lesser extent.

It has been suggested that treatment with drugs possessing PAA such as pindolol, may confer several potential benefits over and above treatment with antagonists devoid of PAA. These claims [19] include the following.

(a) Diminished risk of inducing asthma

Some of the best evidence for this comes from provocation tests with histamine inhalation involving asthmatics taking equipotent cardiac beta-blocking doses of pindolol, propranolol and the selective antagonists metoprolol or atenolol. Treatment with propranolol, but not the partial agonist drug nor the selective blockers, affected histamine responsiveness adversely. Pindolol had the least effect on resting spirometry. However, among individual patients the effect on spirometry did not correlate with histamine responsiveness. Moreover, on pindolol the bronchodilator response to inhaled agonist was inferior to that on atenolol (particularly the small dose of atenolol). These results imply that in asthmatics the greatest advantage of pindolol accrues in the absence of sympathetically induced bronchodilatation, whereas in the presence of airway $beta_2$-receptor stimulation selective antagonism appears more advantageous.

(b) Protection from withdrawal phenomena after abrupt withdrawal?

Abrupt withdrawal of beta-blockade [20] was implicated as possibly causing transient overshoot (lasting about 14 days) in the liability to cardiac ischaemic events (angina, arrhythmias, myocardial infarction and death). Support for this idea was largely based on anecdotal case reports and incidental observations from a single, antianginal crossover trial employing propranolol and placebo [21]. Because the latter was a double-blind investigation, great credence has been placed on its conclusions. However, it should be noted that at least two thirds of the withdrawal periods referred to were not under blind conditions, as they occurred during the open 'no propranolol' period just after the dose-finding phase of the study. By contrast, it was notable that abrupt propranolol withdrawal prior to coronary angiography was not associated with such untoward abrupt events, leading to the suggestion that such withdrawal events did not occur during limitation of activity due to hospitalization or when the period of withdrawal was limited. Furthermore, completely objective data, such as from the numerous double-blind post-infarction secondary prevention trials did not confirm an excess of untoward events after abrupt termination of active drug.

Animal experimentation supported the existence of post-withdrawal hypersensitivity. In man, abrupt withdrawal has been studied experimentally in hypertensive patients without ischaemia [22]. Generally there was no overshoot of the blood pressure. During the first 14 days or so after withdrawal of propranolol, every patient exhibited a heightened heart rate responsiveness to intravenous isoprenaline when compared to the pre-propranolol responsiveness. Some patients experienced palpitation, tremor, sweating or ECG changes coinciding with the time of maximal isoprenaline sensitivity [23]. Prichard's group [23] reported similar findings in healthy volunteers having atenolol or propranolol withdrawn. But after pindolol withdrawal, no such rebound hypersensitivity was encountered. Contrary to these reports, others [24] have been unable to confirm post-propranolol hypersensitivity (heart rate responsiveness) following beta-adrenergically mediated stimuli (i.v. adrenaline and exercise). Not surprisingly, several (often disputed though not mutually exclusive) explanations have been proposed to account for untoward withdrawal events: (1) excessive exertion compared to the pre-treatment state; (2) progression of disease; (3) possible up regulation of beta-receptors; which may not occur in the presence of receptor stimulation, thus accounting for the apparent lack of hypersensitivity after pindolol which has PAA; (4) changes in platelet function; (5) changes in free T_3, platelet stickiness, etc.

The conflicting data from currently available research on beta-blocker withdrawal raise some doubts as to the existence of clinically significant rebound hypersensitivity (particularly a true overshoot). Nevertheless, for ethical reasons, it may be expedient to accord its existence the benefit of doubt. Accordingly, when stopping beta-blockers it is usually accepted that: (1) drugs like pindolol may carry the least risk; (2) dose should be reduced gradually particularly the final decrement (but not at all or very slowly if there are symptoms); and (3) exertion should be minimized.

(c) Advantageous effect on plasma lipids?

In a review of this subject van Brummelen [25] concluded that treatment with beta-blockers excepting sotolol had negligible effect on total plasma cholesterol or low density lipoprotein (LDL). However, apart from those with PAA, beta-blockers (especially non-selective agents) tend to increase plasma triglyceride levels and decrease the levels of so-called 'highly desirable' or high density lipoproteins (HDL). The theoretical disadvantage of the ensuing decreased HDL/LDL ratio is difficult to evaluate. This is because, irrespective of their effect on plasma lipids, they all appear capable of exerting a favourable impact on clinical outcome after myocardial infarction. Interestingly, treatment with drugs possessing PAA such as pindolol, actually increase plasma HDL levels, through a direct or indirect action involving tonic low grade beta-receptor agonism. It remains to be seen whether a clinically significant advantage arises from this effect.

(d) Treatment of orthostatic hypotension due to peripheral autonomic neuropathy?

Study of different categories of postural hypotension [26] and the current approaches to treatment have led to recognition of the importance of venous tone and heart rate in its complex pathophysiology. In patients with peripheral efferent (and afferent) autonomic neuropathy causing severe postural hypotension and symptoms, some workers [27] reported dramatic symptomatic benefits as a result of treatment with pindolol. Within days of initiating regular oral pindolol their patients were rendered capable of standing and walking without 'fainting', the extent of postural hypotension had decreased, and the benefit continued to be felt after several years of treatment. This occurred without a significant change in peripheral resistance, indicating that, on changing to the upright posture there must have been (1) venoconstriction (and decreased venous pooling), and/or (2) increased cardiac rate and contractility (possibly due to venoconstriction and increased venous return). Further reports about such patients (cited in reference [27]) have also confirmed similar beneficial effects from pindolol treatment, but in other forms of autonomic neuropathy with preganglionic efferent denervation, benefit does not seem to ensue. The above-mentioned therapeutic action of pindolol has been ascribed to beta-receptor agonism (due to PAA), occurring in the presence of substantial denervation supersensitivity in the heart, possibly due to beta-receptor up regulation. Indeed, in one patient with autonomic neuropathy, it was shown that cardiac sensitivity (heart rate response) to i.v. isoprenaline and salbutamol had decreased by about 6- and 50-fold respectively, after four weeks of starting regular treatment with pindolol. By the same token, vascular sensitivity 'reduction of mean arterial blood pressure in response to the same beta-agonists' also decreased. The responses in this patient could be taken to suggest a state of heightened cardiac and vascular beta-receptor sensitivity.

Since the benefits of pindolol treatment for the above patients appeared to be sustained even after loss of 'supersensitivity', maintenance of supersensitivity did not seem crucial. However, as vascular beta-receptors are evidently not innervated, it is unclear why denervation supersensitivity should develop. It is also difficult to explain adequately why, in the presence of vascular beta-receptor supersensitivity, pindolol does not give rise to venodilatation sufficient to increase postural symptoms. Moreover, how could pindolol act on the heart to augment cardiac output, if there were a reduction in venous return due to venous pooling? Thus, whilst there may well be denervation alpha-receptor supersensitivity in the vessels of patients likely to respond favourably, beta-receptor 'supersensitivity' *per se* seems insufficient to account for the benefits of pindolol. Alternatively, after commencing regular pindolol therapy, the decreased sensivity to the vasodilator actions of beta-agonists could reflect desensitization rather than loss of supersensitivity. Furthermore, on attaining the upright posture, these patients may still be capable of releasing adrenaline into the circulation. The latter may result in an exaggerated vasodilator response, due to a normal beta-receptor mediated vasodilator response and an absence of the compensatory (alpha-receptor mediated) noradrenergic neural response. In that case, desensitization of blood vessels resulting from the minimal but tonic effect of pindolol therapy might overcome the powerful vasodilator impact of posturally mediated adrenaline release. Moreover, the ensuing improvement in postural symptoms would be sustained over the duration of such therapy. In cases where the neuropathy also affected adrenaline release, no benefit could be expected from pindolol. These and other vexing questions and speculations regarding the role of beta-blockers with and without PAA, in the management of postural hypotension, must await the outcome of further investigations on larger series of patients.

(e)   Provision of beta-blockade without resting bradycardia

When different beta-blockers are administered in doses producing comparable reductions in the tachycardias associated with sympathetic stimulation (e.g. exercise or beta-agonists), it is widely recognized that those without PAA produce trivial or no slowing of resting heart rate by a clinically and statistically significant degree [28]. Whereas there is little doubt that this phenomenon has been widely observed, its clinical usefulness has not been established, since it is not possible to infer that asymptomatic resting bradycardias are necessarily deleterious. Nevertheless, particularly in elderly patients, there may be a case for objectively confirming or refuting the contention that such 'mild' bradycardias are indeed asymptomatic.

Resting and exercise electrophysiological studies [29] in 46 patients using comparable intravenous cardiac beta-blocking doses revealed that pindolol, atenolol, and acebutolol had equivalent depressant activity on AV node conduction. Thus, in patients with sick sinus syndrome and conduction system disorder agents with PAA were unlikely to be safer than the others. It follows that whenever beta-blockade is considered imperative for such patients, pacemakers should be utilized rather than relying on the dubious safety of drugs with PAA.

In a double-blind trial of hypertensive patients treated with pindolol or metoprolol (with and without PAA respectively), both drugs had equivalent antihypertensive effect but after metoprolol resting heart rates were slower and there were lesser reductions in calf vascular resistance [30]. It was concluded that the agent with PAA had an important direct vasodilator component contributing to its antihypertensive action in contrast to the mainly cardiac (central) action of metoprolol.

In patients with coronary artery disease, Taylor and co-workers [15], reported that when intravenous doses of different beta-blockers inhibited exercise tachycardia equally, those with PAA produced lesser reductions in resting heart rate. They also claimed that the latter produced less myocardial depression (as judged by resting and exercise cardiac output, systolic blood pressure and pulmonary artery wedge pressure). This effect of PAA was ascribed to cardiac stimulation and relatively smaller exercise-induced increases in peripheral resistance. However, it is not at all clear whether augmented cardiac contractility is necessarily advantageous in coronary artery disease. Furthermore, before accepting all the conclusions from this between patient, non-blind investigation, it should be noted that four different treatments were compared in only 24 patients.

(f) Diminished risk of peripheral vascular insufficiency

This claim is not well founded as it is based on rather equivocal anecdotal data.

2.5 Lipid solubility

Lack of lipid solubility, reviewed by Shand [31], distinguishes nadolol, atenolol, practolol and sotalol from propranolol. Of these, atenolol is a selective antagonist, practolol has unacceptable toxicity whilst also possessing selectivity and PAA, and sotalol has special electrophysiological properties. Thus, of the non-lipid-soluble beta-blockers, only nadolol and atenolol are currently used in clinical practice and only nadolol differs from propranolol purely on the basis of lipophilicity. Relative water solubility (lipid insolubility) appears to confer beta-blockers with important pharmacokinetic features, many of which may be clinically worthwhile. In contrast to propranolol and other relatively lipophilic drugs (also referred to as hydrophobic or non-polar compounds), the relatively water-soluble (hydrophilic or polar) beta-blockers are largely excreted in the urine and not metabolized by the liver. Moreover, such elimination tends to be much slower than hepatic degradation; the elimination half-life of lipid-soluble agents being about 2–6 hours compared to 7–20 hours for the water-soluble beta-blockers.

These pharmacokinetic attributes of water-soluble beta-blockers result in one major clinically significant advantage over propranolol; namely, they enable infrequent yet effective dosing. As nadolol and atenolol are eliminated relatively slowly, once daily dosing generally maintains plasma drug concentrations within a relatively narrow range. This is not generally possible with the more rapidly eliminated lipid-soluble drugs like propranolol. The latter often require 6–4 hourly dosing in order to provide therapy with drug concentrations that remain within a comparable range (i.e. neither toxic nor ineffectual). The great attraction of drug regimes incorporating single daily dosing is their convenience and acceptability for the majority of patients. As a result, patients may be more willing and able to comply with and benefit from their therapy. When the connection between drug levels and desirable therapeutic activity is remote or weak, it may not be essential to maintain the concentration at or above any given level at all times. In which case, infrequent dosing may be acceptable irrespective of the drug's pharmacokinetics. To some extent, this appears to be the case when beta-blockers are used to treat hypertension. Indeed, equally good control of hypertension can be achieved throughout the twenty-four hours, whether rapidly eliminated drugs such as propranolol are administered twice or four times daily. Single daily dosing however, is less satisfactory. Thus, with respect to the dosing frequency of beta-blockers used to treat hypertension, single daily dosing with nadolol or atenolol offers only a minor advantage over twice daily treatment with other beta-blockers such as propranolol. Many of the other applications of beta-blockers (e.g. treatment of angina or supraventricular tachycardia), involve a much closer correlation between tissue drug concentrations and their desirable actions (cardiac beta-blocking activity). In these instances the ability of single daily doses of nadolol and atenolol to achieve satisfactory benefits throughout a 24 hour period is a distinct advantage.

Lipid solubility or the lack of it, in combination with other physical features such as drug pKa and protein binding may also be linked to pharmacodynamic properties such as selectivity [8], non-lipid solubility appearing to confer selectivity for so-called beta$_1$-receptors. If true, then other factors must be more important in the case of metoprolol which is both selective and lipid soluble, and nadolol which is non-selective and non-lipid soluble. It has also been suggested that the physiochemical/pharmacokinetic properties of non-lipophilic beta-blockers confer several other minor differences which might be of some clinical significance. These include the following.

(a) Lack of hepatic first pass effect reducing the variation in bio-availability after oral dosing?

In contrast to propranolol and other lipid-soluble agents, after nadolol and atenolol are absorbed from the gut, they undergo virtually no metabolism in the liver before reaching the systemic circulation. It has been argued that after oral administration of water-soluble drugs, there might be less interindividual variation in systemic bio-availability than after oral propranolol, since variation cannot arise through changes in hepatic blood flow or liver enzyme activity. These possible advantages have been negated to some extent, due to incomplete bio-availability of both drugs as a result of incomplete absorption from the gut; oral compared to systemic bio-availability of atenolol and nadolol being about 55% and 30% respectively. Conceivably, after oral dosing, variation in absorptive capacity (like variation in first pass effect), could also give rise to considerable interindividual variation in systemic bio-availability. Indeed, after oral nadolol such variable absorption has already been inferred [32].

(b) Absence of drug interactions involving induction or inhibition of liver enzymes or changes in liver blood flow

It has been shown that the systemic bio-availability of oral propranolol but not nadolol or atenolol [33], is drastically increased in individuals receiving cimetidine (a drug which appears to inhibit metabolism and perhaps reduce hepatic blood flow). This is only a minor disadvantage with propranolol, as clinically the dosage is often individualized by titration. Nevertheless, there is a risk of failing to anticipate important changes in bio-availability when other drugs are started or stopped.

(c) Diminished risk from abrupt withdrawal?

As compared to propranolol, nadolol and atenolol are eliminated more slowly and the corresponding beta-blocking activity also decays more slowly. It has therefore been postulated that abrupt termination of dosing might nevertheless constitute more gradual withdrawal of the drug from tissues and diminish the risk of post-withdrawal ischaemic events. Evidence to support this contention is lacking [34].

(d) Drug accumulation in renal failure, but not in hepatic failure

This subject has been reviewed in [31, 35, 36]. Fortunately, correct dosage is usually selected by titration so as to produce the desired beneficial effect with the minimum of drug. Clinically significant renal impairment requiring dosage reduction occurs when the glomerular filtration rate (GFR) is less than 35 ml/min. In general it is sufficient to adjust daily dosage inversely (by reducing individual doses or by increasing the dosing interval) in proportion to the reduction of GFR. In contrast to water-soluble beta-blockers those that are lipid soluble tend to be eliminated by hepatic metabolism and are retained excessively in the presence of hepatic impairment [35]. Nevertheless, in severe renal failure even the dosage of lipid-soluble agents may warrant adjustment, as there is reason to suspect that many such drugs give rise to active metabolites [37] which may be more water soluble and hence more dependent on renal function.

(e) Influence on central nervous system (CNS) activity?

It has long been recognized that individuals receiving beta-blockers may be subject to CNS effects (reviewed by Turner [38]), particularly sleep disturbance, vivid dreams and even hallucinations. Consequently, it has frequently been inferred that treatment with lipid-soluble rather than non-lipid-soluble agents was more likely to give rise to CNS effects, as the former drugs might enter the brain more readily. However, there has been no convincing evidence to suggest that lipid-soluble agents do indeed have a more marked or consistent CNS action. In one recent investigation [39] utilizing psychomotor and psychosensory testing, significant effects were noted after single oral doses of atenolol and nadolol (water-soluble agents) as well as propanolol and diazepam (lipid-soluble drugs). This may be because central nervous system beta-receptors may actually exist within brain water rather than lipid. On the contrary, the beneficial action of beta-blockers in certain types of anxiety (see later) and their effects on psychomotor testing may be attributed to their peripheral action on skeletal muscle [38]. But the subjective responses to beta-blockers [40] and some of the results from psychosensory testing suggest a direct central effect. It must be admitted nonetheless that experimental studies using psychomotor and psychosensory tests in subjects taking a variety of different beta-blockers have yielded conflicting results.

Notwithstanding these issues, according to one double-blind crossover study [41] it has been implied that atenolol's lack of lipid solubility might be associated with a lesser tendency to produce hallucinations than propranolol. In the latter, six patients known to have developed vivid dreams or hallucinations after lipophilic drugs had only one such episode on atenolol compared to 30 on lipophilic drugs (propranolol and meto-prolol). Naturally, the blinding of the patients must be suspect, as drugs previously appearing to cause symptoms may have been recognized. Moreover if the symptoms were due to idiosyncrasy, then any change from the previous drug therapy might be better tolerated irrespective of lipid solubility. No doubt, an enormous trial would have been required to test the hypothesis in patients starting beta-blockers for the first time. Certainly, if a centrally mediated hypotensive action exists, it must account for the hypotensive properties of non-lipid-soluble drugs such as atenolol and nadolol. Experiments [42] in which beta-blocking drugs were infused into the arteries supplying the CNS and the peripheral circulation of cats, did not support a central action for the hypotensive effect of propranolol (but such an action was inferred in the case of alprenolol). Thus, for the majority of beta-blockers, the existence of a centrally mediated hypotensive role can be regarded as subsidiary, at least in cats.

(f) Conservation of renal blood flow?

Both in volunteers and in patients with hypertension there have been claims [43] that, compared to treatment with many beta-blockers includ-ing propranolol, nadolol was less liable to jeopardize renal blood flow. According to some workers propranolol also decreases glomerular filtra-tion rate without a change in plasma creatinine, presumably due to tubular secretion. This possible difference in effect between nadolol and propranolol has not been attributed to lack of lipid solubility. Attention has been drawn to the action on the kidney attributed to nadolol and the renal action of dopamine with which nadolol bears structural similarity. Regrettably, many of these claims have been based on retrospective comparisons, and it was not always possible to ensure that equivalent therapeutic doses of different beta-blockers were being compared. In-deed, there have been many contrary claims [44]. Moreover, it is unclear whether such actions on renal blood flow have any clinically significant influence on renal function in normal subjects or in hypertensives, and what if any influence they have on the evolution of renal impairment in patients with hypertension. Under the circumstances, further studies are required to clarify these issues.

2.6 Coexistent alpha-receptor blocking activity

The physiology and pharmacology of alpha-adrenoceptors in relation to beta-adrenoceptors was reviewed by Gross [45]. It is important to appreciate that either antagonism of *alpha$_1$-receptors*, leading to a reduction in peripheral resistance and reduction in cardiac output due to venous pooling, or stimulation of *alpha$_2$-receptors*, leading to central nervous inhibition of peripheral noradrenaline release, will reduce the blood pressure. Tolerance to the antihypertensive action of traditional alpha-blockers may in part have resulted from their tendency to antagonize both receptor subtypes; the peripheral antihypertensive action thus being opposed by their central action. Reduction in alpha-receptor-mediated arteriolar tone provokes an immediate hypotensive response, whereas reduction in venous tone due to alpha-receptor blockade predisposes to postural hypotension. To date, labetalol is the only well-established and widely marketed beta-blocker also having alpha-blocking activity (predominantly against alpha$_1$-receptors). Nevertheless it is probably appropriate to categorize labetalol principally as a beta-blocker that also exhibits relatively mild alpha-blocking activity (and a correspondingly mild tendency to provoke postural hypotension). Thus, when it exerts a given degree of antihypertensive action due to a combination of beta- and alpha-receptor blocking activity, the associated postural symptoms may be less pronounced than with antihypertensive drugs mediating their effect through alpha-blockade alone, but more pronounced than with treatment utilizing pure beta-blockers.

From a clinical point of view the features which distinguish antihypertensive treatment with the beta- and alpha-receptor blocking drug labetalol from other beta-blockers may be outlined [46, 47] as follows.

2.6.1 ADVERSE EFFECTS AND SIDE EFFECTS

(a) Due to alpha$_1$-receptor blockade

These are especially liable to occur: (1) after large single doses, and thus once daily therapy with a single large dose (e.g. 1 g) may prove unsatisfactory and (2) after moderately large doses (400 mg twice daily) introduced abruptly [47], but are probably less likely if the dose is gradually built up incrementally over several weeks (from about 150 mg daily).

Up to 25% of patients on long-term therapy stop the drug due to symptoms associated with postural hypotension. Side effects due to alpha$_1$-blockade include: light headedness, nausea and vomiting, epigastric discomfort, headaches, nasal stuffiness, scalp tingling, possibly related to piloerection, fluid retention, presumably due to vasodilatation, which often requires diuretics to overcome, and very rarely difficulty with micturition including stranguary. Despite the occurrence of postural hypotension, tachycardia is not pronounced, presumably due to cardiac beta-blockade.

(b) Antinuclear antibodies

According to the experience of Waal-Manning and her colleagues [49] and others they cite, about 20–28% of patients on long-term therapy develop at least weakly positive antibody titres. Although such antinuclear antibodies have long been recognized to develop in patients receiving many beta-blockers, the reported incidence in labetalol-treated patients appears to be rather high. As with other examples of drug-induced lupus, symptomatic illness seems rare, and anti-DNA antibodies (a feature of classical lupus) are notably absent [50].

2.6.2 POSSIBLE ADVANTAGEOUS EFFECTS

(a) Increased antihypertensive activity

Due to its dual mode of action, labetalol is often considered to be more potent than other beta-blockers, and allegedly it is effective in many patients refractory to other antihypertensive drugs. However, it is difficult to evaluate let alone substantiate such claims. A more tangible benefit is the rapidity of its antihypertensive action (presumably due to vascular alpha$_1$-receptor blockade); for which reason it has been utilized to bring about an abrupt reduction in blood pressure in patients presenting with severe hypertension. Such treatment may be given intravenously [51] but occasionally very marked and unpredictable blood pressure reductions may occur. Lest such acute effects produce severe neurological damage, Davies and co-workers [52] using continuous ambulatory blood pressure monitoring have pointed out that even oral labetalol reduces the blood pressure quite rapidly (within 1 hour), but without incurring any marked acute hypotension.

(b) Reduced risk of peripheral vascular insufficiency

Compared to treatment with other beta-blockers, it is alleged that Raynaud's phenomenon and intermittent claudication are less likely to occur during labetalol therapy. Conversely, when Raynaud's syndrome occurs during treatment with pure beta-blockers it may be possible to substitute labetalol without recurrence of symptoms. This relative lack of problems due to peripheral vascular insufficiency presumably reflects the protective effect of alpha$_1$-receptor blockade.

(c) Control of blood pressure surges (or sustained hypertension) mediated through noradrenergic sympathetic stimulation

Amongst beta-blockers, labetalol appears to be uniquely suitable for this purpose on account of its alpha-blocking activity. The whole subject is extensively discussed elsewhere. The theoretical basis for this action is supported by the highly significant correlation between basal plasma levels of noradrenaline (but not adrenaline) and the reduction in blood pressure induced by i.v. labetalol [53].

2.7 Sustained hypertension

The suspicion that asymptomatic moderate to mild hypertension was an independent cardiovascular risk factor was amply confirmed by the Framingham Survey. The Veterans Administration clinical trials together with others [54] have firmly established the benefits of drug treatment; the greatest benefit being in cerebrovascular morbidity and mortality, especially for those with pre-existent target organ damage. Early agents employed to achieve these ends had an unacceptably high incidence of side effects, which led to the acceptance of beta-blockers as important antihypertensive drugs.

The current role of beta-blocking drugs in the treatment of hypertension and the controversies surrounding the possible mechanisms whereby they have antihypertensive activity have been reviewed by Prichard [55]. Traditionally, in the stepped care approach to treatment, step 1 involved therapy with a thiazide diuretic, step 2 involved use of a beta-blocker, which could be followed by combining steps 1 and 2 or further steps entailing use of other agents singly or in combination. Increasingly however, despite their being more expensive, there has been a trend toward using beta-blockers as agents of first choice (step 1). A criticial comparison of the respective clinical benefits, adverse effects and other matters of concern related to diuretics and beta-blockers has been itemized below, and provides some of the reasons for this trend towards using beta-blockers as step 1 alternatives to diuretics. At present, it is not possible to justify an outright preference for using beta-blockers in place of thiazide diuretics.

2.7.1 CONTROL OF HYPERTENSION

According to the ongoing Medical Research Council single-blind placebo controlled trial of mild hypertension [56], fixed dose bendrofluazide (5 mg bd) produced superior blood pressure control (about 5 mm Hg systolic) than titrated dose propranolol therapy. The trial entailed follow-up of more than 20 000 patients for up to 5 years. Paradoxically, a greater proportion of those on diuretics required supplementary treatment (alpha-methyldopa); the difference being clinically and statistically significant.

2.7.2 CLINICAL BENEFITS

Whereas myocardial infarction is the most important cause of death associated with hypertension, the greatest benefit of antihypertensive therapy appears to be a reduction in cerebrovascular complications. Controlled clinical trials published to date do not show unequivocal reductions in the incidence of myocardial infarction, but such trials usually involved antihypertensive drugs other than beta-blockers (e.g. diuretics and/or alpha-methyldopa). Since there is now overwhelming evidence of cardioprotection from post-infarction secondary prevention trials with beta-blockers, it is tempting to speculate that patients who have not had prior myocardial infarction might enjoy a similar beneficial effect (primary protection) during treatment of their hypertension with beta-blockers.

Relatively weak evidence from indirect, non-randomized, non-blind studies provides some grounds for optimism that some benefit may indeed accrue. Thus, Beevers and co-workers [57] performed a retrospective analysis (mean follow-up 44 months) on 920 consecutive hypertensive patients (age <75 years) attending blood pressure clinics. In those without prior strokes, angina or myocardial infarction, vascular complications were less frequent in the 377 individuals who received beta-blockers than the 306 who did not (12.7% versus 16.9%). The risk of angina and myocardial infarction appeared to be reduced the least (6.5% versus 7.3%). By contrast, in the 242 patients with prior vascular complications, treatment with beta-blockers appeared to confer relatively greater benefit with respect to overall vascular complications (16.5% versus 38.3%) as well as cardiac complications (7.3% versus 11.3%). The latter observations were entirely consistent with the known results of post-infarction secondary prevention trials. Furthermore, diuretic therapy per se did not appear deleterious, but rather benefit was exhibited in patients receiving beta-blocker. Definitive evidence concerning these issues must await the results from more formal clinical trials which are currently under way.

2.7.3 ADVERSE EFFECTS LEADING TO WITHDRAWAL

In men, withdrawal from drug treatment due to adverse reactions was equally common after treatment with propranolol and bendrofluazide

[56]. In women the corresponding withdrawal rate was slightly greater after propranolol than the diuretic.

(1) The advantages of propranolol were the lesser liability to impaired glucose tolerance, gout and impotence; the latter two being particularly troublesome in men taking bendrofluazide.

(2) The disadvantages of propranolol were the higher incidences of Raynaud's phenomenon, skin disorders, lethargy and dyspnoea; of which lethargy occurred more frequently in women.

(3) Overall, propranolol suited men marginally better, whereas the thiazide suited women markedly better than propranolol.

2.6.4 BIOCHEMICAL AND OTHER ISSUES

The MRC hypertension trial [56] also provided follow-up data on serum biochemistry of patients after 3 years of treatment on bendrofluazide, propranolol and placebo. The principal changes (summarized in Table 2.1) were: (1) increases in urea and uric acid particularly on thiazide, (2) decreases in potassium after bendrofluazide; and (3) minimal increases in potassium after propranolol. The changes in serum potassium were in line with the known actions of thiazide diuretics and beta-blockers. The extent of the changes were considerably unlikely to be dangerous except in patients on diuretics also receiving cardiac glycosides. Surprisingly, subsidiary studies revealed that with long-term bendrofluazide therapy there was statistically a highly significant correlation between ventricular ectopy and hypokalaemia and curiously also between ventricular ectopy and hyperuricaemia. The clinical significance of the latter correlations remains uncertain.

Table 2.1

Drug treatment	Change in serum biochemical value in mmol/l		
	Urea (3.3—6.7)*	Uric acid (0.24—0.54 men)*	Potassium (3.5—5.0)*
Placebo	+0.2	+0.008	+0.07
Bendrofluazide	+0.6	+0.065	−0.5
Propranolol	+0.35	+0.021	+0.2

* Range of normal values shown in parentheses

In contrast to the MRC trial, a much more sinister view of diuretic-induced potassium depletion was inferred by the investigators of the Multiple Risk Factor Intervention Trial (MRFIT) [58]. These researchers carried out a randomized primary prevention trial involving nearly 13 000 high risk middle-aged men assigned to usual care (UC), or special intervention (SI). The latter group attended at University Clinics directed to the goals of reducing blood pressure, reducing serum cholesterol, and reducing smoking. Paradoxically, both groups had equal mortality rates, despite the SI group having achieved a much greater reduction in risk factors. This apparent lack of benefit from 'risk factor' reduction was ascribed to higher death rates in hypertensive patients with pre-trial ECG abnormalities entering the SI group and receiving potassium-losing diuretics. The report consequently advocated routine potassium sup-plementation with diuretics, or recourse to other antihypertensive drugs such as propranolol (even though the trial had no propranolol-treated patients for comparison). Alternative explanations for the results include (1) a statistical quirk due to multiple subgroup analysis, (2) widespread use of propranolol only in the UC group which may afford some primary protection, (3) incorrect assumptions concerning 'risk factors', or (4) other confounding factors. It has been suggested that the latter include identi-fying patients at risk, notifying patients and their physicians, providing annual follow-up, and higher than anticipated standards of care in the community (UC group). Notwithstanding the MRFIT report, at present there is no convincing case for preferring beta-blockers to diuretics for treating hypertension, nor for routine potassium supplementation with thiazide diuretics unless patients are also digitalized.

2.8 The influence of beta adrenoceptor blockage on surges of blood pressure due to sympathetic stimulation

Goldenberg and co-workers [59] and Barcroft and Starr [60] were the first to elucidate the haemodynamic actions of circulating adrenaline and noradrenaline. They showed that in healthy volunteers, infusion of adrenaline (a potent alpha- and beta-receptor agonist) produced a net reduction in peripheral resistance, as alpha-receptor mediated vasocon-striction in some vascular beds, which was more than balanced out by beta-receptor mediated vasodilatation elsewhere. This was associated with a reduction in diastolic blood pressure, whereas there were increases in systolic blood pressure (beta-adrenoceptor mediated) and heart rate (beta-adrenoceptor mediated and reflex effects). In contrast, infusion of noradrenaline (a more selective alpha-receptor agonist) produced in-creases in peripheral resistance (alpha-adrenoceptor mediated vasocon-striction), and thus diastolic and systolic blood pressure both increased, but heart rate decreased reflexly.

More than a decade later, Prichard and Ross [61] drew attention to a possible adverse effect on blood pressure due to vascular beta-receptor blockade. They described phaeochromocytoma patients in receipt of an alpha-adrenoceptor antagonist (phenoxybenzamine), who experienced increases in lying and standing systolic and diastolic blood pressure (lasting about eight hours) following single 80 mg doses of oral propranolol. Presumably, beta-adrenoceptor-mediated vasodilatation brought about by circulating adrenaline was antagonized, thus unmasking alpha-receptor mediated vasoconstriction producing increased peripheral resistance (increased afterload) and venoconstriction (increased preload). This explanation received support through more controlled studies involving adrenaline infusion in healthy volunteers as well as patients with hypertension [62]. The latter studies confirmed that adrenaline infusion produced a net reduction in peripheral resistance together with a commensurate reduction in diastolic and mean blood pressure, whilst heart rate increased (probably by direct and reflex effects). Both studies also showed that when individuals were pre-treated with propranolol, adrenaline infusion gave rise to increases in peripheral resistance as well as diastolic and mean blood pressures. As with the phaeochromocytoma patients described by Prichard and Ross [61], this was consistent with antagonism of beta-adrenoceptor mediated vasodilatation unmasking alpha-adrenoceptor mediated vasoconstriction. Interestingly, after pre-treatment with metoprolol, a selective antagonist less liable to block beta$_2$-receptor mediated vasodilatation, the haemodynamic responses to adrenaline infusion were akin to those encountered with adrenaline alone.

Other stimuli likely to involve sympathetic activation, viz. isometric hand grip (c.f. lifting a heavy suitcase), brief periods of incremental and steady-state dynamic exercise (c.f. running for a bus), or cold exposure, have been shown to increase diastolic and systolic pressure (except dynamic exercise which only increases systolic pressure); moreover, the presence of selective versus non-selective antagonism made no difference to the pattern of pressor response [63, 64]. Most of these pressor responses are consistent with predominantly neurogenic (noradrenaline mediated) sympathetic stimulation and widespread vasoconstriction. Thus, neurally released noradrenaline, predominantly an alpha-receptor agonist, by virtue of its vasoconstrictor action appears to increase peripheral resistance and thereby increase diastolic and systolic blood pressure. Furthermore, because vascular beta-receptors (as opposed to alpha-receptors) are probably not innervated [27], the minimal beta-receptor agonistic activity of neurally released noradrenaline is unlikely to evoke any clinically significant vasolidation. Consequently whether co-existing beta-blockade was selective (sparing blood vessels) or not, would have little bearing on the ensuing response to sympathetically released noradrenaline at nerve endings.

Beta-adrenergic blocking drugs

By contrast, when circulating adrenaline, a powerful alpha and beta-receptor agonist, was responsible for the pressor response, diastolic pressure fell, at least in the absence of non-selective beta-blockade, whilst systolic pressure and heart rate increased. Moreover, as expected there was a clear difference in the pattern of pressor response depending on whether selective or non-selective beta-blockade was present. Thus, non-selective beta-blockade antagonized beta-receptor mediated vaso-dilation more readily than selective beta-blockade. The resulting diastolic and systolic hypertension appeared to make the action of adrenaline more akin to that of noradrenaline. On the other hand, selective beta-blockade, through relative lack of vascular beta-blocking activity had a trivial influence on the vasodilating action of adrenaline, and as expected interfered very little with the adrenaline effect on peripheral resistance and blood pressure.

It is thus possible to recognize two distinct categories of sympatheti-cally mediated pressor responses involving different humoral transmit-ters. These are:

(1) Responses mediated by neurally released noradrenaline producing increases in systolic and diastolic pressure, which are unaffected by selective or non-selective beta-blockade (except when alpha-blockade is also incorporated e.g. labetolol).

(2) Responses mediated by circulating adrenaline producing increases in systolic and decreases in diastolic pressure. These responses become exaggerated in the presence of non-selective (but not selective) beta-blockade, the diastolic decrease in blood pressure being converted into an increase.

Different provocative manoeuvres may evoke one or other (and rarely both) types of sympathetic pressor response. A tentative classification of the predominant pressor mechanism likely to be involved in the me-diation of a variety of pressor stimuli is provided in Table 2.2 [65].

Remarkably, the category to which each stimulus in Table 2.2 was assigned was not invariably deduced from the presence or absence of an increase in plasma adrenaline concentration. Rather, the physiological and pharmacological characteristics of each pressor response were con-sidered to be more important. For example, five-fold increases in plasma adrenaline and noradrenaline have been recorded during exercise and even larger increases in adrenaline, but not noradrenaline, occur in exercising individuals taking propranolol. Nevertheless, since isometric exercise is accompanied by an increase in both systolic and diastolic pressure and since the extent of the pressor responses is un-affected by selective or non-selective beta-blockade, it is probable that a predominantly neurogenic (noradrenaline mediated) sympethetic

Table 2.2 Pressor stimuli presumed to be sympathetically mediated

Predominantly due to neurogenic noradrenaline release or similar substance	*Predominantly due to circulating adrenaline (or similar substance)*

– cold exposure
– isometric exercise
– dynamic exercise
– smoking and coffee?
– sexual intercourse?
– acute mental stress?
– phenylephrine used as
    topical decongestant
	– phaeochromocytoma?
	– hypoglycaemic attacks
	    (brittle diabetes)
	– schizphrenia?
	– infiltrative local
	    anaesthesia with adrenaline
	– chonidine therapy/
	    withdrawal

Systolic and diastolic BP increase	Increase in systolic but decrease in diastolic BP
HR usually decreased	HR usually increased directly and reflexly
BP surge unaffected by beta-Blockade (non-selective or selective)	Diastolic BP increased during non-selective beta-blockade, but not during selective beta-blockade
Alpha$_1$-blockade (labetolol) may be useful	Alpha$_1$-blockade with labetolol may antagonize BP surge and tachycardia

response is involved. After beta-blockade, the diverse pressor responses to dynamic exercise are more confusing to interpret as the pressor response is mainly systolic, compatible with an effect due to the muscle pump and adrenaline. However, the absence of any difference in pressor response in the presence of selective versus non-selective beta-blockade, suggests that circulating adrenaline is unlikely to have an important role; but the involvement of noradrenergic or yet undefined pressor mechanisms has not been ruled out.

As opposed to what we know about sustained hypertension and its adverse long-term sequelae from the Framingham survey [66] there is no equivalent information as to the clinical significance of sympathetically provoked transient surges in blood pressure as listed in Table 2.2. However, the Framingham survey did find that the entity referred to as 'labile hypertension', assumed to be due to stress provoking sympathetic stimulation, was associated with an adverse prognosis. Similarly,

51

whereas treatment of sustained hypertension is known to be beneficial there have been no controlled studies to indicate whether abolition of acute hypertensive surges is clinically beneficial in terms of preventing life-threatening events such as subarachnoid haemorrhage. However, it is important to view hypertensive surges in an overall context. When mild, infrequent and transient such surges may have little clinical significance. Before inferring that they should all be eliminated or controlled, it is as well to reflect how universally these responses have evolved, and that at such times they may confer some overall benefit to the body.

Nevertheless, in the absence of information to the contrary it seems prudent to adopt a cautious approach and avoid converting purely systolic hypertensive surges into systolic and diastolic surges. Consequently, on an *a priori* basis it appears sensible to prefer selective antagonism or beta- and alpha-blockade rather than simple non-selective antagonism, whenever adrenaline or like substances are liable to enter the circulation in clinically significant amounts. Furthermore, until the precise role of sympathetic stimulation in the pathogenesis of so-called labile hypertension is clarified, indiscriminate treatment of all such patients with non-selective beta-blockers such as propranolol might well be inappropriate.

2.9 Coronary artery disease

The original concept that beta-blockers would be useful in angina due to coronary atheroma, by reducing myocardial oxygen demands, reviewed in the previous edition [1], has been largely confirmed in subsequent work cited in reference [15], and these drugs are the major standby as second-line treatment in the prophylaxis of angina after the acute use of nitrates. However, it is expedient to replace them with the vasodilator calcium antagonists if there are contraindications to beta-blockade or any suggestion of coronary spasm, which may be accentuated by unopposed alpha-activity after beta-blockade [1]. The secondary effects of the beta-blockers (due to ancillary properties) seem to have only a slight effect on the haemodynamic response [15] and the clinical usefulness of the various drugs in this group.

The further suggestion that prompt beta-blockade may limit the size of cardiac infarction (see Reference [15]), has been less well sustained, and it has been difficult to show any improvement in mortality. A recent study [67] showed a reduced incidence of ventricular fibrillation after beta-blockade, but prompt resuscitation prevented a significant reduction in mortality and there was little evidence of reduced infarct size. These findings support the original suggestion of Pantridge (reviewed in Refer-

Pharmacokinetics, dosing frequency and dosage, compliance

ence [1]), that early ventricular fibrillation relied on myocardial adrenergic mechanisms, which could be reduced by beta-blockade, rather than being improved as a secondary effect of reduced infarct size. This concept is supported by the uniform agreement that a variety of beta-blockers, including propranolol [68] produced about a 2% reduction in sudden death over the first year after infarction.

The disappointing response in attempts at reducing infarct size may relate to a misconception about the coronary anatomy. The coronary circulation behaves more like end-arteries, in spite of the profuse superficial large coronary artery anastomoses [69]. Isolated segments of myocardium are supplied by 'discrete capillary loops' [66], so that coronary occlusion produces clearly limited infarction with only minor marginal ischaemic zones which can be saved by intervention. Any major limitation of infarct size must then rely on removal of the causative coronary arterial occlusion, as by thrombolysis. The beneficial effect on ECG current of injury may rely on sparing of the ischaemic subendocardial zone of the infarct itself and elsewhere, where perfusion is made hazardous by the supply by penetrating arteries to the subendocardial plexus and the effect of diastolic cavity pressure on flow in the capillary bed.

Thus, use of beta-blockers after myocardial infarction may be summarized as follows [70]. (1) After recovery, long-term treatment (1–3 years or longer) results in clinically significant benefits in terms of mortality, risk of sudden death, and morbidity, especially in high risk patients. (2) The possible benefits of early intravenous treatment (limitation of infarct size and reduced risk of ventricular fibrillation) remain contentious though recent studies show a certain degree of promise.

2.10 Pharmacokinetics, dosing frequency and dosage, compliance

These interrelated issues are of fundamental importance to the appropriateness of therapy with any drug. Whilst the various ancillary properties of beta-adrenoceptor antagonists, discussed in the preceding edition of this chapter [1], may be of relatively trivial significance to their pharmacodynamic potential, they may nevertheless exert an important, indirect, clinical influence by affecting pharmacokinetics and thus dosing frequency and compliance to therapy. It is evident from Table 2.3 that lipid solubility (which is also associated with a high degree of binding to plasma proteins), confers rapid hepatic degradability, and the attendant pharmacokinetic correlates with lipid solubility are summarized in Table 2.4. The latter lists some commonly used beta-blocking drugs, their routes of elimination, their elimination half-lives, and the commonly advocated dosing schedules for the treatment of hypertension.

53

Table 2.3 Pharmacokinetic features and lipid solubility

Beta-blockers with high lipid solubility	Beta-blockers with low lipid solubility
– rapid elimination, needing more frequent dosing; compliance worse?	– slowly eliminated, enabling less frequent dosing; compliance better?
– hepatic elimination, no accumulation in renal failure alone	– renal elimination, accumulate in renal failure
subject to liver enzyme induction and inhibition	unaffected by liver enzyme induction or inhibition
first pass effect (variable), oral dosage >> IV dosage	no first pass effect oral dosage = I.V. dosage

N.B. Some beta-blockers (e.g. acebutolol, pindolol, timolol) display intermediate properties

Table 2.4 Lipid solubility, elimination characteristics and dosage

	Route of elimination	Elimination $t_{1/2}$ (h)	Oral dosage (mg) for high BP	
Relatively lipid soluble				
Acebutolol	Hepatic/renal	3	up to 200	
Alprenolol	Hepatic	2	up to 400	
Labetolol	Hepatic	4	up to 200	TWICE
Metoprolol	Hepatic	3–4	up to 200	
Oxprenolol	Hepatic	1.5–2	up to 160	
Pindolol	Hepatic/renal	3–4	up to 20	DAILY
Propranolol	Hepatic	2.5–4	up to 160	
Timolol	Hepatic/renal	2.5–4.5	up to 30	
Relatively non-lipid soluble				
Atenolol	Renal	6	up to 100	ONCE
Nadolol	Renal	6–24	up to 240	DAILY
Proctolol	Renal	10–11	NOT RECOMMENDED	
Sotolol	Renal	15–17		

Most of these data were compiled from Martindale [71]. Although the elimination half-lives are quoted from published reports, they should be regarded as approximations only. Wide variations in half life also occur due to age; increasing age tending to reduce both renal and hepatic drug elimination. A number of these agents have very complex dose-dependent pharmacokinetics not strictly described by conventional parameters such as half-life, and some give rise to active metabolites many of which depend on renal elimination. The recommended dosages have been compiled (with modification) from Martindale [71], and the frequency refers to conventional (not sustained release) formulations.

Pharmacokinetics, dosing frequency and dosage, compliance

It has often been argued that the more slowly eliminated non-lipid-soluble agents may be taken less frequently than their more rapidly eliminated lipid-soluble counterparts. Due to less frequent and thus more simplified dosing, compliance to therapy was likely to be enhanced. The spate of recently introduced long-acting (sustained-release) formulations of several well-known beta-blockers was no doubt spawned by the same argument. Implicit in this approach is the notion that tissue drug concentrations correlate closely with pharmacodynamic effects (desirable therapeutic attributes or undesirable toxic actions).

2.10.1 DOSING FREQUENCY IN THE TREATMENT OF HYPERTENSION

The antihypertensive activity of beta-blockers does not appear to conform with the aforementioned premise. On the contrary, such activity is generally acknowledged to be a remote outcome resulting from multiple complex actions [55]. Indeed, plasma concentrations of beta-blockers correlate weakly or not at all with antihypertensive effect [72, 73], possibly because the dose/antihypertensive response relationship rapidly attains a plateau. In keeping with a weak plasma level effect relationship is the suggestion that even with once daily dosing, the antihypertensive benefit of beta-blockers is sustained over 24 hours [74], irrespective of their rate of elimination from the body.

These assertions, however, probably require modification in the light of data available from continuous intra-arterial ambulatory blood pressure monitoring. Compared to traditional once-off methods of indirect blood pressure recording using a sphygmomanometer and cuff, intra-arterial pressure monitoring provides continuous accurate and objective data and is thus more comprehensive and reliable. According to properly controlled studies utilizing these techniques [75], it emerges that, with the more rapidly eliminated agents, when twice daily divided dosing is compared to single daily dosing, high blood pressure is not controlled to the same extent throughout the whole 24 hours; single morning dosing producing adequate control in the morning but inferior though discernible antihypertensive effect in the last 12 hours. More frequent dosing (three or four times daily), offers no further advantage over twice daily dosing. In contrast, it is generally agreed that the more slowly eliminated non-lipid-soluble drugs, such as atenolol and nadolol, as well as sustained-release (long acting) formulations of more rapidly eliminated drugs, provide comparable antihypertensive action over the whole period, whether given once or twice daily. Furthermore, continuous intra-arterial blood pressure monitoring also showed that the hypertensive surges associated with activity are not attenuated by either single or twice daily dosing with long- or short-acting pure beta-blockers [76]. However, such surges are dampened after labetolol treatment (compatible with an alpha-receptor mediated pathogenesis), and surprisingly also after therapy with metoprolol and sotolol.

Thus with respect to the dosing frequency used to treat hypertension:

(1) Short acting (lipid soluble) beta-blockers should be prescribed as two divided doses;

(2) Sustained release formulations of the above beta-blockers may be prescribed once a day; and thus offer only a slight advantage over twice daily dosing, but are generally more expensive than standard formulations;

(3) The more slowly eliminated and longer-acting water-soluble drugs such as atenolol and nadolol, may also be given once daily, and compared to sustained release beta-blockers have the added attractions of (a) being much cheaper (as a rule), and (b) being free from the risk of incomplete absorption, a disadvantage known to occur with sustained release formulations in the past and accepted as one of their inherent characteristics.

2.10.2 DOSAGE REQUIRED TO TREAT HYPERTENSION

In the past there has been an emphasis on using very large doses of beta-blockers to treat unresponsive cases of hypertension. Whereas this may have proved to be necessary in a few patients, it is now realized that in the majority of cases the dose/antihypertensive effect (Fig. 2.1) reaches a plateau after relatively small daily doses [77]. In some cases perhaps, the 'apparent benefit' derived from recourse to massive doses (as described in the past), may have been linked to problems with drug compliance.

2.10.3 DOSING FREQUENCY AND TOTAL DOSAGE TO TREAT ANGINA

In individual patients with effort angina, there appears to be reasonably sound evidence that antianginal activity is closely related to cardiac beta-blocking activity and hence to plasma drug concentration [78] (Fig. 2.2). Not surprisingly, in order to maintain a given degree of antianginal activity at all times, it also appears important to maintain a given plasma drug level. Thus, in comparison to the dosing frequencies recommended for the treatment of hypertension, somewhat more frequent dosing (thrice or four times daily) is advised for the treatment of angina with short-acting drugs [71]. In individual patients who only experience angina at certain times of the day, provision of adequate drug levels

PROPRANOLOL & STANDING BP; Dose/Response (4 wks, n=24)

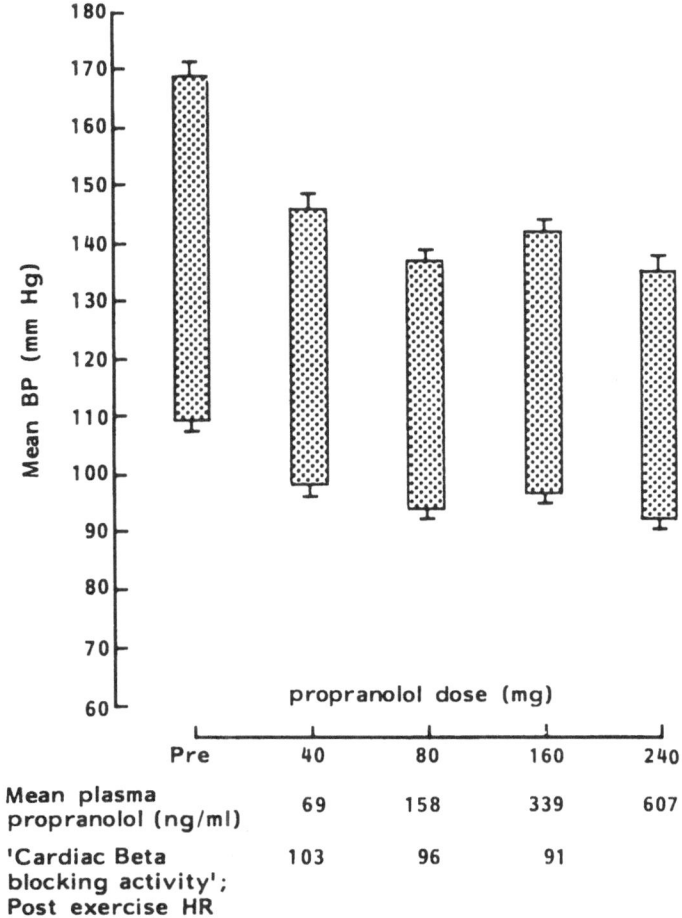

Fig. 2.1 The upper and lower limit of each bar represents systolic and diastolic blood pressure respectively. Despite progressively larger propranolol dosage, plasma propranolol concentrations and cardiac beta-blocking activity (as judged by post-exercise heart rate) virtually a maximum effect on blood pressure was achieved with the smallest dosage (propranolol 40 mg twice daily). (Modified from Fig. 1 of Reference [77] and produced with permission.)

only during the vulnerable period may suffice. In others, probably the majority, as the dosing frequency needs to be greater in order to provide continuous antianginal cover, the slowly eliminated beta-blockers or sustained-release preparations of the rapidly eliminated drugs, offer a

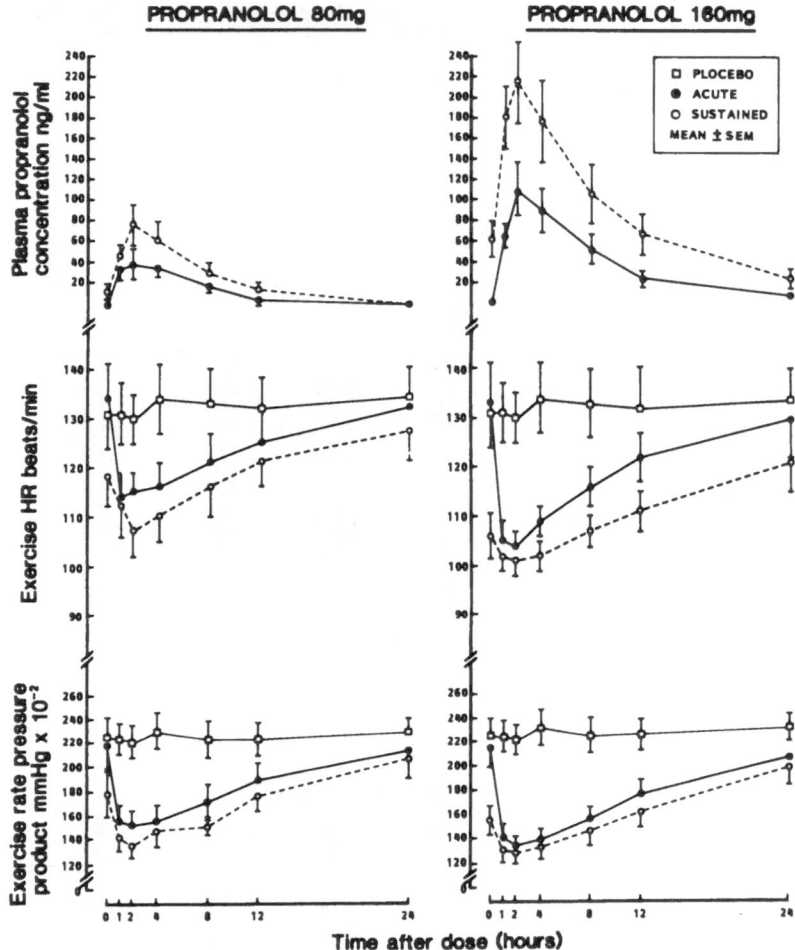

Fig. 2.2 Corresponding plasma propranolol levels were greater after 160 than 80 mg and after sustained (twice daily treatment) than after single acute dosing. Corresponding plasma levels all peaked around 2 hours post-dosing and then gradually decreased. These changes in plasma levels were associated with corresponding reductions in exercise heart rate (HR) and rate pressure product; the latter two parameters being indices of 'antianginal effect'. The results indicate that the antianginal activity of propranolol is closely reflected by the prevailing concentration of propranolol in the plasma. Within the range of plasma propranolol concentrations encountered in this study, the 'antianginal effect' had not reached a plateau. (Modified from Figs 1, 4 and 5 Reference [78] and produced with permission.)

58

somewhat greater advantage. As in the treatment of hypertension, both the slowly eliminated and the sustained release drugs can generally be prescribed once daily, and relative to each other they exhibit precisely the same advantages and disadvantages. It is also evident (Fig. 2.2) that the dose/antianginal effect relationship does not appear to level out in the same way as antihypertensive activity (Fig. 2.1). For this reason and also because there is no precise ideal titratable therapeutic end point, a higher and wider range of total daily dosage is generally prescribed during antianginal as compared to antihypertensive treatment.

2.10.4 COMPLIANCE

Although much has been written about the management of hypertension and compliance with drug treatment there is very little objective data on compliance dealing with drug therapy involving beta-blockers. However, indirect clues concerning this subject do exist.

For example, it is widely believed that there is a large inter-patient variation in propranolol requirements due to a large interindividual variation in propranolol pharmacokinetics [79]. Contrary to the variation in plasma propranolol levels predicted from such data, a highly pertinent and well-designed investigation in 46 diverse hospitalized patients [80], revealed a surprisingly narrow interindividual variation (only up to three fold) in the relationship between meticulously supervised propranolol dosage and the ensuing plasma level in accurately timed blood samples (Fig. 2.3). In contrast to plasma level variations due to interindividual pharmacokinetic differences, slight errors in dosing or sampling times appear liable to produce large plasma level variations. Conversely, the marked interindividual pharmacodynamic variation with respect to anti-arrhythmic actions of beta-blockers [81], (Fig. 2.4) appears to have been neglected hitherto. Presumably, the lower and much more variable plasma levels reported in the past were due to less rigorously conducted studies, in which the possibility of non-compliance by patients was neglected and/or there was lack of attention to the precise time of dosing and blood sampling. As with most forms of unsupervised drug therapy, compliance with beta-blockers is likely to be poor, particularly during long-term treatment for asymptomatic conditions such as hypertension. Under such circumstances, every effort should be directed towards simplifying beta-blocker therapy by utilizing once or twice daily dosing.

2.11 Adverse reactions/drug and non-drug interactions

Beta-adrenoceptor antagonist therapy may result in adverse effects which

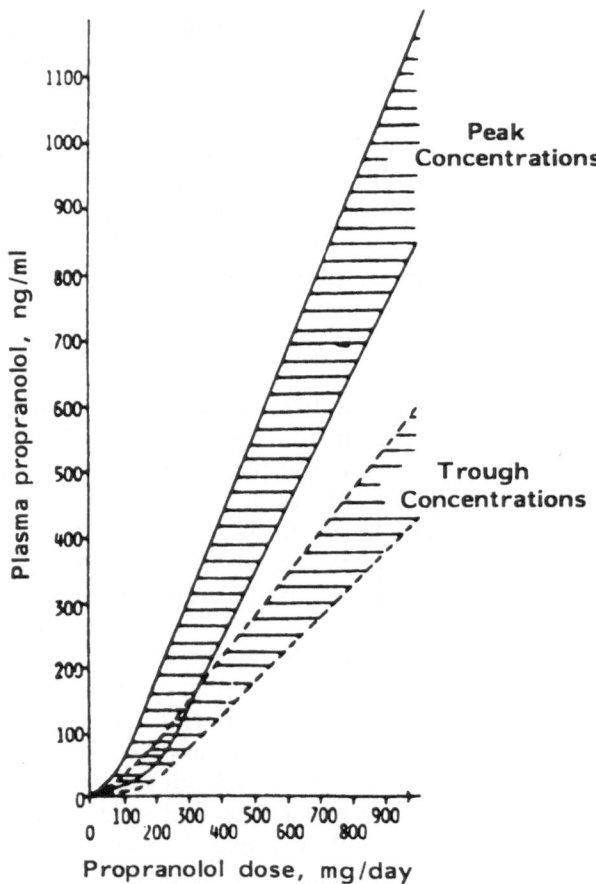

Fig. 2.3 Forty-six hospitalized patients who were heterogenous as to sex, age, body weight, smoking habits, medication they were receiving, and extent of hypertension and ischaemic heart disease had relatively small interindividual variations in steady-state propranolol levels (3-fold on 40 mg per day and 1.3-fold with doses exceeding 600 mg per day). Clearly at high doses individual variation was less than the variation between peak and trough plasma propranolol concentrations. The much-quoted figure of 20-fold variations in steady-state propranolol concentrations was derived from out-patient dosing and the authors [96] admitted that blood sampling to determine propranolol levels took place anywhere between 1 and 3 hours post-dosing. Presumably, the lower and much more variable levels they and others reported in the past were in much less rigorously conducted studies, and would have been due to non-compliance by patients or lack of attention to the time of dosing or blood sampling. (Modified from Fig. 6, Reference [80] and produced with permission.)

can be predicted from their pharmacological properties, viz: hypotension, heart failure, heart block, asthma, exacerbation of

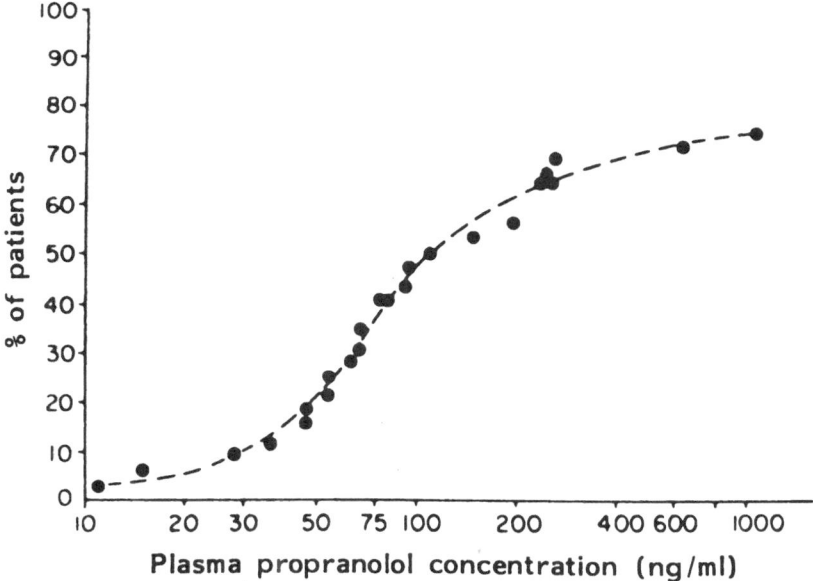

Fig. 2.4 A study of 32 patients with chronic ventricular tachyarrhythimas (VTAs). Cumulative percentage of patients with >70% arrhythmia suppression vs plasma propranolol concentration. Paradoxically, even after arrhythmias were controlled, in a few cases there were recurrences after further increases in drug dose and plasma concentration. The plasma propranolol concentration at which these VTAs were controlled varied over a 1000-fold range. (Modified from Fig. 3, Reference [81]) and produced with permission.)

Raynaud's phenomenon and other symptoms of peripheral vascular insufficiency [82]. Though clinically significant effects due to these are uncommon, they are nevertheless well known and generally it is assumed that such problems only manifest in susceptible individuals and/or after excessive dosage. Unpredictable non-specific side effects occurring uncommonly include: (1) vivid dreams and hallucinations; (2) malaise, impotence, gastrointestinal symptoms and skin rash. The abovementioned predictable and unpredictable adverse effects will not be considered any further.

Non-drug interactions (potential adverse effects) reported with beta-blockers are summarized in Table 2.5, and drug-related pharmacokinetic interactions are summarized in Table 2.6. The clinical significance of many of the pharmacokinetic interactions referred to remains uncertain, partly because dosage is often titrated according to therapeutic response. Also, measurable beta-blocking activity is often proportional to the logarithm of the drug concentration (dosage), so that modest changes in drug concentrations may be relatively unimportant.

Beta-adrenergic blocking drugs

Table 2.5 Non-drug interactions: potential adverse effects

Renal failure – reduces excretion of water-soluble drugs [1]

Advanced age – may increase plasma levels [1]

Precipitation of hepatic encephalopathy – presumably from reduction in cardiac output

Thyrotoxicosis – needs caution as may accentuate thyrotoxic heart failure [1]

Possible precipitation of hypothyroid coma? [83]

Hypoglycaemic stimuli – may potentiate alpha-adrenergic hypertension (see later)

Abrupt withdrawal of beta-blockers – leaves the patient with up-regulated receptors and vulnerable to hypertensive stimuli and exacerbation of angina?

Pregnancy – use in hypertension of pregnancy limited by concern about fetal retardation from reduced placental blood flow and fetal bradycardia from the drugs crossing the placental barrier (see section 2.10.1)

Practolol syndrome [84] – (see section 2.10.2)

Possible hearing loss [85]

2.11.1 PREGNANCY

Treatment of pregnant women with beta-blockers (reviewed in Reference [88]) created considerable controversy when first introduced. This was because retrospective studies as well as case reports implicated them as one factor responsible for (a) premature labour (uterine anti-relaxation activity), (b) intrauterine growth retardation (placental insufficiency), (c) neonatal cardiorespiratory depression, and (d) neonatal hypoglycaemia. These fears have not been realized. On the contrary, considerable cummulative experience from other studies suggests that they produce equivalent benefit to other agents and some of the complications listed above may even be decreased. It is currently believed that beta-blockers have the following advantages over other drugs when used in the treatment of hypertension occurring during pregnancy:

(1) Relatively few side effects
(2) Gradual onset of antihypertensive effect
(3) No postural hypotension
(4) Blood pressure reduced to normal (not low) levels

Fetal cardiac slowing occurs, but does not constitute a clinically significant disadvantage; even monitoring for fetal heart rate changes appears to be valid. There is reason to believe that beta-blockers with partial agonist activity (e.g. pindolol) do not give rise to fetal bradycardia. Compared to other beta-blockers labetolol, which has alpha- and beta-

Table 2.6 Pharmacokinetic drug interactions

Affecting beta-blocker concentration: especially those having high hepatic extraction ratios – propranolol, metoprolol, labetolol

- -

Oral beta-blocker dosage requirement theoretically increased due to liver enzyme induction – accelerated metabolism, e.g. barbiturates, rifampican, thyroxine

Oral beta-blocker dosage requirement theoretically decreased due to liver enzyme inhibition (decreased first pass) or altered liver blood flow, e.g. cimetidine, chlorpromazine? oral contraceptive, hydralazine

Displacement from protein binding, e.g. heparin?
 heparin?

Affecting other drugs:

- -

Reduced dosage requirement of lignocaine and chlorpromazine due to hepatic blood flow reduction by
 – propranolol, metoprolol, labetolol

(Kendal and Beely [82], give details about propranolol and metroprolol but similar considerations probably apply to labetolol). When the dosage is titrated to obtain symptomatic responses, such interactions may not be important, but may have clinical relevance when used prophylactically.

Similarly, pharmacogentic variation affecting timolol and metoprolol hydroxylation (which correlates with debrisoquin hydroxylation phenotype), though it may account for considerable bioavailability and dose-response variation [86], is unlikely to be clinical problem when symptomatic disorders are treated by titrating the dosage after beginning with small doses. Interestingly, about 30% of Chinese subjects appear to be poor metabolizers compared with 9/ of Caucasians [87].

blocking activity, produces a more rapid antihypertensive effect (presumably due to blockade of alpha-receptor mediated arterial and venous dilatation), and has been utilized for this effect in severe hypertension (especially by the i.v. route). However, unlike other beta-blockers which have no vasodilating activity, it is more liable to provoke headaches and postural hypotension (which may be particularly troublesome during pregnancy).

2.11.2 PRACTOLOL SYNDROME

This syndrome (reviewed in Reference [84]) has been encountered after chronic use of practolol but may present within weeks of starting treatment. It is an oculomucocutaneous reaction, which is usually mild and reversible and often only one feature is present. Occasionally, there may be serious sequelae (disfigurement, blindness, gastrointestinal problems needing surgery). There may be involvement of the pleura, pericardium, ear, nose and mouth. Since the syndrome seems unique to practolol, and the latter has been withdrawn from the market, the features of the syndrome are mainly of historical interest. The delay in recognizing these complications of long-term therapy has led to major reappraisal of the way in which post-marketing surveillance for adverse drug reactions is conducted.

2.11.3 COMBINED BETA-BLOCKER/CALCIUM ANTAGONIST TREATMENT

This topic (reviewed in Reference [89]) has generated intense interest and controversy. Both classes of drug when used individually may be regarded as first-line agents for the treatment of angina, and both may be used to treat hypertension. Experimental studies suggest that both may have a cardioprotective action at the subcellular level. To supplement each other's beneficial actions they have been prescribed together, and objective evidence (based on exercise testing, ECGs, and nitroglycerine consumption) indicates that many patients enjoy additive (or even synergistic) benefits. It has also been argued that in some respects both drug classes complement each other, in that calcium antagonists protect individuals at risk of beta-blocker induced coronary or peripheral artery spasm, whereas beta-blockers protect against calcium antagonist induced reflex tachycardia.

There is apprehension that the negative inotropic effects of calcium antagonists and the depressant action on AV conduction and sinus node function produced by verapamil (and diltiazem) may seriously augment the depressant effect of beta-blockers on cardiac contractility and AV conduction. Indeed many case reports of such combination therapy giving rise to fatal and non-fatal heart failure, hypotension AV block and asystole attest to these concerns. It is probable that combination therapy may result in important adverse reactions whenever high doses of beta-blockers are in use and/or there is a past history of myocardial failure or disturbance of cardiac conduction. Combination therapy with verapamil has been estimated to carry a 5–10% risk of such reactions.

Thus, although combination therapy is safe, well tolerated and more likely to provide effective symptomatic relief than either treatment alone, it should nevertheless be used cautiously or avoided altogether when there is a past history of cardiac failure. If AV conduction or sinus node function is suspect beta-blocker combinations with verapamil should be avoided.

2.12 Blood glucose and beta-adrenoceptor blockade

Both in diabetics and non-diabetics, there has been much confusion as to the clinically relevant actions of beta-adrenoceptor blockade on carbohydrate metabolism. Moreover, beta-adrenoceptor blockade also produces subtle effects on the cardiovascular responses to hypoglycaemia. The various issues may be considered under the following headings.

2.12.1   ACTION OF BETA-BLOCKADE ON GLUCOSE TOLERANCE

This subject was reviewed by Kendall [90]. Evidently, treatment with beta-blocking drugs has no influence on the onset of new diabetes, nor is there any clinically significant worsening of established diabetes in patients receiving beta-adrenoceptor antagonists. Nevertheless, it has been claimed that diabetics treated with cardioselective (beta$_1$-selective) drugs have more normal glucose tolerance (and insulin secretion) than when treated with non-selective agents. Such assertions however, were based on only trivial differences and small patient numbers. Conceivably, selective beta-blockers might be less diabetogenic because they tend to spare beta$_2$-receptor mediated insulin release. But one investigation [91], suggests that even selective beta-blockade (with atenolol) blocks salbutamol-induced insulin release (at least partially), indicating that selectivity may not be absolute or that some other mechanism might be involved. Additional therapy with indomethacin blocked the response completely. Notwithstanding the above-mentioned studies it appears unlikely that beta-blockade produces clinically significant impairment of glucose tolerance. It remains to be seen whether such impairment occurs in diabetics or non-diabetics receiving a combination of beta-blocker and non-steroidal anti-inflammatory drug.

2.12.2   INFLUENCE OF BETA-BLOCKADE ON HYPOGLYCAEMIA

Whenever compensatory glucose mobilization from the tissues is inadequate, biochemically and sometimes clinically significant hypoglycaemia is liable to occur after hypoglycaemic provocation. Animal and human experimentation [90, 91] with various alpha- and beta-receptor agonists and antagonists, suggests that these compensatory processes are augmented by sympathetic stimulation, by virtue of alpha- and possibly also beta-receptor mediated glycogenolysis (early response) and beta$_2$-

receptor mediated gluconeogenesis (late response). Not surprisingly, the main endocrine response to hypoglycaemia is an increase in plasma adrenaline, which presumably tends to restore blood glucose through all these various mechanisms. However, such adrenaline release also has secondary effects on the circulation. Thus, beta-adrenoceptor antagonists can interfere with the final outcome in one of at least three ways:

(1) The prodrome of impending hypoglycaemia may be masked, due to inhibition of some of the sympathetically induced peripheral symptoms (tremor and palpitations) but not sweating (which may actually be enhanced). This effect may occur after selective or non-selective drugs, and consequently patients may fail to take their usual counter measures (glucose). Therefore, diabetics receiving hypoglycaemic therapy who are prescribed beta-blocking drugs should be warned to pay special attention to excessive sweating, even in the absence of other symptoms.

(2) Recovery from hypoglycaemia is slowed through inhibition of gluconeogenesis, and it is alleged that hypoglycaemia is more liable to ensue after therapy with non-selective rather than selective antagonists. In the case of labetolol (an alpha- and beta-receptor blocking drug) one can speculate that the hypoglycaemic effect may be compounded due to superadded inhibition of alpha-receptor mediated glycogenolysis, but objective data on this possibility are lacking. The actual difference in the recovery of blood glucose concentration when selective as opposed to non-selective drugs are used, may be marked in some individuals but is generally small. Moreover, some workers studying the influence of insulin on patients given conventionally accepted equivalent cardiac beta-blocking doses of atenolol and propranolol, have even detected more hypoglycaemia on the selective antagonist [92].

(3) Exaggerated hypertensive response in the presence of non-selective blockade, see Table 2.2.

From a consideration of the above-mentioned items, it is clear that diabetics in receipt of hypoglycaemic agents (insulin or sulphonylureas), will be among the most liable to develop such adverse sequelae. Very occasionally however, even non-diabetics receiving beta-blockers may incur clinically significant hypoglycaemia after certain forms of provocation, such as severe exercise [93] and under special circumstances such as end-stage renal failure (see below). These same potentially hypoglycaemic provocations appear to be innocuous in the absence of beta-blockade, presumably due to adequate compensatory glucose mobilization from the tissues.

2.12.3 HYPOGLYCAEMIA IN RENAL FAILURE PATIENTS

End-stage renal disease is a complex and subtle metabolic disturbance, recognized to be an occasional cause of hypoglycaemia even in the absence of beta-blockade [94]. Indeed, the impaired glucose tolerance of diabetics often resolves when the latter develop nephropathy and renal failure. Not surprisingly, the use of beta-blocker therapy in patients with renal failure appears to constitute an additional hypoglycaemic stress. In such patients, the occurrence of hypoglycaemia (lasting days) is well recognized [92], and has been attributed to a combination of (a) glucose omission from the dialysate and (b) impaired compensatory glycaemic responses (due to propranolol therapy). Even when glucose is not missing from the dialysate, treatment with propranolol may induce clinically significant hypoglycaemia in the presence of alternative hypoglycaemic provocation, such as overnight fasting. This hypoglycaemic effect of beta-adrenoceptor antagonist treatment in dialysis patients is likely to be mediated through inhibition of beta-receptor mediated gluconeogenesis referred to earlier, and possibly also through inhibition of glycogenolysis [95].

In keeping with the suggestion that so-called beta$_2$-receptors are involved in such glycaemic responses, a study in haemodialysis patients has shown that the glycaemic response to glucagon challenge was greater in the presence of co-treatment with metoprolol (selective antagonist) as compared to the non-selective drug propranolol [96]. However, in the latter study the superiority of metoprolol in this respect was only evident post-dialysis not pre-dialysis. From this it was inferred that the difference between the two drugs could be due to metoprolol having a dialysable active metabolite (alphahydroxy metoprolol) and not to selectivity. Irrespective of the real explanation behind the difference, the risk of spontaneous hypoglycaemia developing in haemodialysis patients is probably greater during therapy with propranolol rather than metoprolol. The dearth of information regarding hypoglycaemia in renal failure patients treated with the selective antagonist atenolol presumably reflects a reluctance to prescribe this renally eliminated agent in renal impairment.

2.13 Beta-blockers in the management of thyrotoxicosis and anxiety

Many symptoms and signs associated with thyrotoxicosis and anxiety resemble those of sympathetic over-activity, particularly beta-receptor stimulation. This similarity naturally led to the study of beta-adrenoceptor antagonists such as propranolol as a means of alleviating such symptoms. It has since been realized that singly or in combination, many of the manifestations may respond favourably to beta-blockade, whether or not they occur in the presence of florid disease. Most of the favourable experience acquired thus far has been with the non-selective and highly lipid-soluble drug propranolol. Therefore, the guidelines that follow largely refer to propranolol treatment.

2.13.1 THYROTOXICOSIS

The use of beta-adrenoceptor antagonist drugs in hyperthyroidism has been reviewed by Feeley and Peden [97]. It is still not understood how thyrotoxicosis produces symptoms which are also encountered during sympathetic overactivity, nor is it entirely clear why beta-blocking drugs relieve these symptoms. It has long been known that propranolol and several other antagonists give rise to increased plasma concentrations of reversed (biologically inactive) tri-iodothyronine (T_3), but reduce the plasma concentration of active T_3. Nevertheless, antagonists such as oxprenolol and acebutolol which do not affect the deiodination products of thyroxine appear to confer comparable benefits. Currently, there is speculation that the tissues of thyrotoxic patients develop an excess of beta-receptors and thus manifest the features of sympathetic overactivity. Irrespective of their mode of action, beta-blocking drugs have proved to be a very effective adjunct to conventional antithyroid treatment.

For the relief of tachycardia and palpitation, propranolol (pure antagonist) is considered to be superior to pindolol or oxprenolol (drugs with partial agonist activity). Similarly, for the relief of tremor, propranolol (non-selective; $beta_1$- and $beta_2$-receptor antagonist) is considered superior to atenolol or metoprolol (selective; $beta_1$- and $beta_2$-receptor antagonists). In patients with thyrotoxic heart disease administration of propranolol (especially by the intravenous route) should be undertaken very cautiously if at all, lest there is aggravation of heart failure. On the other hand, thyrotoxic atrial fibrillation is relatively resistant to digoxin therapy and, in patients with uncontrolled atrial fibrillation despite digoxin treatment, propranolol therapy is usually very beneficial by virtue of dramatic slowing in the ventricular rate. Conversely when atrial fibrillation appears resistant to digoxin therapy the possibility of thyrotoxicosis should always be considered, in which case propranolol therapy is usually very beneficial by virtue of dramatic slowing in the ventricular rate.

The role of beta-blockers in the treatment of thyrotoxic myopathy remains uncertain. In spontaneous or induced thyrotoxic periodic paralysis (a complication which is evidentiy more common in the Japanese and Chinese than in other races), propranolol therapy appears to be very

Beta-blockers in the management of thyrotoxicosis and anxiety

Table 2.7 Summary of beta-blocker use in thyrotoxicosis

---

1 Indication
   Early control of symptoms during medical treatment with antithyroid drugs or radio-iodine
   Prior to thyroidectomy – reduces preparation time
   Thyrotoxic crisis – given with iodine, steroids, antipyretics etc.
   NB Not recommended as sole agent for long-term medical management; because remissions often incomplete, and activity continues with risk of thyrotoxic bone disease

2 Dosage
   Titration necessary to produce high degree of beta-blockade
   High doses of propranolol (or metoprolol) may be needed because hyperthyroidism increases their metabolism

3 Benefits
   Reductions in: heart rate (palpitation), nervousness, tremor, O_2 consumption, tri-iodothyronine concentration (usually), muscle weakness and hypercalcaemia

4 Precautions
   Omission of dosage peri-operatively may result in thyrotoxic crisis. Fetal bradycardia may occur when used in pregnancy

---

beneficial though at times large doses may be required.

Thyrotoxicosis affects the pharmacokinetics of beta-blocking drugs mainly through enhancing hepatic drug elimination. The dosing implications of this are largely theoretical, since it is common practice to individualize dosage by titration against therapeutic response. The most important considerations relevant to the use of beta-blocking drugs in thyrotoxicosis are summarized in Table 2.7.

2.13.2 ANXIETY

This subject has been reviewed by Tyrer [98] and Turner [38]. Whilst it is well appreciated that propranolol attenuates the peripheral (autonomically mediated) manifestations of anxiety, controlled studies (based on EEG recordings, sleep disturbance, hallucinations, and reaction times) indicate that it also has actions on the central nervous system. Indeed, in one controlled study propranolol was found to be no different from chlordiazepoxide (Librium) in relieving anxiety. However, many of the latter class of drugs appear to be more effective in relieving associated depression and sleep disturbance, whilst beta-blockers appear not to impair performance or produce sedation.

It is widely held that peripheral beta-receptor blockade is the chief

Beta-adrenergic blocking drugs

mechanism by which the anxiolytic action of beta-blockers is mediated. Reasons for this belief include (1) the presence of anxiolytic activity even in doses considered too small to have central effects and (2) anxiolytic effects occurring with non-lipid-soluble agents such as practolol which scarcely enter brain lipid. If true, this explanation supports the hypothesis that, once generated, anxiety frequently becomes self-perpetuating through perception of peripheral (somatic) manifestations. However, there continues to be considerable controversy as to whether chronic anxiety states are generated and perpetuated centrally or through peripheral stimuli, and also as to whether or not the benefits of beta-blockade are conferred through central or peripheral actions.

Currently, beta-adrenoceptor antagonist drugs (particularly propranolol) are acknowledged to be useful agents for treating:

(1) Certain phobic symptoms

(2) Situational anxiety (viz: public speaking, taking examinations, car racing, helicopter training, playing the violin), without appearing to impair performance

(3) Chronic anxiety with predominantly somatic manifestations

Recent concerns regarding withdrawal syndromes following long-term benzodiazepine therapy [98], imply that beta-blockers may need to be evaluated as possible agents of first choice in the treatment of some forms of chronic anxiety.

References

1. Hamer, J. (1979) Beta-adrenergic blocking drugs. In *Drugs for Heart Disease* (Ed. J. Hamer), Chapman and Hall, London, pp. 148–243.
2. *Acta Med. Scand.* (1981) Proceedings on a symposium on adrenoceptor blockade in hypertension. *Acta Med. Scand.*, Suppl. 665, 1–147.
3. Richards, R.A., Robertson, J.I.S. and Prichard, B.N.C. (1982) Proceedings of the third symposium on labetolol – June 1981. *Br. J. Clin. Pharmacol.*, Suppl 1, 13, 1S–141S.
4. Aellig, W.H., Hedges, A., Turner, P. and Waite, R. (1982) Pindolol: the relevance of intrinsic sympathomimetic activity after 12 years of experience. *Br. J. Clin. Pharmacol.*, 13, Suppl. 2, 143S–450S.
5. Breckenridge, A. (1983) Which beta-blocker? *Br. Med. J.*, 286, 1085–8.
6. Zipper, J., Wheeler, R.G., Potts, D.M. and Rivera, M. (1983) Propranolol as a novel, effective spermicide: preliminary findings. *Br. Med. J.*, 287, 1245–6.
7. Patel, L.G., Warrington, S.J. and Pearson, R.M. (1983) Propranolol concentrations in plasma after insertion into the vagina. *Br. Med. J.*, 287, 1237–320.
8. Kumana, C.R. (1978) Selectivity of beta-adrenoceptor agonists and antagonists. In *Recent Advances in Clinical Pharmacology* 1 (eds P. Turner & D. Shand), pp. 31–54.

9. Kumana, C.R. (1979) Selectivity of beta-blockers: Drug aspects. In *Theories and Use of Beta-blockade in Hypertension and Angina*. (ed. R.H. Roberts), pp. 141–56, Symposia Specialists Inc., Miami, Fl. distributed by Year Book Medical Publishers, Chicago.

10. Carruthers, S.G. (1979) Cardioselectivity of beta-blockers: Theoretical aspects in *Theories and Use of Beta-blockade in Hypertension and Angina*. (ed. R.H. Roberts), pp. 125–40, Symposia Specialists Inc., Miami, Fl. distributed by Year Book Medical Publishers, Chicago.

11. McDevitt, D.G. (1978) Beta-adrenoceptor antagonists and respiratory function. *Brit. J. Clin. Pharmacol.*, **5**, 101–6.

12. Perks, W.H., Chatterjee, R.S., Croxson, R.S. and Cruickshank, J.M. (1978) Beta-adrenoceptor antagonists and respiratory function. *Br. J. Clin. Pharmacol.*, **6**, 171.

13. Oh, V.M.S., Kaye, C.M., Warrington, S.J., Taylor, E.A. and Wadsworth, J. (1978) Beta-adrenoceptor antagonists and respiratory function. *Br. J. Clin. Pharmacol.*, **6**, 174–5.

14. Ruffin, R.E., Freith, P.A., Anderton, R.C., Kumana, C.R., Newhouse, M.T. & Hargreave, F.E. (1979) Selectivity of beta-adrenoceptor antagonist drugs assessed by histamine bronchial challenge. *Clin. Pharmacol. Ther.*, **25**, 536–40.

15. Taylor, S.H., Silke, B. and Lee, P.S. (1982) Intravenous beta-blockade in coronary heart disease. *N. Engl. J. Med.*, **306**, 631–5.

16. McDevitt, D.G. (1983) Clinical significance of cardioselectivity. *Drugs*, **25**, Suppl. 2, 219–26.

17. McSorley, P.S. and Warren, D.J. (1978) Effects of propranolol and metoprolol on the peripheral circulation. *Br. Med. J.*, **2**, 1598–600.

18. Hiatt, W.R., Fradl, D.C., Zerbe, G.O. et al. (1984) Selective and non-selective beta-blockade of the peripheral circulation. *Clin. Pharm. Ther.*, **35**, 12–18.

19. Louis, W.J. and McNeil, J.J. (1982) Can ISA compensate for bradycardia due to beta-adrenoceptor blockade?. *Br. J. Clin. Pharmacol.*, **13**, 315S–320S.

20. Kent, R.S. and Shand, D.G. (1981) *Recent Advances in Cardiology*, Vol. 8, *Adrenergic Receptor Regulation*, (ed. J. Hamer), Churchill Livingstone, Edinburgh, ch. 16.

21. Miller, R.R., Olsen, H.G., Amsterdam, E.A. and Mason, D.T. (1975) Propranolol withdrawal rebound phenomenon. Exacerbation of coronary events after abrupt cessation of anti-anginal treatment. *N. Engl. J. Med.*, **293**, 416–8.

22. Nattel, S., Rangno, R.E. and Van Loon, G. (1979) Mechanism of propranolol withdrawal phenomena. *Circulation*, **59**, 1158–64.

23. Prichard, B.N.C., Tomlinson, B., Walden, R.J. and Bhattacharjee, P. (1983) The beta-adrenergic blockade withdrawal phenomenon. *J. Cardiovasc. Pharmacol.*, **5**, Suppl. 1, S56–62.

24. Lindenfeld, J., Crawford, M.H., O'Rourke, A. et al. (1980) Adrenergic responsiveness after abrupt propranolol withdrawal in normal subjects and in patients with angina pectoris. *Circulation*, **62**, 704–11.

25. van Brummelen, P. (1983) The relevance of intrinsic sympathomimetic activity for beta-blocker induced changes in plasma lipids. *J. Cardiovasc. Pharmacol.*, **5**, Suppl. 1, S51–5.

26. Editorial (1981) Management of orthostatic hypotension, *Lancet*, **ii**, 963–4.

27. Man In 'T' Veld, A.J., Boomsa, F. and Shalekamp, M.A.D.H. (1983) Regula-

tion of alpha and beta-adrenoceptor responsiveness. Studies in patients with chronic autonomic failure. *Br. J. Clin. Pharmacol.*, 15 Suppl, 507S–519S.

28. Lohmoller, G. and Stocker, K. (1982) Can ISA compensate for bradycardia due to beta-adrenoceptor blockade? *Br. J. Clin. Pharmacol.*, **13**, 315S–320S.

29. Hombach, V., Braun, V., Hopp, H.W., Gil-Sanchez, D., *et al.* (1982) Electrophysiological effects of cardioselective and non-cardioselective beta-adrenoceptor blockers with and without ISA at rest and during exercise. *Br. J. Clin. Pharmacol.*, **13**, 285S–93S.

30. Hansson, L., Svensson, A., Gudbronolsson, T., *et al.* (1983) Treatment of hypertension with beta-blockers with and without intrinsic sympathomimetic activity. *J. Cardiovasc.Pharmacol.*, **55**, Suppl. 1, 526–9.

31. Shand, D.G. (1983) State of the art: comparative pharmacology of the beta-adrenoceptor blocking drugs. *Drugs*, **25**, Suppl. 2, 92–9.

32. Schafer-Korting, M., Bach, N., Knauf, H. and Mutschler, E. (1984) Pharmacokinetics of nadolol in healthy subjects. *Eur. J. Clin. Pharmacol.*, **26**, 125–7.

33. Kirch, W., Spahn, H., Kohler, H. and Mutschler, E. (1983) Influence of beta-receptor antagonists on pharmacokinetics of cimetidine. *Drugs*, **25**, Suppl. 2, 127–30.

34. Wood, A.J.J. (1983) Beta-blocker withdrawal. *Drugs*, **25**, Suppl. 2, 318–21.

35. Warren, D.J., Waller, D.G. and McAinish, J. (1983) Beta-blockers and renal function. *Drugs*, **25**, Suppl. 2, 108–12.

36. Lebrec, D., Flouvat, B., Decourt, S. and Dupont, C. (1983) Atenolol and liver function. *Drugs*, **25**, Suppl. 2, 147.

37. Balant, L.P. and Fabre, J. (1978) Low dose oral propranolol. *Lancet*, **ii**, 425.

38. Turner, P. (1983) Beta-adrenoceptor blocking drugs and the central nervous systems. *Recent Advances on Clinical Pharmacology*, Vol. 3, Churchill Livingstone, Edinburgh, ch. 11, pp. 223–34.

39. Garvey, A.J., McDevitt, D.G. and Solem, S.A.M. (1984) Comparative study of the psychomotor effects of atenolol, nadolol, propranolol and diazepam in man. *Brit. J. Clin. Pharm.*, **17**. 216P.

40. Betts, T.A. and Alford, C. (1983) Beta-blocking drugs and sleep; a controlled trial. *Drugs*, **25**, Suppl. 2, 268–72.

41. Westerlund, A. (1983) A comparison of the central nervous system side-effects caused by lipophilic and hydrophilic beta-blockers. *Br. J. Clin. Pharmacol.*, 280–1.

42. Offerhaus, L. and Van Zweitan, P.A. (1974) Comparative studies on central factors contributing to the hypotensive action of propranolol, alprenolol and their enantiomers. *Cardiovascular Res.*, **8**, 488.

43. Danesh, B.J.Z., Brunton, J. and Sumner, D.J. (1984) Comparison between short-term renal hemodynamic effects of propranolol and nadolol in essential hypertension: a crossover study. *Clinical Science*, **67**, 243–8.

44. Mueller, J., Byrne, M.J. Van Schalkwyk, J. and Opie, L.H. (1983) Renal impairment in hypertension not improved by nadolol when compared with atenolol. *Drugs*, **25**, Suppl. 2, 146.

45. Gross, F. (1982) The place of alpha-adrenoceptor and beta-adrenoceptor blockade in the treatment of hypertension. *Br. J. Clin, Pharmacol.*, **13**, Suppl. 1, 5S–11S.

46. Breckenridge, A., Orme, M., Serlin, M.J. and MacIver, M. (1982) Labetolol in

essential hypertension. *Br. J. Clin. Pharmacol.*, **13**, Suppl. 1, 37S–9S.

47. Prichard, B.N.C. and Richards, D.A. (1982) Comparison of labetolol with other anti-hypertensive drugs. 'Third Drug' trial – comparative study of antihypertensive agents added to treatment when blood pressure remains uncontrolled by a beta-blocker plus thiazide diuretic. *Br. J. Clin. Pharmacol.*, **13**, Suppl. 1, 41S–7S.

48. McAreavey, D., Ramsey, L.E., Latham, L., McLaren, A.D., Lorimer, A.R., Reid, J.L., Robertson, J.I.S., Robertson M.P. and Weir, R.J. (1984) 'Third drug' trial: comparative study of anti-hypotensive agents added to treatment when blood pressure remains uncontrolled by a beta-blocker plus thiazide diuretic. *Br. Med. J.*, **288**, 106–11.

49. Waal-Manning, H.J. and Simpson, F.O. (1982) Review of long-term treatment with labetolol. *Br. J. Clin. Pharmacol.*, **13**, Suppl. 1, 65S–73S.

50. Hughes, G.V.R. (1982) Hypotensive agents, beta-blockers and drug-induced lupus. *Br. Med. J.*, **284**, 1358–9.

51. Cumming, A.M.M., Brown, J.J., Lever, A.F. and Robertson, J.I.S. (1982) Intravenous labetolol in the treatment of severe hypertension. *Br. J. Clin. Pharmacol.*, **13**, Suppl. 1, 93S–6S.

52. Davies, A.B., Balasubramanian, V., Gould, B. and Raftery, E.B. (1982) Rapid reduction of blood pressure with acute oral labetolol. *Br. J. Clin. Pharmacol.*, **13**, 705–10.

53. Agabitit-Rosei, E., Alicandri, C.L., Beschi, M., Castellano, M., Fariello, R., Montini, E., Muiesa, M.L. Romanelli, G. and Muiesan, G. (1982) The acute and chronic effect of labetolol and the relationship with pretreatment plasma noradrenaline levels. *Br. J. Clin. Pharmacol.*, **13**, Suppl. 1, 87S–92S.

54. Freis, E.D. (1982) The veterans and sequelae. *Br. J. Clin. Pharmacol.*, **13**, 67–72.

55. Prichard, B.N.C. (1982) Propranolol and beta-adrenergic receptor blocking drugs in the treatment of hypertension. *Br. J. Clin. Pharmacol.*, **13**, 51–60.

56. Greenberg, G., Brennan, P.J. and Miall, W.E. (1984) Effects of diuretic and beta-blocker therapy in the Medical Research Council trial. *Am. J. Med.*, **76**, 45–51.

57. Beevers, D.G., Johnston, H., Larkin, H. and Davies, P. (1983) Clinical evidence that beta-adrenoceptor blockers prevent more cardiovascular complications than other antihypertensive drugs. *Drugs*, **25**, Suppl. 2, 326–30.

58. Multiple Risk Factor Intervention Trial Research Group (1982) Multiple risk factor intervention trial: Risk factor changes and mortality results. *J. Am. Med. Assoc.*, **248**, 1465–77.

59. Goldenberg, M., Pines, M.L., Baldwin, E. de B., Greene, D.C. and Roh, L.E. (1948) The hemodynamic response of man to norepinephrine and epinephrine and its relation to the problem of hypertension. *Am. J. Med.*, **5**, 792–806.

60. Barcroft, H. and Starr, I. (1951) Comparison of the actions of adrenaline and noradrenaline on the cardiac output in man. *Clin. Sci.*, **10**, 295–301.

61. Prichard, B.N.C. and Ross, F.T. (1966) Use of propranolol in conjunction with alpha-receptor blocking drugs in phaeochromocytoma. *Am. J. Cardiol.*, **18**, 394.

62. Van Herwaarden, C.L.A., Binkhorst, R.A., Fennis, J.F.M. and Van't Laar, A. (1977) Effects of adrenaline during treatment with propranolol. *Br. Med. J.*, **1**, 1029.

Beta-adrenergic blocking drugs

63. Van Herwaarden, C.L.A., Binkhorst, R.A. and Fennis, J.F.M. (1979) Effects of propranolol and metoprolol on haemodynamic and respiratory indices and on perceived exertion during exercise in hypertensive patients. *Br. Heart J.*, **41**, 99.
64. Morrison, S.C., Kumana, C.R., Rudnick, K.V., Haynes, B. and Jones, N.L. (1982) Selective and non-selective beta-adrenoceptor blockade in hypertension: responses to changes in posture, cold and exercise. *Circulation*, **65**, 1171–7.
65. Kumana, C.R. (1986) Are blood pressure surges associated with sympathetic stimulation aggravated by beta-adrenoceptor antagonist treatment. *Post. Grad. Med. J.*, **62**, 731–5.
66. Miall, W.E. and Chinn, S. (1974) Framingham study: Screening for hypertension: some epidemiological observations. *Br. Med. J.*, **3**, 595.
67. Norris, R.M., Barnaby, P.F., Brown, M.M., Green, G.G., Clark, E.D. Logan, D.L., and Sharp, D.N. (1984) Prevention of ventricular fibrillation during acute myocardial infarction by intravenous propranolol. *Lancet*, ii, 883–6.
68. Pratt, C.M. and Roberts, E. (1983) Chronic beta-blockade therapy in patients after myocardial infarction. *Am. J. Cardiol.*, **52**, 661–4.
69. Factor, S.M., Okun, E.M., Minesi, T. and Kirk, E.S. (1982) The microcirculation of the human heart: end-capillary loops with discrete perfusion fields. *Circulation*, **66**, 1241–8.
70. Norris, R.M. (1985) Beta-adrenoceptor blockers – an update on their role in actue myocardial infarction. *Drugs*, **29**, 97–104.
71. Martindale (1982) Propranolol and other beta-adrenoceptor blocking agents. In *The Extrapharmacopoeia*, 28th edn, Pharmaceutical Press, London, pp. 1324–52.
72. Amery, A., DePlaen, J.F., Lignen, P., McAinish, J. and Reybrouck, T. (1977) Relationship between blood level of atenolol and pharmacologic effect. *Clin. Pharmacol. Ther.*, **21**, 691–9.
73. Hitzenberger, G. (1979) Plasma concentration and antihypertensive effect of beta-blockers. *Cardiology*, **645**, Suppl. 1, 14–19.
74. Scott, A.K., Rigby, J.W., Webster, J., Haeksworth, G.M., Petrie, J.C. and Lovell, H.G. (1982) Atenolol and metoprolol once daily in hypertension. *Br. Med. J.*, **284**, 1514–16.
75. Mann, S., Millar-Crad, M.W., Gould, B.A., Melville, D.I. and Raftery, E.B. (1982) Coital blood pressure in hypertensives: Cephalgia, syncope and the effects of beta-blockade. *Br. Heart J.*, **47**, 84–9.
76. Raftery, E.B. (1983) The effects of beta-blocker therapy on diurnal variation of blood pressure. *Eur. Heart. J.*, **4**, Suppl. D., 61–4.
77. Serlin, M.J., Orme, M.L.E., Baber, N.S. and Sibeon, R.G. (1980) Propranolol in the control of blood pressure: A dose response study. *Clin. Pharmacol. Ther.*, **27**, 586–92.
78. Thadani, U. and Parker, J.O. (1979) Propranolol in the treatment of angina pectoris: Comparison of duration of action in acute and sustained therapy. *Circulation*, **59**, 571–9.
79. Shand, D.G. (1974) Pharmacokinetic properties of the beta-adrenergic blocking drugs. *Drugs*, **7**, 39–47.
80. Walle, T., Conradi, E.L., Walle, U.K., Fagan, T.L. and Gaffney, T.E. (1978) The predictable relationship between plasma levels and dose during chronic

propranolol therapy. *Clin. Pharm. and Thero.*, **24**, 668–77.

81. Woosley, R.L., Kornhauser, D. Smith, R., Roebe, S., Higgins, B., Nies, A.S., Shand, D.G. and Oates, T.A. (1979) Suppression of chronic ventricular arrhythmias with propranolol. *Circulation*, **60**, 819–27.

82. Kendall, M.J. and Beeley, L. (1983) Beta-adrenoceptor blocking drugs: Adverse reactions and drug interactions. *Pharmacol. Ther.*, **21**, 351–69.

83. Murakami, K., Kosania, T., Hyashi, R., Tsushima, M. *et al.* (1982) Myxoedema coma induced by beta-adrenoceptor blocking agent. *Br. Med. J.*, **285**, 543–4.

84. Wright, P. (1979) The practolol adverse reaction and the significance of reactions to other beta-blockers. In *Theories and Use of Beta-blockade in Hypertension and Angina* (ed. R.H. Roberts), pp. 115–23. Symposia Specialists Inc., Miami. Fl., distributed by Year Book Medical Publishers, Chicago.

85. Fololt, R., Lieollious, H. and Aursnes, J. (1985) Beta-blockers and loss of hearing. *Br. Med. J.*, **289**, 1490–2.

86. Lennard, M.S. (1985) Oxidation phenotype and the metabolism and action of beta-blockers. *Klin. Wochenschr.*, **63**, 285–92.

87. Woods, H.F., Lennard, M.S. and Tucker, G.T. (1985) Genetic polymorphism of drug oxidation – ethnic differences. *Proc. SE Asian/Western Pacific Regional Meeting of Pharmacologists* (in press).

88. Lewis, P. (1983) *Clinical Pharmacology and Obstetrics*. John Wright, Bristol, London and Boston, Ch. 9, pp. 100–2.

89. Vanhalwyk, J.L.J., Serruys, P.W. and Hugenholtz, P.G. (1983) Anti-anginal electrophysiologic and hemodynamic effects of combined beta-blocker/calcium antagonist therapy. *Eur. Heart J.*, **4**, Suppl. D, 117–28.

90. Kendall, M.J. (1981) Are selective beta-adrenoceptor blocking drugs an advantage? *J. Roy. Coll. Phys. (Lond.)*, **15**, 33–40.

91. Stornello, M., Di Rao, G., Iachello, B., Pantano, S., Isani, R., and Scapellato, L. (1983) Effects of salbutamol, indomethacin and atenolol on insulin secretion. *Drugs*, **25**, Suppl. 2, 255–6.

92. Ryan, J.R., Lacorte, W., Jan, A. and McMahon, F.G. (1983) Response of diabetics treated with atenolol and propranolol to insulin-induced hypoglycemia. *Drugs*, **25**, Suppl. 2, 256–7.

93. Holm, G., Herlitz, J. and Smith, U. (1981) Severe hypoglycemia during physical exercise and treatment with beta-blockers. *Br. Med. J.*, **282**, 1360.

94. Rutsky, E.A., McDaniel, H.G., Tharpe, D.L. *et al.* (1978) Spontaneous hypoglycemia in chronic renal failure. *Arch. Int. Med.*, **138**, 1364–8.

95. Pun, K.K., Yeung, C.K., Ho, P.W.M., Lin, H.J., Chan, M.K. and Yeung, R.T.T. (1984) Effects of propranolol and haemodialysis on the response of glucose, insulin, C-peptide and cyclic AMP to glucagon challenge. *Clin. Nephrol.*, **21**, 235–40.

96. Pun, K.K., Yeung, C.K. and Yeung, R.T.T. (1985) Effects of propranolol and metoprolol on glucose, cyclic AMP and insulin responses during pharmacological hyperglucosuraemia in haemodialysis patients. *Nephron*, **39**, 175–8.

97. Feeley, J. and Peden, N. (1984) Use of beta-adrenoceptor blocking drugs in hyperthyroidism, *Drugs*. **27**, 425–6.

98. Tyrer, P.J. (1980) Use of beta-blocking drugs in psychiatry and neurology. *Drugs*, **22**, 300–8.

3 Calcium antagonists

JOHN HAMER

3.1 Introduction

In the 20 years since the definition by Fleckenstein [1] of drugs selectively blocking the slow calcium channel in myocardial cells and realization of their clinical usefulness, there has been an outburst of pharmacological research producing new agents in this group. This has led to extensive argument as to which drugs are true calcium channel blockers and which prevent calcium ion entry to the cells by other mechanisms.

The original definition of the slow calcium channel [1] was made on myocardial cells in contrast to the fast sodium channel responsible for depolarization. Calcium ions have a widespread role as intracellular messengers, coupling membrane effects producing calcium ion entry to contraction in muscle cells by binding to a specific protein such as troponin [2], or producing other actions via the versatile intracellular operator protein, calmodulin [3]. An arteriolar vasodilator effect of calcium antagonists on vascular smooth muscle is probably mediated by calmodulin [2,3] and may be potentiated by sympathetic inhibition by an effect of calcium antagonists on the sympathetic ganglia.

The first calcium antagonist to be discovered, verapamil, was an opium alkaloid, chemically analogous to papaverine. Subsequent synthetic calcium antagonists, nifedipine and diltiazem, have a different distribution of actions, competing for a binding site on the calcium channel surface, whereas verapamil acts deeper in the sarcolemma [4] and competes for binding with another group of calcium antagonists, represented in binding studies by cinnarizine, although both binding sites seem to operate on the same channel as do the non-specific blocking effects of other divalent ions such Ni^{2+} and Mn^{2+}. Debate continues [2] as to whether beta-adrenergic calcium entry is through a similar channel or by facilitation of the conventional voltage-operated slow channel [2]. The inotropic effect of digitalis is probably mediated by increased calcium ion entry into the myocardial cells and ouabain is used as an agonist to test the relaxing effect of calcium antagonists.

The slow calcium channel operating in cells less depolarized (about -40mV) than the fully depolarized (about -100mV) cells of working myocardium, seems particularly important in the sino-atrial (SA) and atrioventricular (AV) nodes [2]. In the SA node a secondary effect on pacemaker current tends to slow heart rate and conduction is impaired at the AV node [4]. Although direct injection shows similar effects of the commonly used calcium antagonists, the more potent vasodilator action of nifedipine produces reflexes that reverse the actions on the nodes, so that the rate may even increase [5]. Recent unpublished studies in the denervated heart after cardiac transplantation suggest that the doses used in Reference [5] may have been pharmacological rather than clinical as nifedipine does not appear to depress the SA or AV nodes at the usual therapeutic dose.

The major differences between the calcium antagonists is in their selectivity of action. In general, larger doses are needed for negative intropic effect than for arteriolar vasodilatation and block of the AV node, allowing their selective clinical use for these actions [2]. Of the commonly used drugs, nifedipine is primarily vasodilator, diltiazem slows AV conduction with little other disturbance, and verapamil is intermediate affecting both arterioles and AV node with some negative inotropic action. These differences may be pharmacokinetic from variation in access, or due to differences in penetration into the cells for intracellular calcium antagonistic effects, or represent true differences in sensitivity of the tissues to calcium antagonism [2]. The clinical importance of these drugs has led to the search for better combinations of properties. The position is similar to that produced by the beta-blockers 20 years ago. As in that case the fear is that we will not get the best drugs, but the ones with most commercial advantage. Most clinical experience in angina, hypertension and arrhythmias is with the three main drugs, verapamil and nifedipine, with diltiazem as a relative new-comer. The newer analogues tend to be subject to enthusiastic claims, but have not been fully assessed in relation to the more established calcium antagonists.

Among the useful properties of the calcium antagonists is myocardial protection by preventing calcium overload [6], which is evident as reduced myocardial damage during cardioplegic surgery, and possibly of benefit in reducing cardiac infarction. The drugs seem to act by preventing calcium entry by the slow calcium channel after hypoxic damage to the sarcolemma.

3.2 Clinical pharmacology

In spite of their chemical diversity [7], the calcium antagonists have many pharmacological similarities related to their high lipid solubility. This gives them a large volume of distribution, extensive protein-binding, and clearance mainly by hepatic metabolism and largely dependent on liver blood flow, except in the case of the long-acting less used drugs, perhexiline and lidoflazine, where enzyme capacity seems to be the determinitive factor. Major hepatic metabolism is linked with reduced bioavailability due to first pass effect (less evident for nifedipine [8]), and circulating metabolites may prolong the effect of these drugs. The calcium antagonists tend to increase plasma digoxin levels in combined treatment less by displacement from tissue binding than by interference with renal clearance as seen with quinidine. The effect is most evident with verapamil, but a lesser change is seen with nifedipine [9] and diltiazem.

The different emphasis of site of action is well seen with the three widely used agents, nifedipine, verapamil and diltiazem [8]. As calcium channel blockade is defined as action on the myocardium at low concentration, some negative inotropic effect is inevitable.

Nifedipine is a potent arteriolar vasodilator with little venous effect and the resulting reflex response tends to maintain myocardial contractility and AV node conduction and even to increase heart rate. If these effects are deleterious, as in critical myocardial ischaemia, they can be prevented by combination with a beta-blocker, although caution is needed if there is myocardial failure, as the negative inotropic effect of calcium antagonism is fully expressed when beta-blockade removes any reflex compensation.

Verapamil has potent effects on nodal tissue which seems to rely more on calcium ion than sodium ion currents for its action potential. Verapamil is useful to block tachycardias in the AV node. In angina and hypotension the vasodilator effect is useful and a direct effect on the SA node may prevent reflex tachycardia, so that combination with a beta-blocker is not needed. It may have more direct adverse effect on the myocardium than nifedipine [8].

There is less experience with diltiazem but it seems to have a similar effect to verapamil on AV node conduction, and has been used for coronary spasm. As it has relatively little general haemodynamic effect it now may be the preferred agent for blocking AV nodal tachycardia.

3.3 Myocardial protection

An exciting clinical application of calcium antagonists is the reduction of myocardial damage due to calcium overload during hypoxia [10], well seen during cardioplegic surgery and evident experimentally in the avoidance of the failure of relaxation that eventually produces 'stone heart'. Lidoflazine seems specific in this effect by stabilizing the cell membrane. Talk of 'ischaemic' calcium channels seems unjustified when the evidence is of disintegration of the whole sarcolemma. The effect seems directly correlated with cell calcium content rather than depletion of high energy phosphate stores [6]. A partial effect during hypoxia may relate to loss of high energy phosphate needed to maintain calcium homeostasis, and produce a failure of relaxation similar to that seen in the ischaemic regions in angina [10]. A temperature-dependent effect [11] may account for some variation of the experimental results as the calcium depletion phase of the calcium paradox which produces injury is temperature sensitive, but not the phase of calcium repletion when the injury becomes evident. All calcium antagonists tested were effective at 37°C, but protection cut off below 25°C, probably due to a change in the properties of the calcium channel [11].

There has been hope that a similar effect might be helpful in limiting myocardial damage after infarction. A hypothesis linking local calcium overload to myocardial damage [12] suggests how this can be limited and possibly the risk of fatal ventricular arrhythmias reduced. The suggestion is that intracellular calcium overload can induce a depolarizing inwards sodium current which could produce a current of injury (ST shift on ECG) and also delayed after-potentials triggering ventricular fibrillation. A lesser current of injury (ST shift) after a calcium antagonist might in these circumstances not represent a reduction in infarct size. Studies during induced angina [13] suggest a change in metabolism to fatty acids rather than glucose in the ischaemic tissue after verapamil. The added effect of ischaemia on the calcium channel suggests that unloading by calcium antagonists might be more effective in ischaemia than in normal myocardium [14]. These speculations need the confirmation of clinical trials before calcium antagonists can be recommended for early treatment of myocardial infarction. An apparently well-conducted Danish study showed no suggestion of reduced infarct size after early verapamil [15], though there was an inevitable delay before the patients needed medical attention which may have accounted for the difference from experimental work. Alternatively, some adverse effect of verapamil may be counteracting the expected benefit.

3.4 Ventricular arrhythmias

Experimental work suggests the possibilities of a beneficial effect on the production of ventricular fibrillation by coronary occlusion [16] which might be consistent with the hypothesis outlined above [12]. However, verapamil and related compounds [17] also have antiarrhythmic effects due to block of the fast inwards sodium current (Vaughan Williams Class I action). In a clinical study verapamil was found useful in the prevention of chronic recurrent ventricular tachycardia [18] and it may have a place in the prevention of arrhythmias early in myocardial infarction, as it abolishes ventricular ectopic beats in this situation [19]. It is not clear whether any effect is due to calcium antagonism or to the additional class I effect of this drug.

3.5 Verapamil

The early slow calcium channel blocker, verapamil, was discovered as an opium alkaloid, and is chemically related to papaverine. It is notorious in pharmacology as a 'dirty' drug, i.e. it has many other actions, apart from a high degree of calcium channel block, including the class I fast sodium channel block [17], and alpha-adrenergic antagonism, perhaps by block of calcium-mediated actions in sympathetic terminals concerned with noradrenaline release [20]. Originally introduced for angina, on the basis of a pharmacological obsession with coronary vasodilatation, its main cardiological use has been in the production of AV nodal block to stop or prevent tachycardia involving the AV node [2].

The large first pass effect [21] may be associated with considerable variation in dose. Reduced hepatic clearance on long-term administration [22] may require reduction in dosage. The main metabolite, norverapamil, may also accumulate, and although it may be slightly vasodilator does not seem to contribute to the effect on the AV node [21]. The situation is complicated in liver disease with reduced clearance and less first pass effect accentuated by porto-canal shunting [23].

The situation is complicated by differences between the optical isomers [24] and the greater volume of distribution of the more active (−)-isomer as a calcium antagonist may have given the impression of a qualitative difference in effect.

A major effect of verapamil is the reduction of myocardial contractility [8], but in patients with relatively good left ventricular function this is compensated by the beneficial effect of reduced afterload and the reflex sympathetic stimulation produced by arteriolar vasodilatation [25]. Caution is clearly needed in patients with impaired left ventricular function, and the increased susceptibility of ischaemic myocardial segments to calcium antagonists may add to the effect [25]. Caution is particularly needed when beta-blockers are added to verapamil treatment [26], as apart from summation of the effect on the AV node, reflex myocardial compensation is removed, and propranolol increases the plasma verapamil level [26] with increased adverse effect on myocardial performance.

Higher degrees of AV block are the usual effect of overdose and may occur at therapeutic levels in susceptible subjects. We have produced second-degree Wenckebach block in a normal volunteer [21]. The first-line treatment of overdose is intravenous calcium gluconate [27].

The methoxy derivative of verapamil (D600), named gallapomil, seems similar to its parent compound in experimental studies. Tiapamil with more effect on the fast sodium current seems very similar to verapamil itself [28]. Bepredil is similar, but has more effect on fast sodium current (class I action) and seems particularly active against atrial arrhythmias [29].

3.6 Nifedipine

The type drug of the dihydropyridines [7], nifedipine is thought of as purer calcium antagonist than verapamil and diltiazem [4, 8]. It suffers less from first pass metabolism and there are no active metabolites [30]. As it is relatively selective for arterial vasodilatation [31] with little effect on veins, it may have its best use in coronary spasm and in hypertension. The usual side effects are vasodilator, flush, lethargy, headache, and ankle oedema probably resulting from disturbance of the Starling capillary equilibrium [31] and lack of venodilatation [31], as there is no fluid retention and little response to diuretics [30]. The short half-life after intravenous injection [32] is reflected in the capsules used in angina but is overcome by the use of a slow release tablet (Adalat Retard) in hypertension [32].

As a possible alternative to a beta-blocker in diabetics with angina, there have been no problems reported, but blood sugar fell sharply when nifedipine was stopped in late-onset diabetes [33] and studies of an oral glucose tolerance test in normal volunteers showed a rise in blood sugar and delay of insulin response suggesting that diabetic treatment [33] may need adjustment on nifedipine.

There are several reports of adverse effects such as heart failure or hypotension in patients given nifedipine with a beta-blocker, although the combination seems logical to remove the reflex effects of vasodilatation and to given an additive effect in angina or hypertension. In an objective study [34] in patients with angina on atenolol, at a heart rate fixed by pacing at 100 per minute, nifedipine reduced peripheral resistance and output rose without a rise in left ventricular filling pressure in spite of a reduction in left ventricular dP/dt, suggesting a gain from reduced afterload in spite of the negative inotropic effect, which is usually masked by sympathetic reflex activity. In combination with propranolol in 15 patients with angina there was considerable benefit with improved exercise tolerance [35]. One patient had an excessive fall in blood pressure and angina did not improve, and the authors conclude that in this situation, the nifedipine with its profound hypotensive effect, should be stopped rather than the beta-blocker [35]. Another study [36] has confirmed the additive effect in angina and the combination blocked the pressor response to cold and to mental arithmetic. Any reduction in heart rate was due solely to the beta-blocker as nifedipine had no effect on heart rate [36].

3.7 Newer dihydropyridines

The success of nifedipine has led to a second generation of analogous dihydropyridines [7] in search of pharmacokinetic advantages or different tissue emphasis of effect. Most, like nicardipine [37], are similar in effect to nifedipine, and it would be of little value to list them here. Nitrendipine has a more prolonged effect than nifedipine [38] with a single dose lasting 24 hours but no cumulation over three weeks [38]. It seems promising for the once daily treatment of hypertension. Nimodipine has been used to prevent cerebral vascular spasm in patients with subarachnoid haemorrhage, with the suggestion that it is lipid soluble and should cross the blood–brain barrier [39]. High lipid solubility is a common feature of all the calcium antagonists [7], and it seems likely that the cerebral arteries affected are outside the blood–brain barrier in the subarachnoid space, so this argument seems irrelevant, although nimodipine seems successful in reducing deaths from spasm [39].

In two cases possible differences in distribution of effect may offer advantages. Nisoldipine [7] is said to be an active venous dilator [2] suggesting a nitrate-like effect by venous pooling which may be useful in angina or heart failure. Felodipine [7] is selected for arteriolar vasodilatation without negative inotropic effect. In patients with coronary artery disease, felodipine reduced peripheral resistance and blood pressure with an increase in cardiac output and a slight increase in heart rate, though myocardial oxygen consumption fell [40]. The output increased by 30% when rate was held constant by pacing [40].

3.8 Diltiazem

The newer drug diltiazem is perhaps closer to verapamil than to nifedipine. It is a potent AV nodal blocker with some vasodilator effect but little negative inotropic action [8], so may be the best agent for AV junctional tachycardia. It has a relatively long life and shows cumulation on long-term treatment of diltiazem itself and of the active deacetyl metabolite [41]. A haemodynamic study in normal subjects showed no effect on blood pressure, heart rate, compliance of calf veins, or in the exercise response. A slight fall in blood pressure was interpreted as due to vasodilatation but there was no reflex tachycardia [42]. In general use there are few side effects but AV nodal block may be a problem in susceptible subjects [43].

3.9 The less used calcium antagonists

Many of these drugs have been available for many years and are less used because they are relatively ineffective compared to the more recent specific calcium channel blockers, or suffer from disadvantages of severe toxicity. Many seem to act to prevent calcium entry by mechanisms other than block of the slow calcium channel as in the case of the myocardial protective effect of lidoflazine. Many are also relatively weak slow channel blockers, often competing for the cinnarizine binding sites deep in the sarcolemma rather than for the more superficial sites of action of the dihydropyridines [4]. The toxic arrhythmias, prominent with prenylamine and lidoflazine seem related to prolongation of the QT interval giving rise to recurrent tachycardia, known as 'torsade de pointes', which often degenerates into ventricular fibrillation which may be fatal. It is suspected that this phenomenon is related to prolongation of the myocardial cell action potential, perhaps due to a secondary effect interfering with the repolarizing outwards potassium current, and the risk of this complication seems to be increased by hypokalaemia [30]. The slow pharmacokinetics of perhexiline or lidoflazine may be related to penetration into the cells and prenylamine is known to inhibit calmodulin the intracellular mediator [2]. Many of these drugs have other effects, apart from calcium antagonism which may contribute to their actions, such as block of the fast sodium current (class I action) or metabolic effects (suspected with perhexiline).

3.9.1 PRENYLAMINE

Prenylamine was relatively ineffective in angina and often produces 'torsade de pointes' [44]. The suggestion that risk of torsade could be detected by monitoring QT interval seems impractical as changes may occur unexpectedly in relation to additional influences, such as hypokalaemia, and it has largely been replaced by the conventional calcium antagonists [2].

3.9.2 PERHEXILINE

Perhexiline is very effective in angina, but seems too toxic for ordinary use when other agents are available. Even the observation that the neuro-pathy is related to inherited impaired oxidation [45], and the hepatitis is related to certain HLA groups [46] does not save the situation as detailed screening is impracticable and there are frequent minor changes in nerve conduction [47] and in liver enzymes, suggesting that toxicity is not confined to these groups. The main haemodynamic effect observed is a lower heart rate at a given work load. The mechanism of benefit in angina has caused some discussion [48]. The class I action does not seem powerful enough to account for the dramatic effect and it is a relatively feeble calcium antagonist. There is a suggestion that a myocardial meta-bolic effect may be responsible [48].

3.9.3 CINNARIZINE

Cinnarizine and its analogue flunarizine [49] have mainly been used for peripheral vascular effects in migraine and vertigo. The slow pharma-cokinetics are associated with a cumulative effect. It is thought particular-ly to block receptor-operated effects on the calcium channels [49] suggest-ing its application to migraine.

3.9.4 LIDOFLAZINE

Lidoflazine is, like perhexiline, dramatically effective in angina [50]. Its main use has been for myocardial protection during cardioplegic surgery, where it appears to be well tolerated. It seems to have a stabilizing effect on the cell membrane, preventing calcium influx with relatively little specific effect on the slow calcium channel. So many possible haemody-namic effects are suggested for the benefit in angina [50] as to reduce credibility, and it seems likely that some aspect of myocardial protection is responsible. An attempt to study it objectively on exercise tolerance in angina was abandoned because of serious arrhythmias [51], largely in relation to QT prolongation, and it seems too toxic for widespread use in angina where other alternatives are available.

3.10 AV nodal block

The main antiarrhythmic effect of the calcium antagonists is based on selective block of the AV node to stop or prevent junctional re-entry tachycardias. The cells of the conducting pathway of the AV node rely more on depolarization by calcium ion currents than on sodium ion currents as in the working myocardium [2]. Block of the calcium currents with a calcium antagonist reduces the rate of rise of the action potential in these cells and secondarily slows conduction, as in the corresponding case of block of sodium ion entry in working myocardium, which is the basis of Vaughan Williams class I action. The resulting almost selective block of AV node conduction corresponds to Vaughan Williams class IV antiarrhythmic action.

In clinical use the effect is well seen with verapamil and diltiazem [52], but is little evident with nifedipine [53]. Studies in isolated heart tissue [5] suggested a similar effect of all three drugs, suggesting that the reflex sympathetic response to the more potent vasodilator effect of nifedipine was counteracting a direct effect on the AV node. Recent unpublished work in patients after cardiac transplantation, where the heart is denervated, does not show depression of the AV node on nifedipine at the usual clinical doses. It may be that the much greater vasodilator effect of nifedipine allows the clinical use of doses smaller than those needed to depress the AV node. The differences would then be attributed to a greater vasodilator effect of nifedipine, making it relatively less effective against the AV node. As a corollary nifedipine can be safely used for its vasodilator effect in patients with AV block or in conjunction with beta-blockers [53]. These effects through calcium antagonism in the AV node seem independent of autonomic block of conduction, as shown by the added effect of digoxin, which acts largely by vagal stimulation, after diltiazem [54].

The useful effect of intravenous verapamil selectively to block AV junctional tachycardias with a re-entry process involving the AV node is well known [2] and in frequent use. Also well known is the possibility of adverse effects [26] when verapamil is given in addition to beta-blockade. This is often evident as a fall in blood pressure in relation to bradycardia from the combined effect on the SA node or on AV conduction, or from the adverse effect on myocardial performance as the usual reflex sympathetic compensation is removed. It is important not to regard verapamil as a drug of last resort to be used after beta-blockers have failed to stop an episode of paroxysmal tachycardia. Its role is as a drug of first intention for use when the need for selective AV node block is recognized. A possible further complication is that in patients with the Wolff–Parkinson–White syndrome, block of the AV node may allow rapid conduction of atrial fibrillation (AF) to the ventricle via the anomalous pathway [55]. This was thought to reduce the value of verapamil in the long-term treatment of this subgroup of re-entry AV junctional tachycardias, but not to prevent its use to stop an attack where the risk of AF is unlikely. In the more common varieties of paroxysmal AV junctional tachycardia, verapamil may be considered for long-term use as a prophylactic against attacks [2]. This similar effect of diltiazem on the AV node [52] with its less negative inotropic effect suggest that it may be the calcium antagonist of choice in this situation, through experience as yet is necessarily limited.

The calcium antagonists have similar direct effects [5] on the SA node, producing bradycardia by a secondary effect on the complex pacemaker current [2]. With diltiazem adverse effects such as severe bradycardia were noted in patients with sinus node disease [52] and this should be regarded as a contraindication to the use of diltiazem and verapamil, though presumably nifedipine may be used [53] if a calcium antagonist is required. This effect of verapamil may offer an advantage in preventing reflex tachycardia in the treatment of angina.

Block of the AV node with calcium antagonists is useful in the control of the ventricular rate in AF, and may be used intravenously if AF appears as an acute problem as in myocardial infarction. Chronic AF is well managed with verapamil [56], and may be better than beta-blockade, as the fall in afterload from vasodilatation may improve effort tolerance. Some care is needed in addition of verapamil to digoxin treatment as there is a 60% rise in plasma digoxin, though verapamil itself contributes a major component to the benefit [56]. Regularization of the ventricular rhythm in AF may be seen with verapamil control, but the irregularity is a minor feature of the effect of AF and seems unimportant in practice.

3.11 Angina

The idea of coronary spasm as a cause of angina seems to have a firm hold on pharmacologists and physicians alike, leading to the discovery of the calcium antagonists as coronary vasodilators. The concept was apparently confirmed by the finding of ergonovine-induced focal coronary spasm in Prinzmetal's variant angina [57] but coronary spasm is relatively rare as a cause of the common angina of effort [58]. In most cases effort angina is due to coronary atheroma, and myocardial ischaemia from the increased demands of exercise is an explanation for the relation to effort.

The response to treatment is best considered in terms of the oxygen supply:demand ratio [59] vasodilatation with relief of arterial spasm restoring normal supply, and exercise increasing oxygen consumption and so increasing demand to produce ischaemia. The usual treatments act to reduce demand by a fall in left ventricular work and so in oxygen consumption. Nitrates produce systemic venous dilatation and pooling which reduces venous return and left ventricular volume [59] so that work is reduced although there is probably a component of coronary arterial dilatation which is well seen after direct injection [59].

Beta-blockers act mainly by reducing heart rate during exercise with compensation by greater systemic extraction of oxygen, so that the mixed venous oxygen saturation is reduced with a lower cardiac output, and reduction in contractility plays only a minor part in reducing myocardial oxygen consumption. The effects of calcium antagonists have been difficult to fit into this scheme. The slowing of heart rate with verapamil is relatively slight and is not evident with nifedipine, where arteriolar vasodilatation may reduce left ventricular work by a fall in afterload. A direct effect through interference with excitation–contraction coupling by calcium is suspected [60] and may be regarded as a minor version of the myocardial protective effect discussed earlier. Coronary vasodilatation may play a part as suggested for the nitrates [59].

Coronary spasm as a cause of angina and its relief by nifedipine has been reviewed recently [61]. Spasm is a usual cause of angina at rest and may play a part in some patients with angina of effort, accounting for worsening of provocation, as on exposure to cold or after meals. Failure to respond to, or deterioration after, beta-blockers may be a pointer to coronary spasm [58] as the beta sympathetic is vasodilator in the coronary arteries. In typical Prinzmetal's variant angina with local ST segment elevation, good responses are reported by nifedipine [61] and verapamil [57] with reduction of ST segment shift, though others found no relation to prevention of provocation by ergonovine [62], some having pain with negative tests and others positive tests without pain. Although there are many reports of benefit in Prinzmetal's variant angina [61], there is suspicion that a general coronary vasodilator effect may be independent of spasm [2], due to differences in the mechanism, accounting for some anomalies. A few patients with effort angina not responding to propranolol, suggesting spasm as a basis, were treated effectively with calcium antagonists [58]. Nifedipine has been found useful in patients with unstable angina [63], a heterogenous group with angina at rest, though benefit seems to be mostly confined to those with ST segment elevation, implying either coronary spasm of the Prinzmetal type or the early stages of myocardial infarction where spasm may be a factor, in keeping with the apparent benefit in the rest pain of acute coronary insufficiency where infarction threatens, and the myocardial protective effect may play a part in avoiding myocardial damage, although verapamil had no discernible effect on infarct size in a randomized trial [64].

3.11.1 HAEMODYNAMIC EFFECTS

To interpret the beneficial effects of calcium antagonists in terms of the myocardial oxygen supply:demand ratio, it is necessary to analyse the haemodynamic effects of the calcium antagonists in patients with ischaemic heart disease. A recent review [65] stressed the similarities of the different calcium antagonists with various emphases of effect producing apparent selectivity: verapamil gave more myocardial depression and nifedipine more arterial vasodilatation, with netrendipine even more effective and longer lasting. The main actions relevant to reduced myocardial oxygen consumption were reduced afterload as arterial pressure is reduced by vasodilatation. Reduced myocardial contractility and reduced heart rate, as found with the beta-blockers, are especially evident with verapamil. Calcium antagonists have little effect on venous pooling, which can reduce left ventricular volume after nitrates, but there is a suggestion that nisoldipine may have such an effect [2]. Several studies with nifedipine are in keeping with a reduction in myocardial oxygen consumption as the mechanism of benefit in angina [66]. Improved performance of ischaemic myocardial segments [66] is in keeping with restoration of perfusion as load is reduced. Improvement of impaired relaxation is interpreted as direct reversal of calcium overload [67], as suggested previously [60], but may be merely the effect of reduced myocardial oxygen demand leading to relief of ischaemia as suggested after beta-blockade [68].

Intracoronary injection of nifedipine avoids the peripheral effect of arteriolar vasodilatation [69] and the reflex tachycardia, but does not improve angina as judged by rapid atrial pacing at 6 minutes [69], suggesting that the benefit is due to reduced load. The reflex tachycardia must counteract some of the benefit of reduced afterload, suggesting the combined use of nifedipine with a beta-blocker [36]. A coronary haemodynamic study [70] in patients with demonstrated coronary artery disease, comparing sublingual 20 mg nifedipine and 0.5 mg glyceryl trinitrate showed similar tachycardia and relief of angina. Nifedipine seemed to act here as a coronary vasodilator as coronary flow increased without change in oxygen consumption, though nitrate reduced flow and oxygen consumption as expected from a reduction in load. A vasodilator response to nifedipine raises the possibility of coronary steal with diversion of flow away from ischaemic regions as the more normal arteries dilate.

A reduced myocardial oxygen demand after verapamil [71] is due largely to a lower arterial pressure at any given work load, so that it was not thought necessary to postulate any increase in coronary flow [71]. A haemodynamic study [72] showed a biphasic effect after intravenous verapamil with an early fall in ejection, fraction, and output followed by overshoot, presumably related to the reflex response to vasodilatation. The transient ventricular depression suggests little risk of acute failure in coronary artery disease [72]. The reflex tachycardia is noted to be small with verapamil [13], perhaps because of the direct effect on the sino-atrial node tending to slow the rate. There was no coronary vasodilatation, and the reduction in metabolic work, and therefore in oxygen consumption, was relatively slight [13]. Bagger *et al.* [13] postulate a metabolic switch to more normal substrate utilization with greater uptake of fatty acids and less of glucose which is suppressed in keeping with the finding of decreased lactate release at the point of angina. It is doubtful whether this change represents a metabolic effect of verapamil or a response to improved perfusion of the ischaemic regions as load is reduced. The theory of a metabolic or cardiac protective effect relieving angina is largely related to the dramatic relief produced by the toxic drugs perhexiline [50] and lidoflazine [50].

The different haemodynamic effects of the various groups of drugs used in angina suggests that they might well be used in combination. The use of beta-blockers has long been combined with sublingual glyceryl trinitrate for acute stress and nifedipine may safely be used with beta-blockers in most patients with angina, with an additive effect due to block of the reflex tachycardia [36], though care is needed to avoid combined adverse depressant effects in myocardial disease [34, 35]. The absence of reflex tachycardia with verapamil suggests less gain from combined treatment and a greater risk of adverse myocardial effect.

3.11.2 SIDE EFFECTS

Soon after the introduction of nifedipine, a series of case reports of angina during treatment appeared. The effect was closely related to the time of action of the drug and often occurred with the first dose. Possible causes considered were reduced coronary perfusion from excessive hypotension and coronary steal from vasodilatation in the normal part of the coronary tree, but increased heart rate and cardiac output from the reflex effects is probably responsible in patients with critical myocardial ischaemia. Similar problems may appear at high doses and are overcome by careful adjustment of the dose [73]. Withdrawal of calcium antagonists may produce relapse of angina, especially in patients with coronary spasm [74] but the occurrence of a similar effect in stable angina suggests that a large calcium ion gradient may be established on the antagonists with greater influx on withdrawal.

In diabetes, where calcium antagonists may be used in preference to beta-blockers which remove the warning tachycardia of hypoglycaemic effect, the hyperglycaemia may require re-adjustment of treatment.

An advantage of calcium antagonists over beta-blockers is seen in airways obstruction which is made worse even by cardio-selective beta-blockers. Although there are reports of relief of exercise-induced asthma by verapamil and nifedipine, this is a relatively unusual situation. The bronchodilator effect of calcium antagonists in stable asthma is relatively small [75], but at least this treatment does not have the adverse effect of beta-blockade, and may be the first choice in patients with angina and airways obstruction.

3.11.3 CLINICAL BENEFIT

Many studies show a useful response in angina of effort [2] from nifedipine which may be used with beta-blockers, and verapamil [76] which may be usefully considered as an alternative where beta-blockers are contraindicated, as it has a direct effect slowing the heart rate which replaces much of the effect of beta-blockade. Advantages suggested for verapamil [76] include absence of worsening angina with increasing dose and of rebound angina on withdrawal, presumably as the loss of effect is gradual.

Most studies suggest a comparable effect on angina from calcium antagonists and beta-blockers, and there is some suggestion of tailoring the drugs to prefer verapamil in patients with a low rate response to exercise [77]. Similar considerations apply to verapamil and nifedipine with similar benefit but different side effects [78]. Diltiazem also seems effective in stable angina [79].

Addition of calcium antagonists to beta-blockade has appeal as adding to the unloading by arteriolar vasodilatation, but obviously needs caution if left ventricular function or AV conduction are impaired. A study with propranolol shows an added effect on heart rate, ejection fraction or AV conduction with verapamil, but nifedipine-increased rate and cardiac output has an effect which would be opposed by propranolol [80].

3.12 Hypertension

The demonstration of a specifically greater arteriolar vasodilator response to the calcium antagonist, verapamil, in hypertension [81] has generated controversy between those favouring a fundamental abnormality of handling of calcium in hypertension [82], a prospect of great appeal to the pharmaceutical industry, and the alternative view that the difference relates to the pharmacodynamic response to the two drugs compared, verapamil and sodium nitroprusside on the hypertrophied arterioles in hypertension. After nifedipine treatment, blood pressure fell without change in sodium transport [83]. There is good evidence of hypotensive effect of a fall in plasma calcium [84]. Using blood platelet calcium as a model of vascular smooth muscle behaviour [85], there is a close relation

Calcium antagonists

between free cell calcium and blood pressure and the calcium level falls with the reduction of blood pressure by a variety of treatments, including calcium antagonists, which are no longer specific treatment, and a primary disturbance of sodium transport linked to the elusive natriuretic hormone is rejected [83].

3.12.1 HAEMODYNAMIC EFFECTS

The relaxant effect on vascular smooth muscle is responsible for the reduction in blood pressure and peripheral resistance [85]. Nifedipine has the more powerful peripheral effect, making verapamil seem to have a more cardiac depressant action [85]. Nitrendipine is even more effective as an arteriolar dilator [85]. Reflex control of blood pressure was uneffected by nifedipine [86], so there was no postural hypotension, and renin levels were unchanged [86].

3.12.2 CLINICAL RESPONSE

Both nifedipine and verapamil had satisfactory, comparable effects on blood pressure in hypertension [87] with different side effects, constipation on verapamil, headache and ankle oedema on nifedipine [87]. Caution is needed with addition of other drugs as excessive hypotension is reported with nifedipine and prazosin [2]. The response to calcium antagonists was inversely related to the plasma renin levels before treatment and on verapamil the response was correlated with the age of the patient, suggesting the possible use as first-line treatment in older low-renin patients [87]. Nifedipine is finding a place as a step 3 drug, a vasodilator to follow diuretics and beta-blockers [2] and can be used sublingually or intravenously as an emergency treatment without reducing cerebral blood flow [2]. Verapamil may be particularly useful for hypertension in the elderly, and can be used in patients with airways obstruction. The new more vasodilator dihydropyridine, felodipine, seems likely to be even more effective in hypertension [88].

3.12.3 PULMONARY HYPERTENSION

In addition to the reduction in systemic arteriolar resistance useful to treat hypertension, the calcium antagonists also reduce the elevated pulmonary vascular resistance of pulmonary hypertension due to vasoconstriction of hypertrophied pulmonary arterioles.

As outlined in Chapter 9 there are many haemodynamic problems in attempting to reduce pulmonary vascular resistance with vasodilators. Most of the drugs tried are more effective on the systemic rather than the pulmonary arterioles, so that a fall in systemic rather than the pulmonary arterial blood pressure may limit treatment before the pulmonary hypertension is reduced. The compensatory increase in cardiac output that usually prevents serious hypotension may not occur in the presence of pulmonary hypertension as the cardiac output relies on the performance of the most affected of the two ventricles which operate in series in the intact circulation, so that the left ventricular output cannot rise unless the right ventricle can respond. Even if the output does increase in this situation, the result may be that the pulmonary arterial pressure does not fall in spite of a reduction in peripheral resistance, so there may be little change in the load on the right ventricle, and an inadequate response. Although some success is reported with nifedipine it seems unlikely that this approach will bring an ideal response as a selective effect on the pulmonary circulation is required.

A further problem is seen in the pulmonary hypertension of chronic lung disease, which is based on the hypoxic vasoconstriction that directs blood flow away from underventilated alveoli and ensures an even match of ventilation and perfusion. To overcome this constriction with a vasodilator drug will produce a fall in arterial oxygen saturation [89]. Calcium antagonists can usefully be considered in pulmonary hypertension due to obstructive airways disease as they produce, if anything, a dilator effect on the airways [75], and have been shown to dilate hypoxic pulmonary vasoconstriction in animals. In 13 patients there was partial success with nifedipine in that cardiac output rose slightly as the pulmonary vascular resistance fell, and the slight fall in arterial oxygen saturation was balanced by the rise in cardiac output so that the total oxygen transport was unchanged [89]. The haemodynamic changes are similar to those produced by breathing oxygen which of course will relieve any reduction in arterial oxygen saturation, and improved ventilation and controlled oxygen therapy remain the best approach to treatment by unloading of cor pulmonale in obstructive airways disease, though nifedipine may be helpful. The suggestion that hypoxic vasoconstriction is mediated by calcium ion entry in pulmonary vascular smooth muscle is supported by the similarity of the effects of nifedipine and oxygen therapy [90], which may allow an alternative more convenient approach than continuous oxygen therapy in these patients.

3.13 Myocardial disease

3.13.1 CONGESTIVE HEART FAILURE

The use of calcium antagonists in congestive heart failure was suggested by their vasodilator effects, acting primarily on afterload [91]. Introduced at first in hypertensive heart failure, the fall in blood pressure on nifedipine was associated with an increase in output and secondary fall in left ventricular filling pressure, suggesting improved performance. Verapamil for a similar fall in blood pressure improved output but not filling pressure, in keeping with a greater negative inotropic effect [91]. The observation of coronary microvascular spasm which can be prevented by verapamil as the underlying basis of the hereditary cardiomyopathy of the Syrian hamster suggests that a similar therapeutic approach may be applicable to an early stage of cardiomyopathy in man [92].

The action of calcium antagonists in heart failure is almost entirely arteriolar, so that afterload is reduced without change in preload (Chapter 9). A successful response in failure is usually associated with a rise in cardiac output as peripheral resistance falls so that blood pressure does not fall and there is no reflex sympathetic response to overcome the direct negative inotropic effect on the myocardium. Most attention has therefore been on nifedipine which has relatively little adverse effect on the myocardium.

Nifedipine seemed well tolerated in a group of patients with congestive cardiomyopathy with the expected haemodynamic response and a sustained effect at two months [93]. A series of unpredictable adverse responses [94] have discouraged more widespread use of nifedipine in heart failure. The exact nature of the adverse effect is difficult to determine, but the major feature was a dramatic fall in blood pressure, suggesting a failure to increase cardiac output as the systemic resistance fell with the arteriolar vasodilatation. This finding is in keeping with a negative inotropic effect impairing the myocardial response in the absence of reflex sympathetic effects which may be impaired in failure. As expected the well-controlled patients [93] showed little change in heart rate, but the heart rate is reported as falling in these hypotensive patients [94] and may be the basis of the adverse effect.

Further debate [95] had accepted the negative inotropic effect, as pulmonary oedema has been reported, although paradoxically nifedipine has been used to treat pulmonary oedema, presumably by reducing afterload as nifedipine has little effect on preload. There is a curious suggestion that cardiac output may rise because of an inappropriate increase in venous return. An adverse effect from reduced afterload with little change in preload may possibly be interpreted in this way. The added negative inotropic effect in ischaemic regions [14] may make patients with ischaemic heart disease particularly vulnerable.

The common side effect of ankle oedema in hypertension and angina suggests fluid retention, but is likely to be due to disturbed capillary equilibrium as the calcium antagonists generally have mild diuretic effects.

Verapamil has been tested in patients with heart failure [96] primarily to assess tolerance if it is needed for other purposes. There was little adverse effect suggesting that acute unloading from reduced afterload offset the negative inotropic effect [96]. Diltiazem is also reported as safe in heart failure, producing a slight sodium diuresis [97]. The best therapeutic hope is the new dihydropyridine, felodipine, which has such powerful vascular selectivity that there was no evidence of myocardial depression as the output rose in patients with congestive heart failure [98]. Myocardial oxygen supply improved as coronary flow increased with a fall in oxygen consumption from the reduced afterload [98].

3.13.2 HYPERTROPHIC OBSTRUCTIVE CARDIOMYOPATHY (HOCM)

The problem with HOCM is in some ways the converse of that seen in hypertension and angina. The aim is to reduce myocardial contractility without producing arteriolar vasodilatation. The hypothesis that calcium antagonists will improve diastolic relaxation by reducing sarcoplasmic Ca ion concentration and restrict the primary problem of HOCM has been tested with verapamil and nifedipine and has been applied to the use of nifedipine in other forms of heart failure [99]. Evidence of a primary action on diastolic function is unconvincing and seems unlikely in view of the mechanical effect of the severe hypertrophy. Reduced contractility might be expected to diminish the obstructive element of the disease, but vasodilatation by increasing emptying of the left ventricle will tend to increase the functional outflow obstruction. For this reason verapamil has been most used of the calcium antagonists having most negative inotropic effect, and is often compared with the alternative treatment with a beta-blocker, usually propranolol. Both seem to produce a similar improvement in exercise capacity [100]. Long-term treatment gave evidence of reduction in left ventricular mass and improved the ECG [101]. Verapamil was thought better than propranolol with fewer side effects although the dose of the latter was arbitrarily limited [101].

Some problems are reported with verapamil in HOCM. Increased left ventricular outflow obstruction or negative inotropic effect may produce pulmonary oedema or hypotension from low cardiac output and may be fatal [102]. The effect on the AV node may produce serious bradycardia from higher degrees of heart block [102]. These complications are not surprising in view of the large doses used. More problems might be expected if the suggestion [101] of combination with propranolol were taken up. Combination of nifedipine with propranolol [103] is less dangerous and seems to give satisfactory immediate results with a net reduction in rate, and left ventricular filling pressure fell if initially raised. The ideal drug treatment for HOCM is still under investigation.

Calcium antagonists

References

1. Fleckenstein, A. (1977) Specific pharmacology of calcium in myocardium, cardiac pacemakers and vascular smooth muscle. *Ann. Rev. Pharmaco. Toxicol.*, **17** 149–66.
2. Opie, L.H. (1984) Calcium antagonists. Mechanisms, therapeutic indications and reservations: a review. *Quart. J. Med.*, **53**, 1–16.
3. Tomlinson, S., MacNeil, S., Walker, S.W., Ollis, C.A., Merritt, J.E. and Brown, B.L. (1984) Calmodulin and cell function. *Clin. Sci.*, **66**, 497–507.
4. Braunwald, E. (1982) Mechanism of action of calcium-channel-blocking agents. *N. Engl. J. Med.*, **307**, 1618–27.
5. Kawai, C., Konishi, T., Matsuyama, E. and Okazaki, H. (1981) Comparative effects of three calcium antagonists, diltiazem, verapamil and nifedipine on the sinoatrial and atrioventricular nodes. Experimental and clinical studies. *Circulation*, **63**, 1035–42.
6. Drake-Holland, A.J., and Noble, M.I.M. (1983) Editorial: Myocardial protection by calcium antagonist drugs. *Eur. Heart J.*, **4**, 823–5.
7. Meyer, H., Bossert, F., Wehinger, E., Towart, R. and Belleman, N.P. (1983) Chemistry of calcium antagonists. *Hypertension*, **5**, 112–7.
8. Henry, P.D. (1980) Comparative pharmacology of calcium antagonists: nifedipine, verapamil and diltiazem. *Am. J. Cardiol.*, **46**, 1047–56.
9. Belz, G.G., Aust, P.E. and Munkes, R. (1981) Digoxin plasma concentrations and nifedipine. *Lancet*, i, 844–5.
10. Nayler, W.G., Poole-Wilson, P.A. and Williams, A. (1979) Hypoxia and calcium. *J. Mol. Cell Cardiol.*, **11**, 683–706.
11. Baker, J.E. and Hearse, D.J. (1983) The temperature-sensitivity of slow channel calcium blockers in relation to their effect on the calcium paradox. *Eur. Heart J.*, **4**, Suppl. H, 97–103.
12. Clusin, W.T., Buchbinder, M. and Harrison, D.C. (1983) Calcium overload 'injury' current, and early iscahemic cardiac arrhythmias – a direct connection, *Lancet*, i, 272–4.
13. Bagger, J.P., Toftegaard-Nielsen, T. and Hennigsen, P. (1983) The effect of verapamil on myocardial exchange of free fatty acids, citrate lactate and glucose in coronary artery disease. *Eur. Heart J.*, **4**, 406–14.
14. Smith, H.J., Goldstein, R.A., Griffith, J.M., Kent, K.M. and Epstein, S.E. (1976) Regional contractility: selective depression of ischemic myocardium by verapamil. *Circulation*, **54**; 629–35.
15. The Danish study group on verapamil in myocardial infarction (1984) Verapamil in acute myocardial infarction. *Eur. Heart J.*, **5**, 516–28.
16. Brooks, W.W., Verrier, R. and Lown, B. (1980) Protective effects of verapamil on vulnerability to ventricular fibrillation during myocardial ischaemia and reperfusion. *Cardiovasc. Res.*, **14**, 295–302.
17. Winslow, E., Marshall, R.J. and Hope, F.G. (1983) Comparative effects of fast and slow ion channel blocking agents on reperfusion-induced arrhythmias in the isolated perfused rat heart. *J. Cardiovasc. Pharmacol.*, **5**, 928–36.
18. Mason, J.W., Swerdlow, C.D. and Mitchell, L.B. (1983) Efficacy of verapamil in chronic, recurrent ventricular tachycardia. *Am. J. Cardiol.*, **51**, 1614–17.
19. Fazzini, P.F., Marchi, F., Pucci, P., Ledda, F. and Mugelli, A. (1979) Effects

of verapamil on ventricular premature beats of acute myocardial infarction. *Am. Heart J.*, **98**, 816–18.

20. van Zweiten, P.A., van Meel, J.C.A. and Timmermans, P.B.M.W.M. (1983) Pharmacology of calcium entry blockers: interaction with vascular alpha-adrenoceptors. *Hypertension*, **5**, 118–17.

21. Johnston, A., Burgess, C.D. and Hamer, J. (1981) Systematic availability of oral verapamil and effect on PR interval in man. *Brit. J. Clin. Pharmacol.*, **12**, 397–400.

22. Shand, D.G., Hammill, S.C., Aanonsen, L. and Pritchett, E.L.C. (1981) Reduced verapamil clearance during long-term oral dministration. *Clin. Pharm. Ther.*, **30**, 701–3.

23. Somogyi, A., Albrecht, M., Kleims, G., Schafter, K. and Eichelbaum, M. (1981) Pharmacokinetics, bioavailabilities, and ECG response to verapamil in patients with liver cirrhosis. *Br. J. Clin. Pharmacol.*, **12**, 51–60.

24. Eichelbaum, M., Mikas, G. and Vogelgesang, B. (1984) Pharmacokinetics at (+)- (−)- and (±)-verapamil after intravenous administration. *Br. J. Clin. Pharmacol.*, **17**, 453–8.

25. Vlietstra, R.E., Farias, M.A.C., Frye, R.L., Smith, H.C. and Ritman, E.L. (1983) Effect of verapamil on left ventricular function: a randomized placebo-controlled study. *Am. J. Cardiol.*, **51**, 1213–17.

26. Packer, M., Meller, J., Medina, N., Yushak, M., Smith, H., Holt, J., Guererro J., Todd, G.D., McAllister, R.G. and Gorlin, R. (1982) Hemodynamic consequences of combined beta-adrenergic and slow calcium channel blockade in man. *Circulation*, **65**, 660–8.

27. Woie, L. and Storstein, L. (1981) Successful treatment of suicidal verapamil poisoning with calcium gluconate. *Eur. Heart J.*, **2**, 239–42.

28. Gmeiner, R. and Ng, C.K. (1981) Effect of tiapamil in the Wolff–Parkinson–White syndrome. *J. Cardiovasc. Pharmacol*, **3**, 237–50.

29. Flammang, D., Waynberger, M., Jansen, F.H., Paillet, R. and Courmel, Ph. (1983) Electrophysiological profile of bepridil, a new anti-anginal drug with calcium blocking properties. *Eur. Heart J.*, **4**, 647–54.

30. Maclean, D. and Feely, J. (1983) Calcium antagonists, nitrates, and new antianginal drugs. *Br. Med. J.*, **286**, 1127–30.

31. Robinson, B.F., Dobbs, R.J. and Kelsey, C.R. (1980) Effects of nifedipine on resistance vessels, arteries and veins in man. *Br. J. Clin. Pharmacol*, **10**, 433–8.

32. Raemsch, K.D. and Sommer, J. (1983) Pharmacokinetics and metabolism of nifedipine. *Hypertension*, **5**, II18–II24.

33. Charles, S., Ketelslegers, J.-M. Buysschaert, M. and Lambert, A.E. (1981) Hyperglycaemic effect of nifedipine. *Br. Med. J.*, **283**, 19–20.

34. Joshi, P.I., Dalal, J.J., Ruttley, M.S.J., Sheridan, D.J. and Henderson, A.H. (1981) Nifedipine and left ventricular function in beta-blocked patients. *Br. Heart J.*, **45**, 457–9.

35. Opie, L.H. and White, D.A. (1980) Adverse interaction between nifedipine and beta-blockade. *Br. Med. J.*, **281**, 1462.

36. Harris, L., Dargie, H.J., Lynch, P.G., Bulpitt, C.J. and Krikler, D.M. (1982) Blood pressure and heart rate in patients with ischaemic heart disease receiving nifedipine and propranolol. *Br. Med. J.*, **284**, 1148–51.

37. Iliopoulou, A., Turner, P. and Warrington, S.J. (1983) Acute haemodynamic

effects of a new calcium antagonist, nicardipine, in man. A comparison with nifedipine. *Br. J. Clin. Pharmacol.*, **15**, 59–66.

38. Hansson, L., Andren, L., Oro, L. and Ryman, T. (1983) Pharmacokinetic and pharmacodynamic parameters in patients treated with nitrendipine. *Hypertension*, **5**, II25–II28.

39. Allen, G.S., Ahn, H.S., Preziosi, T.J., Battye, R., Boone, S.C., Chou, S.N., Kelly, D.L., Weir, B.K., Crabbe, R.A., Lavik, P.J., Rosenbloom, S.B., Dorsey, F.C., Ingram, C.R., Mellits, D.E., Bertsch, L.A., Boisvert, D.P.J., Hundley, M.B., Johnson, R.K., Strom, J.A. and Transou, C.R. (1983) Cerebral arterial spasm – a controlled trial of nimodipine in patients with subarachnoid hemorrhage. *N. Engl. J. Med.*, **308**, 619–24.

40. Tweddel, A.C., Johnsson, G., Pringle, T.H., Murray, R.G., and Hutton, I. (1983) The systemic coronary haemodynamic effects of felodipine in patients with coronary heart disease. *Eur. Heart J.*, **4**, 699–705.

41. Smith, M.S., Verghese, C.P., Shand, D.G. and Pritchett, E.L.C. (1982) Pharmacokinetic and pharmacodynamic effects of diltiazem. *Am, J. Cardiol.*, **51**, 1369–74.

42. Valette, H. and Apoil, E. (1980) Haemodynamic effects of dilitiazem in healthy volunteers. *Br. J. Clin. Pharamcol.*, **10**, 623–4.

43. Hossack, K.F. (1982) Conduction abnormalities due to diltiazem. *N. Engl. J. Med.*, **307**, 953–4.

44. Grenadier, E., Keidar, S., Alpan, G., Marmor, A. and Palant A. (1980) Prenylamine-induced ventricular tachycardia and syncope controlled by ventricular pacing. *Br. Heart J.*, **44**, 330–4.

45. Shah, R.R., Oates, N.S., Idle, J.R., Smith, R.L. and Lockhart, J.D.F. (1982) Impaired oxidation of debrisoquine in patients with perhexiline neuropathy. *Br. Med. J.*, **284**, 295–9.

46. Dawes, F. and Moulder, C. (1982) Perhexiline hepatitis and HLA B8. *Lancet*, **ii**, 109.

47. Sebille, A. (1978) Prevalence of latent perhexiline neuropathy. *Br. Med. J.*, **i**, 1321–2.

48. Horgan, J.H., O'Callaghan, W.G. and Tee, K.K. (1981) Therapy of angina pectoris with low-dose perhexiline. *J. Cardiovasc. Pharmacol.*, **3**, 566–72.

49. Holmes, B., Brodgen, R.N., Heel, R.C., Speight, T.M. and Avery, G.S. (1984) Flunarizine. A review of its pharmacodynamic and pharmacokinetic properties and therapeutic use. *Drugs*, **27**, 6–44.

50. Towse, G. (ed.) (1980) Myocardial protection and exercise tolerance: the role of lidoflazine a new anti-anginal agent. *Roy. Soc. Med. Int. Congr. Symp. Series*, **29**.

51. Hanley, S.P. and Hampton, J.R. (1983) Ventricular arrhythmias associated lidoflazine: side-effects observed in a randomized trial. *Eur. Heart J.*, **4**, 889–93.

52. Valette, H., Barnay, C., Lopez, M., Hebert, J.L., Gallet, M., Apoil, E., Moyse, D. and Medvedowsky, J.L. (1983) Effect of intravenous diltiazem on sinus node function and atrioventricular conduction in patients. *J. Cardiovasc. Pharmacol.*, **5**, 62–6.

53. Rowland, E., Evans, T. and Krikler, D.M. (1979) Effect of nifedipine on atrioventricular conduction as compared with verapamil. Intracardiac- electrophysiological study. *Br. Heart J.*, **42**, 126–7.

54. Mitchell, L.B., Jutzy, K.R., Lewis, S.J., Schroeder, J.S. and Mason, J.W. (1982) Intracardiac electrophysiological study of intravenous diltiazem and combined diltiazem-digoxin in patients. *Am. Heart J.*, **103**, 57–66.

55. Harper, R.W., Whitford, E., Middlebrook, K., Federman, J., Anderson, S. and Pitt, A. (1982) Effects of verapamil on the electrophysiologic properties of the accessory pathway in patients with the Wolff–Parkinson–White syndrome. *Am. J. Cardiol.*, **50**, 1323–30.

56. Lang, R., Klein, H.O., DiSegni, E., Gefen, J., Sareli, P., Libhaber, C., David, D., Weiss, E., Guerrero, J. and Kaplinsky, E. (1983) Verapamil improves exercise capacity in chronic atrial fibrillation: double-blind crossover study. *Am. Heart J.*, **105**, 820–5.

57. Johnson, S.M., Mauristen, D.F., Willerson, J.T. and Hillis, L.D. (1981) A controlled trial of verapamil for Prinzmetal's variant angina. *N. Engl. J. Med.*, **304**, 862–6.

58. Yasue, H., Omote, S., Takizawa, A., Nagao, M., Miwa, K. and Tanaka, S. (1979) Exertional angina pectoris caused by coronary arterial spasm: effects of various drugs. *Am. J. Cardiol.*, **43**, 647–52.

59. Editorial (1984) Nitrates and angina. *Lancet*, i, 998–9.

60. McIlwraith, G.R., Kidner, P.H. and Oram, S. (1980) Effect of nifedipine on exercise tolerance in angina pectoris. *Br. Heart J.*, **44**, 335–341.

61. Lown, B. (ed.) (1979) Symposium on nifedipine and calcium flux inhibition in the treatment of coronary arterial spasm and myocardial ischemia. *Am. J. Cardiol.*, **44**, 779–844.

62. Winniford, M.D., Johnson, S.M., Mauritson, D.R. and Hillis, L.D. (1983) Ergonovine provocation to assess efficacy of long-term therapy with calcium antagonists in Prinzmetal's variant angina. *Am. J. Cardiol.*, **51**, 684–8.

63. Gerstenblith, G., Ouyang, P., Achuff, S.C., Bulkley, B.H., Becker, L.C., Mellits, E.D., Baughman, K.L., Weiss, J.L., Flaherty, J.T., Kallman, C.H., Llewellyn, M. and Weisfeldt, M.L. (1982) Nifedipine in unstable angina. A double-blind randomized trial. *N. Engl. J. Med.*, **306**, 885–9.

64. Thuesen, L., Jorgensen, J.R., Kvistgaard, H.J., Sorensen, J.A., Vaeth, M., Jensen, E.B., Jensen, J.J. and Hagerup, L. (1983) Effect of verapamil on enzyme release after early intravenous administration in acute myocardial infarction: double blind randomised trial. *Br. Med. J.*, **286**, 1107–8.

65. Lehmann, H.-U., Hochrein, H., Witt, E. and Mies, H.W. (1983) Hemodynamic effects of calcium antagonists. *Rev. Hypertension*, **5**, I166–I173.

66. Zacca, N.M., Verani, M.S., Chahine, R.A. and Miller, R.R. (1982) Effect of nifedipine on exercise-induced left ventricular dysfuntion and myocardial hypoperfusion in stable angina. *Am. J. Cardiol.*, **50**, 689–95.

67. Serruys, P.W., Hooghoudt, T.E.M., Reiber, J.H.C., Slager, C., Brower, R.W. and Hugenholtz, P.G. (1983) Influence of intravenous nifedipine on left ventricular function, coronary vasomotility and myocardial oxygen consumption. *Br. Heart J.*, **49**, 427–41.

68. Dagenais, G.R., Moisan, A., Marquis, Y., Davies, R.O. and Blouin, S. (1976) Effects of practolol on exercise tolerance, and cardiac haemodynamics and metabolism in patients with coronary artery disease. *Cardiovasc. Res.*, **10**, 25–36.

69. Schazenbacher, P., Liebau, G., Deeg, P. and Kochsiek, K. (1983) Effect of intravenous and intracoronary nifedipine on coronary blood flow and

myocardial oxygen consumption. *Am. J. Cardiol.*, **49**, 442–6.

70. Stone, D.L., Stephens, J.D. and Banim, S.O. (1983) Coronary haemo-dynamic effects of nifedipine. Comparison with glyceryl trinitrate. *Br. Heart J.*, **49**, 422–6.

71. Rouleau, J-L., Chatterjee, K., Ports, T.A., Doyle, M.B., Hiramatsu, B. and Parmley, W.W. (1983) Mechanism of relief of pacing-induced angina with oral verapamil: reduced oxygen demand. *Circulation*, **67**, 94–100.

72. Klein, H.O., Ninio, R. Oren, V., Lang, R., Sareli, P., DiSegni, E. David, D., Guerrero, J. and Kaplinsky, E. (1983) The acute hemodynamic effects of intravenous verapamil in coronary artery disease: assessment of equilibrium-gated radionuclide ventriculography. *Circulation*, **67**, 101–10.

73. Deanfield, J. Wright, C. and Fox, K. (1983) Treatment of angina pectoris with nifedipine: importance of dose titration. *Br. Med. J.*, **286**, 1467–70.

74. Subramanian, V.B., Bowles, M.J., Khurmi, N.S., Davies, A.B., O'Hara, M.J. and Raftery, E.B. (1983) Calcium antagonist withdrawal syndrome: objective demonstration with frequency-modulated ambulatory ST-segment monitor-ing. *Br. Med. J.*, **286**, 520–1.

75. Editorial (1983) Calcium-channel blockers and asthma. *Thorax*, **38**, 481–5.

76. Packer, M. and Frishman, H. (eds) (1982) Symposium on verapamil therapy for angina pectoris. *Am. J. Cardiol.*, **50**, 881–912, 913–28, 1153–95.

77. Bowles, M.J., Subramanian, V.B., Davies, A.B. and Raftery, E.B. (1981) Comparison of antianginal actions of verapamil and propranolol. *Br. Med. J.*, **282**, 1754.

78. Subramanian, V.B., Bowles, M.J., Shurmi, N.S., Davies, A.B. and Raftery, E.B. (1982) Randomized double-blind comparison of verapamil and nifedi-pine in chronic stable angina. *Am. J. Cardiol.*, **50**, 696–703.

79. Wagniart, P., Ferguson, R.J., Cheitman, B.R., Achard, F., Benacerraf, A., Delanguenhagen, B., Morin, B., Pasternac, A. and Bourassa, M.G. (1982) Increased exercise tolerance and reduced electrocardiographic ischemia with diltiazem in patients with stable angina pectoris. *Circulation*, **66**, 23–8.

80. Winniford, M.D., Markham, R.V., Firth, B.G., Nicod, P. and Hillis, L.D. (1982) Hemodynamic and electrophysiologic effects of verapamil and nifedi-pine in patients on propranolol. *Am. J. Cardiol.*, **50**, 704–10.

81. Robinson, B.F., Dobbs, R.J. and Bayley, S. (1982) Response of forearm resistance vessels to verapamil and sodium nitroprusside in normotensive and hypertensive men: evidence for a functional abnormality of vascular smooth muscle in primary hypertension. *Clin. Sci.*, **63**, 33–42.

82. de Wardener, H.E. and MacGregor, G. (1983) Sodium efflux and essential hypertension. *Lancet*, i, 185–6.

83. Heagerty, A.M., Bing, R.F., Thurston, H. and Swales, J.D. (1983) Calcium antagonists in hypertension: relation to abnormal sodium transport. *Br. Med. J.*, **287**, 1405–7.

84. Bianchetti, M.G. Beretta-Piccoli, C., Weidmann, P., Link, L., Boehringer, K., Ferrier, C. and Morton, J.J. (1983) Calcium and blood pressure regulation in normal and hypertensive subjects. *Hypertension*, **5**, I157–I165.

85. Erne, P., Bolli, P., Burgisser, E. and Buhler, F.R. (1984) Correlation of platelet calcium with blood pressure. Effect of antihypertensive therapy. *N. Engl. J. Med.*, **310**, 1084–8.

86. McLeay, R.A.B., Stallard, T.J., Watson, R.D.S. and Littler, W.A. (1983) The

effect of nifedipine on arterial pressure and reflex cardiac control. *Circulation*, **67**, 1084–90.

87. Erne, P., Bolli, P., Bertel, O., Hulthen, L., Kiowski, W., Muller, F.B. and Buhgler, F. (1983) Factors influencing the hypotensive effects of calcium antagonists. *Hypertension*, **5**, II97–II102.

88. Andersson, O., Bengtsson, C., Elmfedt, D., Haglund, K., Hedner, T., Seideman, P., Sjoberg, K.H., Stromgren, E., Aberg, H. and Ostman, J. (1984) Short-term effects of felodpine, a new dihydropyridine, in hypertension. *Br. J. Clin. Pharmacol.*, **17**, 257–63.

89. Simmonneau, G., Escourrou, P., Duroux, P. and Lockhart, A. (1981) Inhibition of hypoxic pulmonary vasoconstriction by nifedipine. *N. Engl. J. Med.*, **304**, 1582–5.

90. Kennedy, T.P., Michael, J.R., Huang, C.-K., Kallman, C.H., Zahka, K., Schlott, W. and Sommer, W. (1984) Nifedipine inhibits hypoxic pulmonary vasoconstriction during rest and exercise in patients with chronic obstructive pulmonary disease. A controlled double-blind study. *Am. Rev. Resp. Dis.*, **129**, 544–51.

91. Guazzi, M.D., Cipolla, C., Sganzerla, P., Agostoni, P.G., Fabbiocchi, F. and Pepi, M. (1983) Clinical use of calcium channel blockers as ventricular unloading agents. *Eur. Heart J.*, **4**, Suppl A, 181–7.

92. Factor, S.M. and Sonnenblick, E.H. (1982) Editorial. Hypothesis: is congestive cardiomyopathy caused by a hyperactive myocardial micro-circulation (microvascular spasm)? *Am. J. Cardiol.*, **50**, 1149–52.

93. Bellocci, F., Ansalone, G., Santarelli, P., Loperfido, F., Scabbia, E., Zecchi, P. and Manzoli, U. (1983) Oral nifedipine in the long-term management of severe chronic heart failure. *J. Cardiovasc. Pharmacol.*, **4**, 847–55.

94. Brooks, N., Cattell, M., Pidgeon, J. and Balcon, R. (1980) Unpredictable response to nifedipine in severe cardiac failure. *Br. Med. J.*, **281**, 1324.

95. Alves, L.E. and Rose, E.P. (1982) Use of nifedipine in older patients and patients with congestive heart failure. *Am. J. Med.*, **72**, 462, 472.

96. Ferlinz, J. and Citron, P.D. (1983) Hemodynamic and myocardial performance characteristics after verapamil use in congestive heart failure. *Am. J. Cardiol.*, **51**, 1339–45.

97. Kinoshita, M., Kusukawa, R., Shimono, Y., Motomura, M., Tomonaga, G. and Hoshino, T. (1979) The effect of diltiazem hydrochloride upon sodium diuresis and renal function in chronic congestive heart failure. *Arzneim. Forsch.*, **29**, 676–81.

98. Timmis, A.D., Campbell, S., Monaghan, M.J., Walker, L. and Jewitt, D.E. (1984) Acute haemodynamic and metabolic effect of felodipine in congestive heart failure. *Br. Heart J.*, **51**, 445–51.

99. Given B.D., Lee, T.H., Stone, P.H. and Dzau, V.J. (1985) Nifedipine in severely hypertensive patients with congestive heart failure and preserved ventricular systolic function. *Arch. Intern. Med.*, **141**, 281–5.

100. Rosing, D.R., Kent, K.M., Maron, B.J. and Epstein, S.E. (1979) Verapamil therapy: a new approach to the pharmacological treatment of hypertrophic cardiomyopathy. II Effects on exercise capacity and symptomatic status. *Circulation*, **60**, 1208–13.

101. Kaltenbach, M., Hopf, R., Kober, G., Bussmann, W.-D., Keller, M. and Petersen, Y. (1979) Treatment of hypertrophic obstructive cardiomyopathy

Calcium antagonists

with verapamil. *Br. Heart J.*, **42**, 35–42.
102. Epstein, S.E. and Roising, D.R. (1981) Verapamil: Its potential for causing serious complications in patients with hypertrophic cardiomyopathy. *Circulation*, **64**, 437–41.
103. Landmark, K., Sire, S., Thaulow, E., Amile, J.P. and Nitter-Hauge, S. (1982) Haemodynamic effects of nifedipine and propranolol in patients with hypertrophic obstructive cardiomyopathy. *Br. Heart J.*, **48**, 19–26.

4 Antianginal vasodilators

L.H. OPIE and U. THADANI

To explain the mode of action of antianginal vasodilators (Table 4.1), requires first a reasonable hypothesis for the production of angina; secondly, an understanding of the vascular contractile mechanism and its metabolic and neurogenic control; and, thirdly, the way in which these vasodilators interact with their receptors or binding sites to produce clinical effects. On the background of such knowledge, a more rational approach to the principles (Table 4.2) and practice of the use of anti-anginal vasodilators can be formulated. This chapter will deal chiefly with the nitrates and the calcium antagonists (= calcium channel blockers); effects on the circulation as well as on the heart will be emphasized.

Table 4.1 Possible mechanisms of antianginal vasodilators

Possible mode of action	Agents	Comments
Inhibition of contractile mechanism	Nitrates	Dilate chiefly veins and coronary arteries; May act by enhancing myocyte cyclic GMP
Inhibition of calcium ion entry	Calcium antagonists	Act both as coronary artery and general arteriolar vasodilator
Enhanced formation of adenosine	Dipyridamole	Not clinically used as antianginal agent; Probably causes 'coronary steal'
Inhibition of neurogenic vasoconstriction	$Alpha_1$ $Alpha_1+$ $Alpha_2$ antagonists	Not generally useful not even as antagonists in coronary spasm

Antianginal vasodilators

4.1 Production of angina pectoris

4.1.1 OXYGEN SUPPLY VS DEMAND

A useful hypothesis is that angina pectoris can be caused whenever the myocardial oxygen demand exceeds the supply to cause myocardial ischaemia. Factors likely to precipitate angina of effort are all those that increase the oxygen demand in the face of a supply limited by coronary artery disease (Table 4.2). During exercise, the increase of heart rate and blood pressure may consistently precipitate effort angina at a constant double (rate × pressure) product, while an increase of heart rate (together with some rise of blood pressure) is probably the major factor in emotion-provoked angina. Sometimes exercise precipitates angina at a variable (rate × pressure) product, when it is thought that a variable added component of coronary spasm (see later) is present.

4.1.2 CORONARY STENOSIS [1]

Increasing coronary stenosis has two ultimate effects: there is the direct effect decrease in the perfusion pressure, and an indirect effect of tissue ischaemia which causes contractile failure, thereby increasing the left ventricular end-diastolic pressure which in turn compresses subendocardial tissue and reduces coronary perfusion [2, 3]. Of the total coronary flow, 85% occurs in diastole; the remaining 15% occurs in systole but only in the epicardial zone [4]. In subendocardial tissue, blood flow in systole stops as the pressure within the left ventricle rises, increasing the vulnerability of the subendocardial zone to ischaemia.

To reduce coronary flow by stenosis requires a very large reduction of the arterial lumen [5]. The most important factor is the severity of the stenosis and the consequent increase in resistance to blood flow across the stenosis [6]. The resistance increases by a power of four as the radius decreases (Poiseuille's Law) so that reducing the internal diameter from 80 to 90% dramatically elevates the resistance [6]. Resting flow is not affected till the stenosis is very severe, so that one estimate is that a 70% reduction of internal diameter with a 90–95% fall in luminal area is required for basal coronary flow to fall [5]. In response to stimuli causing maximal vasodilation, flow starts not to achieve maximal values when the internal diameter is reduced beyond 30% and the internal luminal area by over 50%. For a given severity of stenosis, the longer the stenotic segment, the more marked the effects of any given degree of occlusion.

For any given degree of *fixed coronary stenosis*, there are complex additional factors such as the degree of turbulence across the stenosis and added changes in vascular tone or spasm which may decrease the flow as the demand rises during exercise, which is called *dynamic stenosis* [7]. In

104

Table 4.2* Principles of therapy of angina pectoris

1 *Reduction of oxygen demand*
   - reduce heart rate by beta-blockade (also some calcium antagonists)
   - reduce afterload by beta-blockade, calcium antagonists and by control of hypertension
   - reduce metabolic demand by calcium antagonists, beta-blockade
   - reduce preload by nitrates
2 *Increase oxygen supply*
   - coronary vasodilators (calcium antagonists, nitrates)
   - promote growth of collaterals (? exercise)
   - change anatomy of coronary disease (coronary artery bypass grafting, angioplasty, laser techniques)

* Modified from [1]

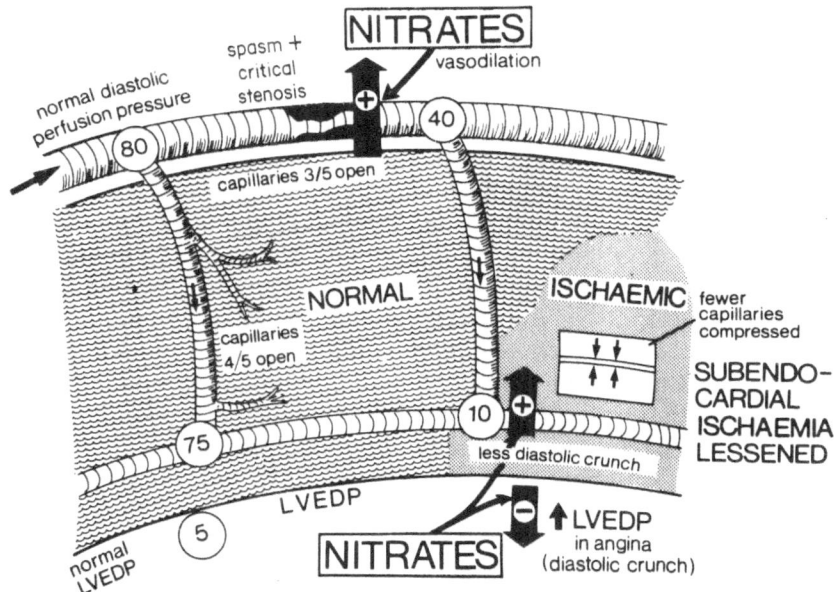

Fig. 4.1 When a patient with a critical stenosis exercises, subendocardial ischaemia and temporary left ventricular failure accompany the onset of anginal pain. Alternatively, angina at rest can develop if there is super-added coronary spasm. Nitrates bring relief by increasing the diameter of large coronary arteries, by relaxing spasm, and chiefly by reducing left ventricular end-diastolic pressure (LVEDP). For evaluation of the importance of 'diastolic crunch', see Reference [2], from which this Figure is modified with permission. © Opie, 1986.

severe stenosis, the post-stenotic pressure can fall below a critical value of about 50 mmHg, required for normal vasodilator autoregulation [6]. The failure of compensatory vasodilation further robs the already ischaemic myocardium of blood flow. Severe subendocardial or even transmural ischaemia causes left ventricular failure, by increasing the intracavity pressure, and further decreases the actual perfusion (driving) pressure across the stenosis. Here a useful concept is that angina pectoris has the haemodynamic features of acute left ventricular failure [2]; the abruptly elevated left ventricular end-diastolic pressure causes a 'diastolic crunch' (Fig. 4.1).

4.1.3 CORONARY ARTERY SPASM

The concept that coronary spasm can be clinically significant dates back at least to the time of Lewis. Yet proof of this hypothesis had to await the pioneering studies of Maseri and his group at Pisa [8]. Focal spasm is thought to occur chiefly in the large epicardial arteries and is frequently superimposed on anatomical stenosis. Clinically, coronary spasm is thought to have a wide range of expression, varying from asymptomatic ST-deviations on the electrocardiogram to transmural ischaemia with severe chest pain at rest and the typical ST-segment elevation of Prinzmetal's angina. There are two explanations for the association of spasm and organic stenosis. First, platelet thrombi may form at the stenotic site to liberate vasoconstrictive agents such as thromboxane A_2 [9] and white cells may liberate leukotrienes. Secondly, coronary atheroma damages the vascular endothelium with loss of the endothelial relaxing factor, which is required for the action of some vasodilators. Thus endothelial damage may mute some physiological vasodilatory influences to allow an excess of vasoconstrictive stimuli. By such mechanisms the arteries are thought to become sensitized to vasoconstrictive alpha-adrenergic stimuli and to potential circulating vasoconstrictors such as histamine [10]; and especially thromboxane A_2 [9]. Also, some factors normally acting as coronary vasodilators can become vaso-constrictive in the presence of endothelial damage; an example is cholinergic stimulation.

Coronary artery spasm frequently occurs at night, in part because decreased body metabolism leads to an increase of blood pH and an increased ionized calcium concentration in the blood; the latter change promotes spasm [11]. Parasympathetic vasoconstrictor stimuli, which normally are not very strong, may also play a part at night when parasympathetic tone is highest; this probability is strongest in the presence of a damaged endothelium.

VASCULAR SMOOTH MUSCLE

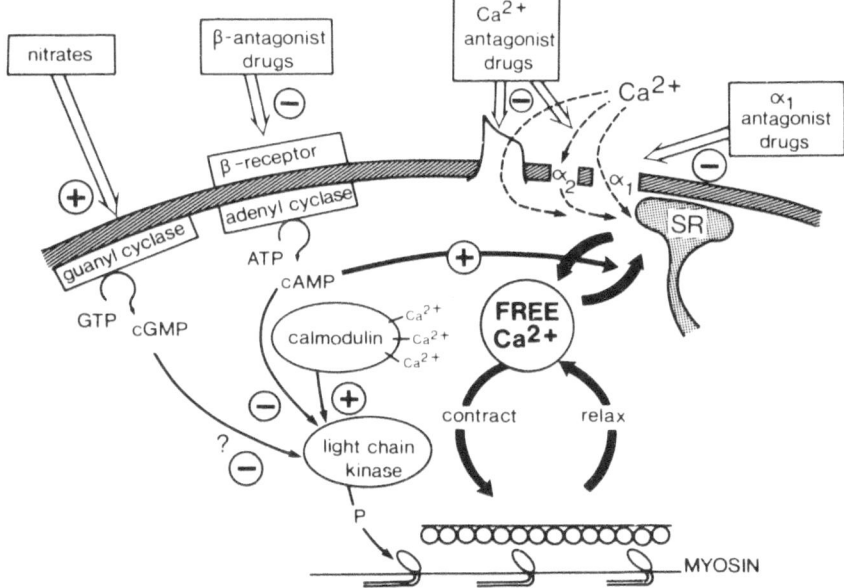

Fig. 4.2 Proposed molecular mechanisms for vascular smooth muscle contraction, showing the cellular effects of nitrates and the contrasting cellular effects of calcium antagonists and beta-adrenergic receptor antagonist drugs. Calcium antagonists, by decreasing the cytostolic free calcium ion concentration in vascular smooth muscle, decrease calmodulin activity to decrease the activity of myosin light chain kinase. These processes lessen the phosphorylation of myosin light chain which is required for vascular smooth muscle contraction, so smooth muscle relaxes. Beta antagonists (a) allow a high cytosilic calcium by decreasing uptake of calcium ions into the sarcoplasmic reticulum and (b) lessen the inhibition by cyclic AMP of the phosphorylation of the myosin light chains. Both effects increase smooth muscle contraction. In addition, unopposed alpha-adrenergic mediated vascular spasm worsens the vasoconstrictive effect of beta-adrenergic antagonists. Modified from [1]. © Opie, 1986.

4.2 Calcium and regulation of vascular smooth muscle tone

To understand the mechanism of vasodilator action requires a review of smooth muscle contraction mechanisms (Fig. 4.2). Many of the events are similar to those described in the cardiac contraction cycle: the entry of calcium, the (presumed) calcium-induced calcium release from the sarcoplasmic reticulum, the rise in cytosolic free calcium ion concentration, the interaction of calcium with the myosin ATPase, the subsequent uptake of calcium into the sarcoplasmic reticulum, and the discharge of excess calcium via calcium exit channels as in the heart [12].

4.2.1 VASCULAR SMOOTH MUSCLE VS MYOCARDIUM

Three important differences between vascular smooth muscle and the myocardium are: (1) due to the tonic nature of the peripheral arteriolar contracture, there should be a sustained level of free ionized calcium or another mechanism must come into play to sustain tone; (2) due to the lessened force of contraction that needs to be developed, the peak intracellular calcium concentration reached should be less; and (3) there must be a major difference between heart and peripheral smooth muscle in response to the stimulation of the beta-adrenergic receptor, because beta-stimulation causes the heart to contract and peripheral vessels to dilate. In peripheral vascular muscle, calcium ions also regulate the myosin–actin interaction by a mechanism which is different from that in the heart because troponin C is absent from vascular smooth muscle. According to the *phosphorylation hypothesis* [12], calcium ions interact with calmodulin to promote phosphorylation of the light chains of the myosin heads (Fig. 4.2).

4.2.2 LATCH MECHANISM

Vascular contraction is maintained for long periods with little use of ATP, since the contractile mechanism has no ejection work to do as in the case of the myocardium. Rather, contraction needs to be sustained and varied to allow vascular smooth muscle tone to help to regulate the coronary flow. A 'latch mechanism' is described [13], whereby once myosin and actin are joined, they latch on to each other and fail to relax until a further signal is applied. This latch mechanism involves crossbridges which are not phosphorylated, the *latchbridges*, which are slowly cycling in contrast to the rapidly cycling, usual type of crossbridge which can be phosphorylated. How calcium regulates latchbridges is still not known.

4.2.3 CALCIUM CHANNELS IN SMOOTH MUSCLE

It may be that there are two types of calcium channels in vascular smooth muscle.

(a) Depolarization-operated channels (DOCs)

These are found in smooth muscle as well as heart muscle. In smooth muscle, they have also been termed potential sensitive channels [14]. To maintain arterial tone, intermittent spontaneous autonomic nervous discharges are required. Such discharges could either directly operate the DOCs, or could intermittently release noradrenaline to activate receptor-operated channels (ROCs). Experimentally a clear role for DOCs is shown in the case of a potassium-induced contracture. It is on such potassium-induced contractures that the calcium antagonist agents have been shown to act by Fleckenstein [15]. The fact that calcium antagonists act to dilate smooth muscle and to reduce peripheral vascular resistance, suggests that either the DOCs are of basic importance in setting the level of peripheral smooth muscle tone or the receptor operated channels act via the DOCs. Electrophysiological evidence stresses the role of the membrane potential, and hence of the DOCs, in regulating vascular tone [16].

(b) Receptor-operated channels (ROCs)

These respond to agonists, the chief being noradrenaline. Serotonin and angiotensin may also operate on ROCs. The depolarization-operated channels are inhibited by calcium antagonists in the vascular beds throughout the body, whereas in only some vascular beds are there receptor-operated channels which are sensitive to calcium antagonism. For example, nimodipine blocks the depolarization-operated channels in the saphenous artery but leaves the serotonin-induced contraction unchanged; whereas in the basilar artery nimodipine inhibits both ROCs and DOCs [17].

4.2.4 PHASIC AND TONIC COMPONENTS OF VASCULAR CONTRACTION

Smooth muscle has two components to its contraction: phasic and tonic. In peripheral vascular smooth muscle, the tonic component regulates peripheral vascular resistance, and is sensitive both to the noradrenaline and calcium contents of the extracellular fluid. Electrophysiological evidence stresses the role of the membrane potential in regulating vascular tone [16].

4.2.5 METABOLIC AND HUMORAL VASODILATION

Adenosine is generally accepted as the major factor in the metabolic regulation of the coronary circulation. The breakdown of high-energy phosphate compounds leads eventually to the production of adenosine by the action of the enzyme 5'-nucleotidase [18]. Adenosine is broken down by adenosine deaminase when it enters the circulation. Inhibition of this enzyme, for instance by dipyridamole, increases coronary vasodilatation in a diffuse unselective way which does not relieve angina, perhaps because of steal in normal parts of the coronary vascular bed.

Antianginal vasodilators

Potassium released from damaged cells can act as a vasodilator perhaps by modulation of noradrenaline release from sympathetic nerve terminals. There is a suggestion [19] that *ATP* released from damaged cells or purinergic nerve terminals can have a vasodilator effect.

Prostaglandins are released into coronary venous blood in angina [20] suggested that E-type prostaglandins may be physiological vasodilators which are increased by nitrate treatment [21], and may mediate the coronary vasodilator effect of bradykinin [22].

Histamine generally produces vasodilation through H_1 and H_2 receptors. H_1 receptors, acting independently of adenylate cyclase, appear to mediate coronary vasoconstriction [10] especially in the presence of coronary atherosclerosis [23].

4.2.6 NEUROGENIC REGULATION

The major neurogenic control of vascular smooth muscle is through sympathetic alpha-receptors by release of noradrenaline from sympathetic terminals or by the effects of circulating catecholamines [24]. The effect on smooth muscle tone in the resistance vessels is mediated by regulation of calcium ion entry via the receptor-operated channels.

The action of the postjunctional alpha$_1$-receptor is modulated by prejunctional influences, which may be cholinergic, alpha$_2$- or beta-adrenergic. The normal vasodilator mechanism is probably this cholinergic (muscarinic) inhibition of noradrenaline release (Fig. 4.3) or by direct action in the presence of endothelial relaxing factor [25]. Low levels of stimulation are facilitated by prejunctional beta-receptors which augment the release of noradrenaline for vasoconstriction. At higher levels of stimulation, prejunctional alpha$_2$-receptors inhibit noradrenaline release [26].

In peripheral vessels the antagonist vasodilatory effect of beta$_2$-receptors is produced by circulating catecholamines, not by sympathetic nervous stimulation [27]. In the conscious dog vasodilation of the major coronary artery appears to be mediated by beta$_1$-receptors, probably by the overriding effect of beta$_1$-mediated increase in metabolic demand [28].

Part of the vasoconstrictor effect is mediated by post-junctional alpha$_2$-receptors (Fig. 4.1), and these have been identified in the human peripheral vascular bed [29]. It is proposed [30] that calcium antagonists act by inhibition of those alpha$_2$-receptors to cause vasodilation. Variations in receptors (Fig. 4.1), and these have been identified in the human peripheral vascular bed [29]. It is proposed [30] that calcium antagonists act by inhibition of those alpha$_2$-receptors to cause vasodilation. Variations in

Calcium and regulation of vascular smooth muscle tone

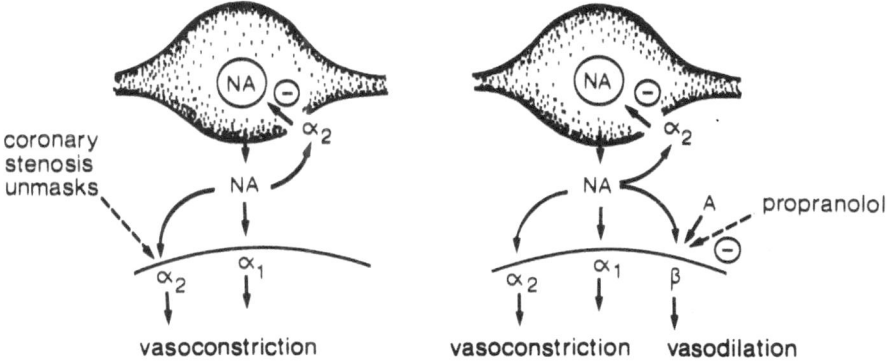

Fig. 4.3 Role of presynaptic and postsynaptic alpha- and beta-receptors in regulation of vascular smooth muscle tone. Note that sympathetically mediated vasoconstriction may be important in genesis of coronary artery spasm. Noradrenaline (NA), released from the varicosities of the terminal nerve-endings, is thought to cause vasoconstriction by two types of post-synaptic alpha-adrenergic receptors, alpha$_1$ and alpha$_2$. The current proposal is that increasing coronary stenosis unmasks alpha$_2$-mediated vasoconstriction, whereas beta-adrenergic blockade by propranolol inhibits vasodilation mediated by noradrenaline and circulating adrenaline (A) to allow unopposed vasoconstriction which is alpha$_2$-mediated. The further concept that calcium antagonists act to inhibit alpha$_2$-induced vasoconstriction is shown in Fig. 4.2. For general concept of the role of alpha$_2$-mediated inhibition of noradrenaline release, see Reference [26]. (Modified from [1].) © Opie, 1986.

4.2.7 CYCLIC NUCLEOTIDES

In general cyclic AMP and cyclic GMP are thought to have opposing intracellular effects analogous to the chinese 'Yin-Yang' philosophy. For myocardial contraction there is little evidence of a major role for cyclic AMP [32]. In the case of the slow response action potential cyclic AMP increases the probability of the calcium channel being open, and cyclic GMP has an opposing effect.

In contrast in vascular smooth muscle both cyclic nucleotides (AMP and GMP) appear to cause vascular relaxation. Cyclic AMP does not open the calcium channels in vascular smooth muscle as it does in the myocardium, but may inhibit the activation of myosin ATPase [12] and mediate the uptake of calcium by the sarcoplasmic reticulum of vascular smooth muscle [33] to produce beta-adrenergic relaxation.

Cyclic GMP is also vasodilatory in vascular smooth muscle in opposition to the 'Yin-Yang' hypothesis. It may inhibit the entry of calcium ions as in nodal tissues [32], alter myosin phosphorylation, or accelerate the uptake of calcium ions by the sarcoplasmic reticulum [33]. The

111

cholinergic vasodilatory effect may be mediated by cyclic GMP if the vascular endothelium is intact to provide endothelial relaxing factor [34]. When the endothelium is destroyed as by coronary artery disease acetylcholine is vasoconstrictor [35, 11], providing a mechanism for vasoconstriction in the presence of coronary artery disease.

4.3 Pharmacological vasodilators – possible sites of action

4.3.1 EFFECTS ON CIRCULATION

Pharmacological vasodilators are a complex category of agents, acting on the coronary or peripheral circulation by multiple and diverse mechanisms among which are: prejunctional neuromodulation (e.g. inhibition of formation of angiotensin or serotonin), calcium channel antagonism, beta-stimulation, formation of the vasodilatory cyclic nucleotide, cyclic GMP, and (possibly) alpha-receptor antagonism. Theoretically, vasodilators can act on different parts of the vascular tree; for example, nitrates act on the veins and large coronary arteries, but only slightly on the peripheral arterioles, the major site of the peripheral vascular resistance, whereas hydralazine acts on the peripheral arterioles. Different calcium antagonists also have different sites of vasodilator activity. Thus verapamil acts chiefly on coronary arteries and only has lesser effects on the peripheral arterioles, whereas nifedipine acts on both coronary arteries and peripheral arterioles. The reason for these anatomical differences is still unknown. Yet it is these different mechanisms and sites of action that allow for *selective regional vasodilation*, so that a venodilator allows reduction of the preload on the heart, an arteriolar dilator reduces the afterload and a coronary vasodilator relieves chiefly coronary spasm. It should be noted that afterload reduction by itself, as achieved by hydralazine, is not a procedure which is usually regarded as antianginal. Hence the major anatomical sites of action of antianginal vasodilators are the venous and/or coronary vascular beds.

4.3.2 CELLULAR EFFECTS

At a cellular level, vasodilators also have different possible modes of action. Some inhibit the slow channel in the vascular myocyte. These include the calcium antagonists, alpha$_1$-adrenergic antagonists, adenosine, and agents such as nitrates which increase cyclic GMP in the vascular myocyte. Other potential vasodilators decrease the phosphorylation of myosin by increasing tissue cyclic AMP levels; agents acting here include the beta$_2$-agonists, histamine and forskolin [33]. Such agents have not yet been shown to have a definitive effect on the coronary circulation. A controversial and still unproven site of vasodilator action is by enhancing the dephosphorylation of myosin [33], which is a possible theoretical result of an increasing level of cyclic GMP in the vascular smooth muscle cell [36]. The effect of pharmacological vasodilators may be governed by the presence of the endothelial relaxing factor.

4.3.3 ENDOTHELIAL RELAXING FACTOR

An intact endothelium is an important regulator of the vascular smooth muscle response [25, 35] and is required for the vasodilating effects of some agents enhancing intramyocyte cyclic GMP, such as acetylcholine. In contrast, nitrates act independently of the endothelium to vasodilate directly [25]. Hence nitrates are vasodilators even in the presence of coronary artery disease, whereas the release of acetylcholine at muscarinic receptors could cause either vasodilation when the endothelium is healthy, or vasoconstriction when the endothelium is damaged. The endothelial relaxing factor is an unstable humoral agent, which is neither a lipoxygenase derivative nor a free radical [36].

4.4 Nitrates: mechanisms of action

Nitrates have been used for angina pectoris since 1867, when Lauder Brunton in Edinburgh, Scotland, successfully tried amyl nitrite, to 'lessen the arterial tension', in a patient with nocturnal angina. But in 1933 Sir Thomas Lewis held that the effect of amyl nitrite was probably due mainly to its powerful dilatation of the coronary vessels, rather than to its effect in lowering the blood pressure. Emphasis swung back to the peripheral effect of nitrates when Gorlin and co-workers [37] found that overall coronary blood flow was unchanged by nitroglycerine. Further support for a prime peripheral effect came with the observation that angina of effort was consistently precipitated by a certain value of the double product, heart rate times blood pressure, an index of the myocardial oxygen demand [38].

Three newer observations again emphasize the cardiac effects of nitrates. First, in animal preparations nitrates can cause vasodilatation in the ischaemic zone, and do so more effectively than verapamil [39]. Second, in man, increase in coronary vascular tone may be a major factor in precipitating chest pain, even in some patients with angiographically proven coronary artery disease, and nitrates are very effective against vasospastic angina and angina at rest. Thirdly, direct angiographic measurements show that nitrates act powerfully to increase the arterial diameter at the site of coronary artery stenosis [3, 7]. Yet the peripheral haemodynamic effects of nitrates cannot be ignored. It is now clear that long-acting nitrates have long-lasting haemodynamic effects, reducing the afterload, but especially the preload of the heart.

4.4.1 ACTION OF NITRATES ON THE CIRCULATION

In relation to the oxygen supply to ischaemic myocardium, a distinction must be made between antianginal and vasodilator properties. Nitrates redistribute blood flow along collateral channels and from epicardial to endocardial regions (Fig. 4.1). By reducing left ventricular end-diastolic pressure, nitrates increase the transmyocardial coronary arterial pressure gradient and facilitate subendocardial blood flow. Thus, nitrates are 'effective' vasodilators for angina; but dipyridamole and many other vasodilators are not, and may increase angina by diverting blood from the ischaemic area, creating a 'coronary steal' effect [40].

Effects of nitrates on the oxygen demand are even more important than effects on the oxygen supply. Nitrates increase the venous capacitance causing pooling of blood in the peripheral veins and in the splanchnic vascular bed, thereby causing a reduction in ventricular volume, which reduces myocardial oxygen demand. The fall in arterial pressure will furthermore reduce myocardial oxygen demand, although this is accompanied by a reflex increase in heart rate. The latter effect increases myocardial oxygen demand but can be abolished by beta-adrenergic blockade. The beneficial effect of nitrates in congestive heart failure also depends on venodilatation.

4.4.2 INTRACELLULAR MODE OF ACTION OF NITRATES
(Fig. 4.2)

One important recent theory is that nitrates (like nitroprusside) activate guanylate cyclase, presumably by formation of the nitric oxide free radical, thereby increasing cyclic GMP in vascular smooth muscle [41]. The end result is that calcium ion entry via the slow channel is inhibited [32] or that the state of myosin phosphorylation is altered [36]. If nitrates and nitroprusside share the same molecular mechanism [41], then it is not clear why nitrates dilate chiefly the major and nitroprusside the small coronary arterioles, nor why nitrates are chiefly venodilators whereas nitroprusside is a combined arteriolar and venodilator. Nitroglycerine may be a more effective antianginal agent than nitroprusside because (a) nitroglycerine is more potent in its effect on the large coronary arteries than on the smaller resistance vessels, and (b) nitroglycerine drops the arterial pressure less, so that there may be less danger of underperfusion of the ischaemic myocardium [42].

The 'cyclic GMP theory' explains the development of partial tolerance to the effects of nitrates by impaired formation of intracellular cyclic GMP [43]. The alternate theory that nitrates help the formation of vasodilatory prostaglandins [21] is less likely because the antianginal and vasodilatory effects of nitrates are preserved despite pretreatment with the potent prostaglandin inhibitor indomethacin [44]. Nitrates also differ in their site of action from adenosine, which acts on the small intramural vessels which possess the adenosine receptors that regulate most of the coronary resistance. Nitrates increase coronary flow to the ischaemic myocardium when the large coronary arteries are the site of vasoconstriction.

4.5 Nitrates: clinical implications

4.5.1 NITRATES FOR ANGINA

Nitrates remain the basis of therapy for all forms of angina (Tables 4.3 and 4.4), whether precipitated by effort or coronary spasm. In angina of effort, sublingual short-acting nitrates can abort the attack. In angina at rest and unstable angina, oral nitrates (both short-acting and long-acting) have long been used, but there is surprisingly little objective evidence of their efficacy.

Recently intravenous nitrates have been shown to be effective. In Prinzmetal's angina at rest, caused by coronary artery spasm, nitroglycerine is given for acute attacks and long-acting nitrates for prophylaxis;

Table 4.3* Proposed step-care for angina of effort

---

1 General therapy: History and physical examination to exclude valvular disease, anaemia, hypertension, thromboembolic disease, and heart failure. Check risk factors for coronary artery disease (smoking, hypertension, blood lipids)

2 Nitrates, short or long-acting given intermittently as needed to control pain

3 Intermittent short and long-acting nitrates plus beta-adrenergic blocker

or

4 Intermittent short and long-acting nitrates plus calcium antagonist

or

5 Intermittent short-acting nitrates plus calcium antagonist plus beta-blocker

6 Intermittent short- and long-acting nitrates plus beta-blockade plus calcium antagonist.

7 Failure to respond to medical therapy and/or left main stem lesion requires bypass surgery

---

* Modified from [1].

combination with calcium antagonists (verapamil, diltiazem, nifedipine) is usual (Table 4.4).

4.5.2 LONG-ACTING NITRATES

The 'nitrate controversy' relates to the long-held opinion that the long-acting nitrates have few truly long-lasting effects [45]. Long-acting nitrates are to some extent back again in favour because with high doses there are long-lasting haemodynamic effects over 3 months in congestive heart failure, where the venous effect is better maintained than the arterial [46]. It is now well accepted that single doses of long-acting nitrates can confer longer protection against angina than can single doses of sublingual nitroglycerine. The probable explanation is the formation of the long-acting hepatic metabolites, isosorbide 5-mononitrate and isosor-

Table 4.4 Proposed step care for angina at rest – 'Spontaneous angina'

1 *General therapy*
Bed rest, preferably in hospital
Treat pain (morphine if needed). Nasal oxygen
Evaluate for heart failure, valve disease, anaemia, hypertension, and thromboembolic disease
Rule out myocardial infarction present or past

2 *Relieve presumed coronary spasm*
Intravenous nitroglycerine or oral nitrates, short and long-acting
If no relief:
  add calcium antagonists
  – intravenous or oral verapamil
  – sublingual or oral nifedipine
  – oral diltiazem

3 *Reduce oxygen demand*
If tachycardia
  – beta-blockade or diltiazem
If hypertension
  – beta-blockade or calcium antagonists

4 *Combination therapy*
Nitrates plus calcium antagonists plus beta-blockade (needs careful clinical evaluation especially for side-effects)
NB: Beta-blockade may aggravate coronary spasm

5 *Reduce thrombotic process*
  i Antiplatelet agents, e.g. low dose aspirin
  ii heparin – consider use to avoid venous thrombosis in severely ill patients

bide 2-mononitrate. Mononitrates are now being developed as long-acting nitrates in their own right (Table 4.5).

4.5.3 LEFT VENTRICULAR FAILURE AND MYOCARDIAL INFARCTION

In acute pulmonary oedema from various causes, including acute myocardial infarction, nitroglycerine can be strikingly effective. There is, however, some risk of precipitous falls in blood pressure and unexpected tachycardia or bradycardia. Intravenous nitroglycerine with a very short duration of action may allow best titration of dose against clinical effects. In patients with acute myocardial infarction, it would be safest to give nitrates only to those who have obvious left ventricular failure, although there is growing evidence that 'infarct size' and even ventricular arrhythmias can be reduced by nitrates. For optimum haemodynamic control, intravenous nitrates are best.

4.5.4 SPECIFIC NITRATE PREPARATIONS

(a) Short-acting nitrates: sublingual nitroglycerine

Although very well established in the therapy (for doses see Table 4.5) and diagnosis of angina of effort nitroglycerine may be ineffective – sometimes because the patient has not received proper instruction.

When angina starts, the patient should rest in the sitting position (standing promotes syncope, lying enhances venous return and heart work) and take sublingual nitroglycerine (0.3–0.6 mg) every 3 minutes until the pain goes or 4 to 5 tablets have been taken.

(b) Intravenous nitroglycerine

Nitroglycerine for intravenous use is now available in most countries; elsewhere it can be prepared from sublingual tablets in sterile conditions with special attention to purity.

In selected and monitored patients with acute myocardial infarction, nitroglycerine, when infused at rates of 0.6–12.0 mg/h decreased the left ventricular filling pressure and the arterial pressure [48]. The cardiac output, however, was virtually unchanged; in other words, nitrates acted primarily as venodilators. Similar doses also decreased ventricular premature beats. In unstable angina pectoris, a similar dose of nitroglycerine also effectively reduced the number of ischaemic episodes without being more effective than oral isosorbide dinitrate which was combined with nitroglycerine ointment [49]. All the doses of intravenous nitroglycerine refer to preparations which require dilution in sterile water

Table 4.5* Doses of nitrate preparations

Compound	Route	Preparation and dose	Duration of effects
Amyl nitrate	Inhalation for diagnosis	2–5 mg	10 s – 10 min
Nitroglycerin (trinitrin, TNT)	(a) Sublingual	0.3–1.5 mg as needed Tablets: usually 0.5 mg or 0.6 mg	1.5 min–1 h; peak blood levels at 2 min with half-time of 7.5 min
	(b) Percutaneous	2% ointment 15×15 cm or 12.5–40 mg	3–4 h
	(c) Transdermal		
	i) Nitrodur	2%; 5 mg/cm^2; 5–20 cm^2 26–104 mg	Initial reports up to 24 h; not confirmed in recent studies
	ii) Transderm-nitro	2%; 2.5 mg/cm^2; 10–20 cm^2 25–50 mg	
	iii) Nitrodisc	2%; 2mg/cm^2; 8–16 cm^2 16–32 mg	
	(d) Oral; sustained release	2.6 mg, 1–2 tablets thrice daily	8–12 h
	(e) Intravenous	0.6–12.0 mg/h when urgent 0.1 mg bolus (care with lower dose for new sets)	During infusion and 30 min post-infusion; haemodynamic benefit in AMI with LV failure

Drug	Route	Dose	Effect/duration
Isosorbide dinitrate (=sorbide nitrate)	(a) Sublingual	5-15 mg	Up to 60 min
	(b) Oral*	5-80 mg 4-6 hourly (top dose 480 mg daily)	Exercise time raised for 2-8 h (see text for tolerance)
	(c) Chewable	5 mg as single dose	Exercise time raised for 2 min-2.5 h
	(d) Oral; sustained release*	40 mg once or twice daily	2-6 h free from angina
	(e) Intravenous	1.25-5.0 mg/h (care: adsorbed onto tubing)	Effective for repetitive attacks of angina at rest
Isosorbide-5-mononitrate	Oral; sustained release	10-40 mg 2-4 times a day	6-10 h
Pentaerythritol tetranitrate	(a) Sublingual	10 mg as needed	45 min
Erythrityl tetranitrate	(a) Sublingual	5-10 mg as needed	10-45 min
	(b) Oral	10-30 mg thrice daily, chew before swallowing	Effects begin after 20-30 min

AMI = acute myocardial infarction; LV = left ventricle

* Duration of haemodynamic effects has been most closely studied, but there is good correlation between such effects and antianginal action.

* Modified from [45] and [98].

or saline before administration. About 20–80% of the nitroglycerine can be adsorbed onto the polyvinyl tubing usually used for intravenous administration; specially prepared infusion sets eliminate the problem of adsorption of the drug but correspondingly lower rates of infusion are probably going to be needed.

(c) Nitroglycerine paste

Prolonged release can be obtained from nitroglycerine paste (i.e. ointment) applied to the skin of the chest. Usually oral isosorbide dinitrate is the long-acting agent of choice, but the paste may be better in acute myocardial infarction because it can be wiped off in the event of an adverse reaction. Following application of paste, absorption from different sites and in different individuals is highly variable. Paste has to be applied every 4 to 6 hours and is messy.

(d) Cutaneous discs

Transcutaneous delivery systems in various patch sizes (5–30 cm^2) containing 2–5 mg/cm^2 nitroglycerine in different vehicles permits the release of nitroglycerine over a 24-hour period. Therapeutic benefit for up to 24 hours has been reported in only one study [50]. However, several recent studies have shown that transdermal nitroglycerine patches do not provide prophylaxis against exertional angina for 24 hours [51, 52]. In a placebo controlled study, weekly angina frequency and exercise duration on the treadmill was similar after placebo and nitroglycerine patch [53]. Furthermore, it has been shown that Nitrodisc 8 cm^2 and 40 cm^2 did not increase exercise duration as much as did one tablet of sublingual nitroglycerine [52]. At present, the evidence for the use of transdermal patches or discs of nitroglycerine or isosorbide ointment for the treatment of angina is not impressive [54]. However, in patients with congestive heart failure, nitroglycerine patches have produced prolonged salutary effects. The unexplained and striking contrast between the dramatic commercial success of nitroglycerine patches and their limited proven efficacy is reviewed by Abrams [54]. There are many explanations, including the psychological advantage to a patient of trying a new and convenient preparation. Transdermal isosorbide dinitrate, only recently studied, is effective for eight hours in acute therapy but tolerance develops after only 7–10 days of sustained therapy [55].

(e) Long-acting nitrates

An important question is whether regular therapy with long-acting nitrates gives long-lasting protection against angina. In an important placebo-controlled study, exercise duration improved significantly for 6 to 8 hours after single oral doses of 15–120 mg isosorbide dinitrate, but for only 2 hours when the same doses were given repetitively four times daily [47] (Table 4.5). The development of tolerance occurred, despite higher plasma isosorbide dinitrate concentrations during sustained therapy than those of actute therapy. Thus the antianginal effects of long-term therapy with long-acting nitrates are attenuated.

(f)   The new mononitrates

Isosorbide dinitrate is normally subject to a variable and major first-pass hepatic metabolism to mononitrates, including the 2- and 5-mononitrates both of which have major systemic and coronary vascular effects [56]. In a double-blind three-way cross-over study in eleven female volunteers, isosorbide-5-mononitrate 30 mg was more potent than sustained-release isosorbide dinitrate 20 mg, as judged by acute effects on the finger plethysmogram [57]. There have only been a few clinical reports comparing the mononitrate with the dinitrate preparations as far as effects on angina pectoris are concerned. One such study [58] showed that the mean incidence of attacks during the mononitrate therapy was lower than during medication with slow release dinitrate or with placebo. The additional nitroglycerine consumption per patient was lower during the treatment with the mononitrate than with the slow release isosorbide dinitrate. Such comparisons obviously have to be extended and confirmed. What is particularly difficult to know is whether optimum doses of both preparations were used. The mononitrate preparation is rapidly absorbed and excreted by the kidney partially unchanged and partially as an inactive glucuronide metabolite, with an elimination half-life of 4–6 hours. Its clinical efficacy correlates with its plasma concentration, being about 8 hours for 20 mg dose with the dosage being 20–40 mg three times daily [59].

Because of long half-life and near complete bioavailability after oral administration, isosorbide-5-mononitrate is considered by some to be the nitrate preparation of choice. Placebo-controlled studies have shown that after 20 and 40 mg isosorbide-5-mononitrate, exercise tolerance increased and ST segment depression was less than with placebo [60]. These workers reported that smaller doses (20 mg) administered two or three times a day did not lead to development of tolerance. However, in a recent placebo-controlled study, 50 and 100 mg of sustained release preparation of isosorbide-5-mononitrate increased exercise duration at 4 but not at 20 and 24 hours despite high plasma concentrations of isosorbide-5-mononitrate [61]. This study suggests that rapid attenuation of antianginal effects also develops with slow release formulations of isosorbide-5-mononitrate. Furthermore, even with the ordinary formulation, tolerance develops when larger doses of isosorbide-5-mononitrate are used [62]. Therefore, present evidence suggests that isosorbide-5-mononitrate also suffers from the defect of the development of tolerance with continued use.

4.6 Problems in the use of nitrates

4.6.1 ISOSORBIDE DINITRATE VERSUS NITROGLYCERINE

A choice that must frequently be made is whether to use short-acting nitroglycerine or long-acting nitrates such as isosorbide dinitrate, or whether to use a combination. In stable angina pectoris, 0.4 mg nitroglycerine sublingually increased the exercise time for 1 hour, whereas a single dose of 30 mg isosorbide dinitrate increased the exercise time to angina for 3 hours [63]. For the patient requiring protection for several hours, long-acting nitrates, whether taken sublingually, orally, or by paste, have obvious advantages [47]. However, for the patient requiring rapid relief of angina or protection from threatened angina, sublingual nitroglycerine acts quickest.

4.6.2 TOLERANCE TO NITRATES

Studies in animals and in man have clearly demonstrated that tolerance to circulatory effects of nitrates and to headaches develops rapidly and is both dose and time-dependent [64]. Partial attenuation of antianginal effects during long-term therapy with isosorbide dinitrate has been well documented by some but not by other investigators [64]. The cellular mechanism of these effects may be by decreased formation of cyclic GMP [43]. Recent studies suggest that continuous delivery of nitrates whether by transdermal route or by oral route leads to rapid development of tolerance to the antianginal effects even within 24 hours [51, 55, 61]. Such tolerance has been reported with transdermal preparations of nitroglycerine or isosorbide dinitrate, with isosorbide ointment, with oral isosorbide dinitrate, and with the slow release formulation of isosorbide-5-mononitrate. Therefore, we recommend intermittent or pulse therapy with long-acting nitrates rather than continuous therapy. Alternatively, it may be necessary temporarily to increase the dose of isosorbide dinitrate to 480 mg daily [65]. There are already some reports suggesting that intermittent therapy with small doses of isosorbide dinitrate 20–30 mg or with isosorbide-5-monitrate 20 mg administered twice daily prevents the development of tolerance [62]. However, further studies are needed to substantiate these claims.

4.6.3 NITRATE CROSS-TOLERANCE

Cross-tolerance is the phenomenon whereby patients receiving sustained chronic therapy with isosorbide dinitrate may have a diminished acute response to therapy with nitroglycerine or sublingual isosorbide [66]. In practice, long-acting and short-acting nitrates are frequently combined. In patients already receiving isosorbide dinitrate, addition of sublingual nitroglycerine gave a further small (10%) therapeutic effect, and it was concluded that no nitrate cross-tolerance was found [66]. When judged by the hypotensive effect, however, both sublingual nitroglycerine and sublingual isosorbide dinitrate have effects which are rapidly attenuated during chronic therapy with oral isosorbide dinitrate. Why the acute antianginal effect of both sublingual nitroglycerine and sublingual isosorbide is retained even in the presence of proven nitrate tolerance is unclear [66]. One proposed explanation is that the surge of blood levels during acute administration brings about the added beneficial effect.

4.6.4 LONG-TERM PROPHYLAXIS OF ANGINA

A different question is whether sustained therapy with long-acting nitrates gives long-lasting protection against angina. In one study, isosorbide dinitrate 20 mg three times daily for 1 month had no effect on the number of anginal attacks, on the usage of nitroglycerine, or on the exercise time [67]. Furthermore, 14 of 32 patients could not tolerate isosorbide at a dose of only 10 mg three times daily. In another study, however, a long-acting preparation of isosorbide dinitrate (sustained release capsules) 40 mg every 8 hours for 1 month improved the exercise time on a multistage treadmill test by 24%, 6 hours after the dose; there was neither nitrate cross-tolerance nor self-tolerance [68].

Improvement in exercise tolerance for up to 3 hours during acute and for up to 5 hours during sustained therapy with isosorbide dinitrate has been reported [63]. In an important placebo-controlled study, exercise duration improved significantly for 6 to 8 hours after single oral doses of 15–120 mg isosorbide dinitrate, but for only 2 hours when the same doses were given repetitively four times daily [47]. The development of partial tolerance to the antianginal effects during sustained therapy occurred, despite higher plasma isosorbide dinitrate concentrations during sustained therapy than those of acute therapy [47].

4.6.5 INTRAVENOUS NITRATES

The problem here may be very new – the doses required may be much lower when using the new sets which are designed to avoid adsorption onto the polyvinyl tubing.

4.6.6 FAILURE OF NITRATE THERAPY

Causes of failure are: (a) increasing severity of angina or development of nitrate-resistant myocardial ischaemia; (b) development of tolerance to nitrates; (c) loss of potency of tablets; (d) incorrect route of administration (some sublingual preparations should not be taken orally, and vice versa); (e) arterial hypoxaemia, especially in chronic lung disease (caused by increased venous admixture); and (f) non-compliance, usually because of headaches. Nitrates are more effective if taken before the expected onset of pain. In some patients nitrates are less effective than is expected due to tachycardia; then, combined treatment with beta-blockade should give better results. Another possibility is a wrong initial diagnosis, because nitrates sometimes relieve the pain of oesophageal spasm and renal or biliary colic.

4.7 Calcium antagonists for angina pectoris

4.7.1 BASIC PROPERTIES OF CALCIUM ANTAGONISTS

Besides their diversity of action, the major calcium antagonists (verapamil, nifedipine, diltiazem) do share common properties. All can, in the appropriate experimental conditions, have the following effects: (a) inhibition of contractile activity; (b) inhibition of conduction through the atrioventricular node; (c) inhibition of smooth muscle contraction. At an electrophysiological level, all these agents decrease the entry of calcium ions by the slow channel as shown by voltage-clamp studies on myocardial tissue. They all inhibit excitation–contraction coupling in smooth muscle and the slow responses provoked by cyclic AMP when the fast channel is blocked. The common denominator to all the above effects is inhibition of transmembrane calcium influx. It is for this reason that there are alternative names including calcium channel blockers. In electrophysiological terms there is also true calcium antagonism of the blockade, so that it is acceptable to use one of the several terms for this category of agents.

Inhibition of the slow inward current is now widely regarded as the critical property common to all calcium antagonists and explains one of the current names, viz. 'calcium entry blocking agents'.

The initial and classical calcium antagonist effect obtained by Fleckenstein was the decreased inotropic effect of verapamil [15], antagonized by the injection of calcium salts [1]. It is now known that the tissue most sensitive to verapamil is not the myocardium but the atrioventricular node, and that therapeutic effects can be found at concentrations which have no apparent effect on the sinus node nor on myocardial contractility; hence the effective use of verapamil in supraventricular tachycardias. Unexpectedly, the inhibitory effect of the atrioventricular node is only partially antagonized by an increased extracellular calcium, whereas the inhibitory effect on the sinus node is not at all antagonized by calcium. These differences argue for the concept of varying properties of the slow calcium channel in various tissues. Hence, Nayler proposes [69] that there are three different types of calcium channels in different tissues – Class I in the myocardium, Class II in the vasculature and Class III in nodal tissue. Alternatively, the same calcium channel in different tissues could have different binding sites for the various drugs, or the drug-binding site interaction could vary.

4.7.2 PROPERTIES OF CALCIUM ANTAGONISTS OF VALUE IN ANGINA PECTORIS

The major anatomical site of action of calcium antagonists relevant to their antianginal effect is vascular arterial smooth muscle. It is not clear why calcium antagonists in general act more powerfully on vascular smooth muscle than on the myocardium, nor why the major vascular site of action is the arterial rather than the venous vascular bed. From the point of view of angina pectoris, the major effects of calcium antagonists are (a) to cause peripheral vasodilation, thereby unloading the heart; (b) to dilate the coronary arteries, thereby relieving dynamic stenosis. Sometimes, as in the case of verapamil, an additional factor may be the negative inotropic effect. Here it is useful to bear in mind that the direct negative inotropic effect of the calcium antagonists is antagonized by indirect positive effects, achieved by peripheral vasodilation. Judging by the anti-hypertensive effects it is nifedipine that has the major effect as a peripheral arterial vasodilator, whereas in the case of the coronary arteries all the three 'first-generation' calcium antagonists (nifedipine, verapamil and diltiazem) are probably equally active. It is important to note that these clinical generalizations are not based on strictly comparable trials with measurements of blood levels and various dose–response curves. Each of the three major calcium antagonists, by virtue of its vasodilatory properties, has been used with some success not only in angina of effort but also in angina at rest (Fig. 4.4) and in Prinzmetal's variant angina as well as in mixed angina. Whereas some other peripheral vasodilators caused a marked reflex tachycardia, in the case of calcium antagonists the heart rate is either unchanged (verapamil), falls (dilitiazem), or rises slightly

Antianginal vasodilators

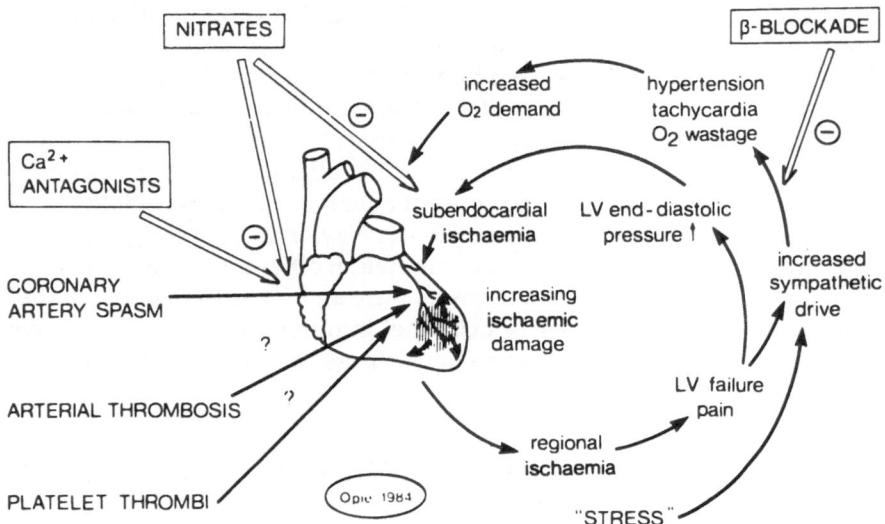

Fig. 4.4 Hypothetical events during angina at rest, supposing that the initial event is coronary artery spasm or another temporary obstructive process such as arterial thrombosis or platelet agglutination. Nitrates, as intravenous nitroglycerine or a combination of oral and sublingual or in disc form, are usually used as first-line agents in angina at rest. Calcium antagonists, like nitrates, may relieve coronary spasm. Beta-adrenergic blockade will not relieve (and may aggravate) coronary spasm, although it will relieve secondary hypertension and tachycardia. In clinical practice, nitrates, calcium antagonists and beta-blockade are frequently combined in the therapy of severe angina at rest, provided that careful attention is paid to drug interactions and side effects. From [1]. © Opie, 1986.

(nifedipine). These variable effects on the heart rate may be explained by the balance between the peripheral vasodilation causing a reflex tachycardia and a variable direct negative chronotropic effect on the SA node. Such a contrast between the peripheral and direct myocardial effects has been well studied in the case of nifedipine [70].

4.7.3 CELLULAR EFFECTS OF CALCIUM ANTAGONISTS

In the myocardium it is clear that the major effect of the calcium antagonists is on the calcium channel and not on an intracellular site. In vascular smooth muscle, voltage-clamping is a difficult technique; hence proof of the effect on the slow inward current has been more difficult to obtain. Nevertheless, it is widely assumed that the major site of action of calcium antagonists is on the calcium channel of the vascular myocyte, as in the

126

case of the myocardial cell. A puzzle is that the influx of $^{45}Ca^{2+}$ is not inhibited by verapamil, nifedipine or diltiazem [71]. Possibly an interaction with calmodulin may explain at least part of the inhibition of contraction of vascular smooth muscle by calcium antagonist drugs.

4.8 Verapamil

Verapamil was introduced for angina pectoris as a calcium antagonist agent with vasodilator properties. More recently its major use has been for supraventricular tachycardias, especially re-entrant tachycardias involving the atrioventricular node. Even more recently, verapamil has been re-studied for its effects in angina of effort and angina at rest, where it is a remarkably effective agent. In chronic stable angina, verapamil increases exercise capacity on treadmill, reduces the amount of nitroglycerine consumed, and the degree of ST-segment depression during exercise. It also prevents the ischaemic consequences of atrial pacing and supine bicycle exercise (lactate production, fall in ejection fraction, development of wall motion abnormalities).

4.8.1 CHRONIC STABLE ANGINA

High-dose verapamil (120 mg three times daily) was as effective against angina as propranolol 100 mg three times daily, whereas verapamil had no effect on lung function [67]. Recent studies have confirmed the antianginal efficacy of verapamil in chronic stable angina; it is comparable to that of beta-blockers [72]. Verapamil appears to have less effect on the rate × pressure product at rest as well as having less effect during exercise than does beta-blockade, despite equivalent antianginal effectiveness. It is thus possible that at least in part the action of verapamil may be mediated by an increase of coronary blood flow. The differing action of beta-blockers and verapamil (and other calcium antagonists) provides the rational basis for combination therapy. Such combination therapy appears safe except in patients with myocardial dysfunction or conduction system disease.

4.8.2 UNSTABLE ANGINA

Two studies have recently confirmed the role of verapamil in unstable angina. In angina at rest (but with episodes of angina only lasting up to 15 minutes), 80 mg every 4 hours, followed by 80 mg three to five times a day, were very effective in relieving pain and correcting electrocardiographic changes [73]. Similar findings have been reported [74] in a

Antianginal vasodilators

double-blind, placebo-controlled study in patients admitted with features of unstable angina to a coronary care unit.

4.8.3 PRINZMETAL'S VARIANT ANGINA

In Prinzmetal's variant angina, verapamil is also effective (as are all the major calcium antagonists). There have been anecdotal reports in the past, but a double-blind placebo-controlled study [75] showed that verapamil in conventional oral doses significantly reduced nitroglycerine consumption, the number of ischaemic episodes on 24-hour Holter recordings, and the number of angina attacks. In a subsequent study, verapamil (average dose: 70 mg/day, 3–4 divided doses) was found to be equipotent; the side effects with nifedipine were not serious, but limited the dose in 7 of 27 patients.

4.8.4 ACUTE MYOCARDIAL INFARCTION: FOLLOW-UP

In patients with angina pectoris after myocardial infarction, verapamil may be considered on its merits. However, unlike beta-blockade, verapamil does not reduce the incidence of sudden death or of re-infarction [76].

4.9 Nifedipine

Besides its established efficacy in Prinzmetal's angina, nifedipine is effective against angina of effort [77] and against pacing-induced angina [7]. Whereas nitrates do not benefit pacing-induced angina when given into the coronary arteries, nifedipine does so even when given as a very small dose (0.1 mg of a special intravenous preparation) which has no detectable peripheral effect [78]. The dual mechanism is first by vasodilation of the coronary vessels including widening of the stenotic site [7, 70], and secondly by a favourable influence on myocardial metabolism [79]. When given normally by the oral or sublingual route, afterload reduction is an important component of its mechanism. Careful dose titration is required to ensure that an excessive peripheral effect does not over-reduce blood pressure, thereby occasionally worsening angina of effort and unstable angina.

A recent double-blind trial showed that nifedipine should not be given routinely in a dose of 20–30 mg every 6 hours to patients with unstable angina as it might sometimes worsen the clinical outcome [80]. Presumably excess hypotension and/or tachycardia and/or 'coronary steal' was occurring in the absence of careful dose titration. Of interest was the benefit achieved over placebo when nifedipine plus propranolol were compared with conventional therapy (including nitroglycerine and isosorbide dinitrate); in contrast, nifedipine was less effective than isosorbide when given in the absence of propranolol [80].

4.10 Diltiazem

The main indications are the ischaemic syndromes; its role in other cardiocirculatory disorders (e.g. hypertension, hypertrophic cardiomyopathy, and Raynaud's phenomenon) remain to be elucidated. In a small double-blind cross-over study in patients with Prinzmetal's variant angina, 240 mg/day of diltiazem significantly reduced the number of episodes of pain and the amount of nitroglycerine consumed [74]. The short-term response generally predicted the long-term response at 16 months [81]. In a multicentre, randomized controlled cross-over study, 19% of patients on 120 mg of diltiazem daily became pain free, whereas at 240 mg daily, 30% became pain free, in the majority the frequency of angina was reduced [82].

4.10.1 CHRONIC STABLE ANGINA

Diltiazem is also effective in chronic stable angina. Two recent multicentre, double-blind, placebo-controlled trials have demonstrated that the drug significantly decreases anginal frequency and nitroglycerine consumption, while increasing total exercise duration and the time of onset of angina [83, 84]. One trial showed that high-dose diltiazem (360 mg daily) in divided doses was as effective as propranolol in relieving angina pectoris [85]. In the doses used in these studies, the drug was safe with no effect on PR or QRS intervals of the ECG. Side effects necessitating discontinuation of diltiazem have been very rare, but may become more frequent with the higher dose (360 mg daily) that may be required for an optimum antianginal effect. As with verapamil and nifedipine, the dose of diltiazem is an important determinant of the therapeutic response.

4.11 Newer calcium antagonists

The newer calcium antagonists include agents of the dihydropyridine group (felodipine, nicardipine, others), verapamil-like agents (tiapamil) and mixed agents such as bepridil. In a large placebo-controlled multicentre study, bepridil (200–400 mg) once a day improved exercise tolerance and reduced angina frequency in patients with stable angina pectoris [86]. Apart from agents such as nimodopine which are thought to act more specifically on the cerebral vascular bed, all the other agents should have antianginal potential.

4.12 Other potential antianginal agents

4.12.1 MOLSYDOMINE

This agent acts by release of vasodilator metabolites formed during first-pass liver metabolism. The conventional dose is 2 mg twice daily. Thus far molsydomine has not yet been introduced into widespread clinical practice although some preliminary reports are encouraging.

4.12.2 PERHEXILENE

This agent has complex actions, with both antianginal and antiarrhythmic activities. Although a calcium antagonist, additional quinidine-like properties make the true classification difficult. It also differs from other calcium antagonists by not having an acute effect against Prinzmetal's angina. Experimentally, there is a nitrate-like effect with redistribution of blood flow to the subendocardial zones. It has especially been used as an antianginal agent when beta-blockade and nitrates fail, but in view of the very serious side effects now recognized, other calcium-antagonist agents should be tried first.

4.12.3 PRENYLAMINE

Prenylamine has an antianginal effect (dose 40–200 mg thrice daily) which may be explained by calcium antagonism and a general antiadrenergic effect. Although less effective than perhexilene, prenylamine is safer in the therapy of angina pectoris. Like other Ca^{2+} antagonists, it causes facial flushing and dizziness. In addition hypotension and myocardial depression may be troublesome, so lower doses are needed in the presence of beta-blockade.

4.12.4 LIDOFLAZINE

Lidoflazine is also viewed as a calcium antagonist by some workers, as it decreases smooth muscle tone and tends to inhibit atrioventricular conduction. It has antianginal properties in control studies, but the full clinical response often takes some weeks or months. Also, the effects may continue for some time after treatment is stopped, which may indicate cellular accumulation of lidoflazine. 'This lack of immediate response greatly limits the usefulness of lidoflazine, especially when a quick benefit is desired' [59].

4.12.5 PHOSPHODIESTERASE INHIBITORS

Phosphodiesterase inhibitors, such as the methylxanthines, are occasionally classified as coronary vasodilators and are sometimes still used for that purpose. Their complex additional effects on intracellular calcium fluxes have prevented general use of these agents for conditions such as angina pectoris. Furthermore, clinical trials have not shown any pronounced efficacy.

4.12.6 ALPHA-1 ADRENERGIC BLOCKING AGENTS

Prazosin has a site of action on the veins and peripheral arterioles; yet it is not used as an antianginal agent. Thus far there has been only equivocal evidence that prazosin also inhibits coronary vascular alpha-receptors, which may explain why prazosin is not effective in vasospastic angina. When the patient is already receiving prazosin therapy for hypertension, then the addition of nitrates for angina requires careful dose titration to avoid syncope or hypotension.

Labetalol is a combined alpha beta-blocker, with a more powerful effect on the beta than on the alpha-receptors. The alpha-receptors involved are the alpha$_1$-vascular receptors, as in the case of prazosin. The alpha$_1$ inhibitory effects are strong enough to ensure that the arterial pressure of hypertensive patients rapidly comes down within minutes in response to intravenous labetalol, whereas the conventional beta-blockers take hours for their initial effect even when given intravenously. With oral dosing, the added vasodilatory effect is much less, and not yet of added proven therapeutic benefit when compared with conventional beta-blockade. In patients with combined hypertension and angina, it was originally thought that the added alpha-blocking qualities of labetalol might give added antianginal properties [87], but a recent double-blind and as yet unpublished study compared atenolol with labetalol and failed to show any specific advantage for labetalol when using the latter in a total dose of 400 mg.

Phenoxybenzamine is a powerful alpha-blocking agent said to be inhibitory on both alpha$_1$ and alpha$_2$-receptors, but especially on the alpha$_1$-vascular receptors. It is classically used in the therapy of phaeochromocytoma, not in angina.

Indoramin is an alpha-adrenergic receptor blocker and also possesses cardio-inhibitory properties. It is a potent hypotensive agent, but its role in improving exercise tolerance in patients with stable angina pectoris remains controversial.

Antianginal vasodilators

Phentolamine is another powerful inhibitor of both alpha$_1$ and alpha$_2$ receptors so that complex effects can be expected. Alpha$_1$-blockade results in the expected vasodilation. Alpha$_2$-presynaptic blockade removes the 'alpha$_2$-brake' on release of noradrenaline, so that there is enhanced release of noradrenaline from the varicosities into the synaptic cleft, with positive inotropism and tachycardia, which are not useful in the therapy of angina, although there have been some reports of successful therapy.

4.12.7 DIPYRIDAMOLE

For long this agent has been known to be a potential coronary vasodilator; yet in practice it is seldom used for angina pectoris. The reason appears to be that 'effective' coronary vasodilation by nitrates apparently dilates chiefly the large epicardial vessels, bringing blood to both ischaemic and non-ischaemic zones, whereas dipyridamole by dilating the small intramural arterioles 'steals' blood from the non-ischaemic zone. Whether this explanation is valid or not, dipyridamole is not generally seen to be an antianginal vasodilator.

4.13 Which agent for which type of angina?

4.13.1 ANGINA OF EFFORT

(a) Nitrates

In angina of effort, first-line therapy is still sublingual nitroglycerine (Fig. 4.1). Where this proves ineffective, the conventional strategy has been to add long-acting nitrates or beta-blockers. Nitrates are now presented in both discs and ointments for transdermal absorption and in new guises such as the mononitrates. Recent data suggest that transdermal delivery systems of nitroglycerine, isosorbide ointment, and slow-release oral preparations of isosorbide-5-mononitrate do not exert antianginal effects for 24 hours and rapid attentuation of effects occurs within 24 hours. Even with ordinary formulations of isosorbide dinitrate and isosorbide-5-mononitrate, tolerance develops with continued therapy especially when these agents are used four times a day. Therefore, we currently do not use transdermal or slow-release oral preparations of long-acting nitrates but utilize minimum effective doses of isosorbide dinitrate 15–30 mg or isosorbide-5-mononitrate (20–40 mg) two or three times a day. Intermittent or pulsed therapy may help to prevent the development of tolerance. Otherwise, the doses may need adjusting upwards to a maximum of 480 mg of isosorbide dinitrate daily [65]. However, even with low doses,

132

headaches may be troublesome in some 20–30% of the patients and alternative therapy is often indicated.

By contrast, when calcium antagonists are used for long-term vasodilator therapy tolerance does not seem to develop, so that one of the authors [88, 89] favours a switch to this type of agent for chronic vasodilator therapy of effort angina. However, it should be emphasized that most of the presently available calcium antagonists are arterial rather than venous dilators; hence, they do not directly reduce the preload. Hence, chewed sublingual nifedipine can act rapidly to relieve angina of effort, though probably not as quickly as the short-acting nitrates.

For acute therapy in patients with frequent or unstable angina, or angina at rest, long-acting nitrates give hours of relief rather than the minutes offered by nitroglycerine. There is as yet no convincing evidence of much therapeutic difference between established preparations such as oral isosorbide and the new discs and ointments.

(b) Calcium antagonists

Calcium antagonists, having fewer serious side effects than beta-blockers, must be taken three times a day. Each of the three major calcium antagonists has its advocates and arguments for it. Diltiazem has few side effects and its negative inotropic effect is slight. Verapamil is an agent well known to many cardiologists by virtue of its long-established effect on supraventricular arrhythmias, but it may have more of a negative inotropic effect than diltiazem. In patients with pre-existing nodal (sinus or atrioventricular) disease, the added inhibitory effect of verapamil may be serious. Nifedipine seems to have more side effects, but these relate chiefly to vigorous vasodilation and are seldom serious, in contrast to the potential of beta-blockade for serious side effects. Patients treated for angina of effort are frequently going to have combination therapy, and some workers argue that nifedipine is the safest agent for combination with beta-blockade. *What is now becoming clear is that patients react very differently to different agents* and one patient may tolerate one calcium antagonist better than another. Therefore a certain amount of individual exploratory dosing and trial and error approach is usually required.

(c) Beta-adrenergic blockers

Despite the inroads made by calcium antagonists, beta-blockers remain the drugs most frequently combined with short- and long-acting nitrates for effort angina. It is surprising how many clinicians still prescribe propranolol four times a day when an excellent slow-release preparation is available. Even conventional propranolol need be given no more than twice daily for angina pectoris. A relatively cardioselective agent such as atenolol has the advantage of prolonged antianginal effects and also lessens the hazard of bronchospasm. The benefits of intrinsic sympatho-mimetic activity in a beta-blocker remain to be proven, although agents with this property (such as pindolol, acebutolol and oxprenolol) are the logical choice in patients with resting bradycardia or impaired peripheral circulation, or in elderly patients where contractility is potentially already depressed.

(d) Step care of angina of effort

Having started with short-acting and long-acting nitrates, and taking into account the possible development of tolerance, the second step is a combination of nitrates with either calcium antagonists or beta-blockers; this combination may be better tolerated and more effective than the combination of a beta-blocker with sustained dosage of isosorbide be-cause of the problem of nitrate tolerance. In apparent contrast to this recommendation, a double-blind study showed that the acute addition of nifedipine (10 mg), isosorbide dinitrate (5–30 mg), or verapamil (120 mg) all equally improved exercise time in patients already receiving sustained and apparently optimum doses of propranolol [90]. There were great differences in individual responses and side effects, making it hard to generalize. In that study only acute effects of these three drugs were evaluated and it was only propranolol that was given as sustained therapy. Comparative studies during long-term therapy with combina-tion beta-blockers plus long-acting nitrates versus beta-blockers plus calcium antagonists are urgently needed.

A rough idea of equivalent doses of nitrates, beta-blockers and calcium antagonists can be obtained by comparing the effects of acute oral administration of 80 mg propranolol, 120 mg diltiazem, 20 mg nifedipine and 0.6 mg of sublingual nitroglycerine [91]. All agents increased exercise tolerance, although propranolol was least effective and the calcium antagonists most effective with nitroglycerine in between. The peak effect came on at 3 hours for each drug (exception sublingual nitroglycerine), but was also found at 1 hour for nifedipine and 8 hours for diltiazem; nitroglycerine was only tested at 20 minutes. Thus for speedy relief of angina, nitroglycerine is better than calcium antagonists. Unfortunately the effects of sublingual nifedipine were not evaluated.

Although in most patients verapamil and diltiazem can be safely combined with beta-blockers, troubles occasionally arise from further negative inotropic effects (verapamil) and from depression of heart rate and conduction (diltiazem); with either agent there may be additive inhibitory effects on the atrioventricular node. Therefore, for combina-tion with a beta-blocker we recommend nifedipine, provided that there is careful monitoring to avoid excessive hypotension.

A common belief is that 'maximum' therapy of angina of effort consists of a beta-blocker, isosorbide, and nifedipine. When acutely added to propranolol, with 20 mg isosorbide, the triple combination is somewhat less effective than the double [92], presumably because too much vasodilation reduces the coronary perfusion pressure (Fig. 4.1). Therefore, 'maximum therapy' is probably beta-blocker plus nifedipine or beta-blocker plus intermittent long-acting nitrates, with short-acting nitrates as needed. However, such studies cannot directly be extrapolated to the situation of a patient receiving sustained therapy with a combination of agents.

4.13.2 SPONTANEOUS ANGINA AND UNSTABLE ANGINA

Intravenous nitroglycerine or intermittent therapy with long-acting nitrates such as high doses of isosorbide or nitroglycerine ointment applied every six hours at different sites are usually effective in the management of patients with unstable and spontaneous angina [49]. 'The extremely short duration of action of intravenous nitroglycerine permits delicate titration in these fragile patients' [93]. If an episode of angina is accompanied by tachycardia or a rise in blood pressure, addition of a beta-blocker to nitrate therapy is often warranted and usually beneficial in controlling angina. However, many patients with unstable angina do not have tachycardia while in some or even most of these patients, increased coronary vascular tone may play an important role in precipitating angina. Since beta-blockers can sometimes promote coronary artery spasm, these agents are losing popularity as basic therapy for angina at rest, so that they are now almost invariably combined with nitrates or calcium antagonists in the management of patients with spontaneous angina. If angina at rest is not accompanied by tachycardia, we prefer not to use a beta-blocker but instead use either calcium blocker alone or the combination of a calcium blocker and nitrates. However, if such a patient is already on a beta-blocker, we recommend continuation of therapy for fear of the withdrawal syndrome.

Calcium antagonists are now widely seen as first-line treatment for angina at rest and unstable angina, especially when a vasospastic component is suspected. Whether they are truly more effective than intravenous nitrates is not yet known; a recent study stressed the possible danger of using continuous high-dose nifedpine in threatened infarction [94]. Combination treatment is frequently used in unstable angina, on the theoretical grounds that calcium antagonists add to the dilating effects of nitrates on 'dynamic' stenotic lesions [7], provided that hypotension with poor coronary perfusion is avoided.

Angina at rest may be accompanied by left ventricular failure, which is commonly regarded as a contraindication to treatment with verapamil.

135

Antianginal vasodilators

Yet relief without ill-effects is found when verapamil is given cautiously to patients with congestive heart failure – evidence that the benefits of peripheral vasodilation may outweigh the direct negative inotropic effects in these circumstances. In severe angina at rest the pain may be such as to rule out gradual increases of dose; then, if there is any question of clinical cardiac failure, nifedipine or diltiazem is preferred to verapamil.

4.13.3 MIXED ANGINA

In patients having the features both of effort-induced and spontaneous angina, it would be logical to combine beta-blockade with calcium antagonists or to use calcium antagonists as first-line therapy. There are, as yet, few studies on this problem which would require separate analysis of the two components to the anginal attacks.

4.14 Summary

Among vasodilating antianginal drugs, nitrates remain the major therapeutic standby. Both short and long-acting forms are widely used, and the recent introduction of transcutaneous discs and the mononitrates has added to the potential number of preparations available. The major problem in the use of nitrates relates to the possibility that repetitive prophylactic use leads to tolerance and lessened efficacy, requiring enhanced doses for the same effect. When nitrates by themselves fail, it is conventional to add beta-blockade. More recently the calcium antagonist agents have come to be seen as agents of choice above beta-blockade, because of their capacity to relieve both angina of effort and angina induced by coronary spasm and the fewer contraindications to their use. Therefore it is equally permissible to add calcium antagonists to nitrates as second-line therapy, instead of using beta-blockade. As third-line therapy, combinations of nitrates, calcium antagonists and beta-blockade may be used when such combination therapy is carefully monitored. Because calcium antagonists do not on present evidence, it seems, develop any tolerance with prolonged use, they may well come to replace the prophylactic use of long-acting nitrates in patients with angina.

The general recommendation [95] is *to keep the dose of nitrates as low as possible to avoid tolerance.* Many studies in which tolerance seems not to have occurred employed nitrate-free intervals before exercise test [95], and intermittent treatment may well be the best answer. It seems likely that tolerance is due to depletion of sulphydryl groups at the receptor site and can be corrected or prevented by treatment with a sulphydryl donor, such as N-acetylcysteine [96], though this approach needs clinical testing. The new drug molsydomine acts in the same way as the nitrates by stimulation of guanylate cyclase, but avoids tolerance as it is independent of the presence of cysteine [97]. The haemodynamic effects are similar to those of the nitrates.

Acknowledgement

Sections 4.4, 4.4.1, 4.5.2, 4.5.4 and 4.6.4 are modified with permission from [45] and [98].

References

1. Opie, L.H. (1986) *The Heart. Physiology, Metabolism, Pharmacology and Therapy*, Grune & Stratton, London and Orlando.
2. Parratt, J.R., Marshall, R.J. and Ledingham, I. (1980) Interventions for improving blood flow, oxygen availability and the balance between oxygen supply and demand in the acutely ischaemic myocardium. *J. Physiol., Paris*, 76, 791.
3. Brown, B.G., Bolson, E., Petersen, R.B., Pierce, C.D. and Dodge, H.T. (1981) The mechanisms of nitroglycerin action: stenosis vasodilatation as a major component of the drug response. *Circulation*, **64**, 1089–97.
4. Winbury, M.M. and Howe, B.B. (1979) Stenosis: regional myocardial ischemia and reserve. In *Ischemic Myocardium and Antianginal Drugs* (eds M.M. Winbury & Y. Abiko), Raven Press, New York, pp. 55–76.
5. Gregg, D.E. and Bedynek, J.L. (1978) Compensatory changes in the heart during progressive coronary artery stenosis. In *Primary and Secondary Angina Pectoris* (eds A. Maseri, G.A. Klassen & M. Lesch), Grune & Stratton, New York, pp. 3–11.
6. Klocke, F.J. (1983) Measurements of coronary blood flow and degree of stenosis: current clinical implications and continuing uncertainties. *J. Am. Coll. Cardiol.*, 1, 31–41.
7. Lichtlen, R., Engel, H.-J. and Rafflenbeul, W. (1984) Calcium entry blockers, especially nifedipine in angina of effort: possible mechanisms and clinical implications. In *Calcium Antagonists and Cardiovascular Disease* (ed. L.H. Opie), Raven Press, New York, pp. 221–36.
8. Maseri, A., L'Abbate, A., Pesola, A., Ballestra, A.M., Marzilli, M., Maltinti, G., Severi, S., de Nes, D.M., Parodi, O. and Biagini, A. (1977) Coronary vasospasm in angina pectoris. *Lancet*, i, 713–17.
9. Tada, M., Kuzuya, T., Inoue, M., Kodama, K., Mishima, M., Yamada, M., Inui, M. and Abe, H. (1981) Elevation of thromboxane beta$_2$ levels in patients with classic and variant angina pectoris. *Circulation*, **64**, 1107–15.
10. Bristow, M.R., Ginsburg, R. and Harrison, D.C. (1982) Histamine and the human heart: the other receptor system. *Am. J. Cardiol*, **49**, 249–51.
11. Yasue, H. (1984) Coronary artery spasm and calcium ions. In *Calcium Antagon-*

ists and Cardiovascular Disease (ed. L.H. Opie), Raven Press, New York, pp. 117–28.

12. Adelstein, R.S. (1983) Regulation of contractile proteins by phosphorylation. J. Clin. Invest., 72, 1863–6.

13. Murphy, R.A. and Gerthoffer, W.T. (1984) Cell calcium and contractile system regulation in arterial smooth muscle. In Calcium Antagonists and Cardiovascular Disease (ed. L.H. Opie), Raven Press, New York, pp. 75–84.

14. Bolton, T.B. (1979) Mechanisms of action of transmitters and other substances on smooth muscle. Physiol. Rev., 59, 606–718.

15. Fleckenstein, A., (1971) Specific inhibitors and promoters of calcium action in the excitation–contraction coupling of heart muscle and their role in the prevention of production of myocardial lesions. In Calcium and the Heart (eds P. Harris, L.H. Opie), Academic Press, London & New York, pp. 135–88.

16. Hermsmeyer, K., Trapini, A. and Abel, P.W. (1981) Membrane potential dependent tension in vascular muscle. In Vasodilation (eds P.R. Vanhoutte & I. Leusen), Raven Press, New York, pp. 273–84.

17. Towart, R. (1981) The selective inhibition of serotonin-induced contractions of rabbit cerebral vascular smooth muscle by calcium-antagonistic dihydropyridines. An investigation of the mechanism of action of nimodipine. Circ. Res., 48, 650–7.

18. Berne, R.M. and Rubio, R. (1980) Coronary circulation. In Handbook of Physiology. The Cardiovascular System. 1. The Heart (ed. R.M. Berne), American Physiological Society, Bethesda, Maryland, pp. 873–952.

19. Clemens, M.G. and Forrester, T. (1980) Appearance of adenosine triphosphate in the coronary sinus effluent from isolated working rat heart in response to hypoxia. J. Physiol., 312, 143–58.

20. Berger, H.J.L., Cohen, L.S. & Wolfson, S. (1977) Cardiac prostaglandin release during myocardial ischemia induced by atrial pacing in patients with coronary artery disease. Am. J. Cardiol., 39, 481–6.

21. Marcillio, E., Reid, P.R., Dubin, N., Ghodgaonkar, R. and Pitt, B. (1980) Myocardial prostaglandin release by nitroglycerin and modification by indomethacin. Am. J. Cardiol., 45, 53–7.

22. Needleman, P., Key, S.L., Denny, S.E., Isakson, P.C. and Marshall, G.R. (1975) Mechanism and modification of bradykinin-induced coronary vasodilation. Proc. Natl. Acad. Sci., 72, 2060–3.

23. Shimokawa, H., Tomoike, H., Nabeyama, S., Yamamoto, H., Araki, H. and Nakamura, M. (1983) Coronary artery spasm induced in artherosclerotic miniature swine. Science, 221, 560–2.

24. Murray, P.A., Lavallee, M. and Vatner, S.F. (1984) Alpha-adrenergic-mediated reduction in coronary blood flow secondary to carotid chemoreceptor reflex activation in conscious dogs. Circ. Res., 54, 96–106.

25. Vanhoutte, P.M. and Rimele, T.J. (1982–1983) Role of the endothelium in the control of vascular muscle smooth muscle. J. Physiol., Paris, 78, 681–6.

26. Heyndrickx, G.R., Vilaine, J.P., Moerman, E.J. and Leusen, I. (1984) Role of prejunctional alpha$_2$-adrenergic receptors in the regulation of myocardial performance during exercise in conscious dogs. Circ. Res., 54, 683–93.

27. Russell, M.P. and Moran, N.C. (1980) Evidence for lack of innervation of beta$_2$-adrenoceptors in the blood vessels of the gracilis muscle of the dog. Circ. Res., 46, 344–52.

28. Vatner, S.F. and Hintz, T.H. (1983) Mechanism of constriction of large coronary arteries by beta-adrenergic mechanisms in the conscious dog. *Circ. Res.*, **51**, 56–66.

29. Jie, K., van Brummelen, P., Vermey, P., Timmermans, P.B.M.W.M. and van Zwieten, P.A. (1984) Identification of vascular postsynaptic alpha$_1$ and alpha$_2$ adrenoceptors in man. *Circ. Res.*, **54**, 447–52.

30. van Meel, J.C.A., de Jonge, A., Kalleman, H.O., Wilffert, B., Timmermans, P.B.M.W.M. and van Zwieten, P.A. (1981) Ventricular smooth muscle contraction initiated by postsynaptic alpha$_2$-adrenoceptor activation is induced by an influx of extracellular calcium. *Eur. J. Pharmacol*, **69**, 205–8.

31. Colucci, W.S., Gimbrone, M.A. Jr and Alexander, R.W. (1984) Regulation of myocardial and vascular alpha-adrenergic receptor affinity. Effects of guanine nucleotides, cations, estrogen and catecholamine depletion. *Circ. Res.*, **55**, 78–88.

32. Opie, L.H. (1982) Review: Role of cyclic nucleotides in heart metabolism. *Cardiovasc. Res.*, **16**, 483–507.

33. Gerthoffer, W.T., Trevethick, M.A. and Murphy, R.A. (1984) Myosin phosphorylation and cyclic adenosine 3′, 5′-monophosphate in relaxation of arterial smooth muscle by vasodilators. *Circ. Res.*, **54**, 83–9.

34. Furchgott, R.F. (1983) Role of endothelium in responses of vascular smooth muscle. *Circ. Res.*, **53**, 2–3.

35. Rapoport, R.M., Draznin, M.B. and Murad, F. (1983) Endothelium-dependent vasodilator and nitrovasodilator-induced relaxation may be mediated through cyclic GMP formation and GMP-dependent protein phosphorylation. *Nature*, **306**, 174–6.

36. Griffith, T.M., Edwards, D.H., Lewis, M.J., Newby, A.C. and Henderson, A.H. (1984) The nature of endothelium-derived vascular relaxant factor. *Nature*, **308**, 645–7.

37. Gorlin, R., Brachfeld, N., MacLeod, C. and Bopp, P. (1959) Effect of nitroglycerin on coronary circulation in patients with coronary artery disease or increased left ventricular work. *Circulation*, **19**, 705–18.

38. Robinson, B.F. (1967) Relation of heart rate and systolic blood pressure to the onset of pain in angina pectoris. *Circulation*, **35**, 1073–83.

39. Forman, R., Eng, C. and Kirk, E.S. (1983) Comparative effect of verapamil and nitroglycerin on collateral blood flow. *Circulation*, **67**, 1200–4.

40. Fam, W.M. and McGregor, M. (1964) Effect of coronary vasodilator drugs on retrograde flow in areas of chronic myocardial ischemia. *Circ. Res.*, **15**, 355–65.

41. Gruetter, C.A., Gruetter, D.Y., Lyon, J.E., Kadowitz, P.J. and Ignarro, L.J. (1981) Relationship between cyclic guanosine 3′, 5′-monophosphate formation and relaxation of coronary arterial smooth muscle by glyceryl trinitrate, nitroprusside, nitrite and nitric oxide: Effects of methylene blue and methemoglobin. *J. Pharmacol. Exp. Ther.*, **219**, 181–6.

42. Macho, P. and Vatner, S.F. (1981) Effects of nitroglycerin and nitroprusside on large and small coronary vessels in conscious dogs. *Circulation*, **64**, 1101–7.

43. Keith, R.A., Burkman, A.M., Sokoloski, T.D. and Fertel, R.H. (1982) Vascular tolerance to nitroglycerine and cyclic GMP generation in rat aortic smooth muscle. *J. Pharmacol. Exp. Therap.*, **221**, 525–31.

44. Thadani, U. and Kellerman, D. (1983) Interaction of indomethacin and nitroglycerine on hemodynamics and excercise tolerance in patients with angina

pectoris. Z. Kardiol., **72** (Suppl. 3), 35–9.

45. Opie, L.H. and Thadani, U. (1984) Nitrates. In *Drugs for the Heart* (ed. L.H. Opie), Grune & Stratton, Orlando, pp. 23–37.
46. Leier, C.V., Huss, P., Magorien, R.D. and Unverferth, D.V. (1983) Improved exercise capacity and differing arterial and venous tolerance during chronic isosorbide dinitrate therapy for congestive heart failure. *Circulation*, **67**, 817–22.
47. Thadani, U., Fung, H.-L., Darke, A.C. and Parker, J.O. (1982) Oral isosorbide dinitrate in angina pectoris: Comparison of duration of action and dose–response relation during acute and sustained therapy. *Am. J. Cardiol.*, **49**, 411–19.
48. Flaherty, J.T., Come, P.C., Baird, M.G., Rouleau, J., Taylor, D.R., Weisfeldt, M.L., Greene, H.L., Becker, L.C. and Pitt, B. (1976) Effects of intravenous nitroglycerin on left ventricular function and ST segment changes in acute myocardial infarction. *Br. Heart J.*, **38**, 612–21.
49. Curfman, G.D., Heinsimer, J.A., Lozner, E.C. and Fung, H.-L. (1983) Intravenous nitroglycerin in the treatment of spontaneous angina pectoris: A prospective, randomized trial. *Circulation*, **67**, 276–82.
50. Thompson, R.H. (1983) The clinical use of transdermal delivery devices with nitroglycerin. *Angiology*, **34**, 23–31.
51. Parker, J.O. and Fung, H.L. (1984) Transdermal nitroglycerin in angina pectoris. *Am. J. Cardiol.*, **54**, 471–6.
52. Reichek, N., Priest, C., Zimrin, D., Chandler, T. and St John Sutton, M. (1984) Antianginal effects of nitroglycerin in patches. *Am. J. Cardiol.*, **54**, 1–7.
53. Crean, P.A., Ribeiro, P., Crea, F., Davies, G.J., Ratcliffe, D. and Maseri, A. (1983) Continuous transdermal nitroglycerin administration in the treatment of chronic angina pectoris (Abstr). *Circulation*, **168** (Suppl III), III–405.
54. Abrams, J. (1984) The brief saga of transdermal nitroglycerin discs: Paradise lost? *Am. J. Cardiol.*, **54**, 220–4.
55. Parker, J.O., van Koughnett, K.A. and Fung, H.-L. (1984) Transdermal isosorbide dinitrate in angina pectoris: Effect of acute and sustained therapy. *Am. J. Cardiol.*, **54**, 8–13.
56. Wendt, R.L. (1972) Systemic and coronary vascular effects of the 2- and 5-mononitrate esters of isosorbide. *J. Pharmacol Exp. Ther.*, **180**, 732–42.
57. Abshagen, U. and Sporl-Radun, S. (1981) First data on effects and pharmacokinetics of isosorbide-5-mononitrate in normal man. *Eur. J. Clin. Pharamcol.*, **19**, 423–9.
58. Muller, G., Hacker, W. and Schneider, B. (1983) Intra-individual comparison of the action of equal doses of isosorbide-5-mononitrate, slow-release isosorbide dinitrate and placebo in patients with coronary heart disease. *Klin. Wochenschr.*, **61**, 409–16.
59. Maclean, D. and Feely, J. (1983) New Drugs. Calcium antagonists, nitrates, and now antianginal drugs. *Br. Med. J.*, **286**, 1127–29.
60. Tauchert, M., Jansen, W., Osterspey, A., Fuchs, M., Hombach, V. and Hilger, H.H. (1983) Hemodynamic effects of 5-isosorbide mononitrate during acute and chronic administration. In *Nitrates and Nitrate Tolerance in Angina Pectoris* (eds M. Kaltenbach and G. Kober), Steinkopff, Darmstadt.
61. Thadani, U., Hamilton, S., Teague, S., Brady, D. and White, B. (1984) Slow

release isosorbide-5-mononitrate for the treatment of angina pectoris: plasma concentration effect relationship (Abstr). *Circulation*, **70** (Suppl), II–190.

62. Tauchert, M., Jansen, W., Osterspey, A., Fuchs, M., Hombach, V. and Hilger, H.H. (1983b) Dose dependence of tolerance during treatment with mononitrates. *Z. Kardiol.*, **72** (Suppl. 3), 218–28.

63. Danahy, D.T., Burwell, D.T., Aronow, W.S. and Prakash, R. (1977) Sustained hemodynamic and antianginal effect of high dose oral isosorbide dinitrate. *Circulation*, **55**, 381–7.

64. Thadani, U. (1984) Nitrates for angina pectoris. A critical review of therapeutic efficacy and tolerance. *Hertz*, **3**, 123–36.

65. Schneider, W.U., Bussman, W.-D., Stahl, B. and Kaltenbach, M. (1984) Dose–response relation of antianginal activity of isosorbide dinitrate. *Am. J. Cardiol.*, **53**. 700–5.

66. Dalal, J.J. and Parker, J.O. (1984) Nitrate cross-tolerance: Effect of sublingual isosorbide dinitrate and nitroglycerin during sustained nitrate therapy. *Am. J. Cardiol.*, **54**, 286–8.

67. Livesley, B., Catley, P.F., Campbell, R.C. and Oram, S. (1973) Double-blind evaluation of verapamil, propranolol and isosorbide dinitrate against a placebo in the treatment of angina pectoris. *Br. Med. J.*, **1**, 375–8.

68. Lee, G., Mason, D.T. and DeMaria, A.N. (1978) Effects of long-term oral administration of isosorbide dinitrate on the antianginal response to nitroglycerin. Absence of nitrate cross-tolerance and self-tolerance shown by exercise testing. *Am. J. Cardiol.*, **41**, 82–7.

69. Nayler, W.E., Dillon, J.S. and Daly, M.J. (1984) Cellular sites of action of calcium antagonists and beta-adrenoceptor blocks. In *Calcium Antagonists and Cardiovascular Disease* (ed. L.H. Opie), Raven Press, New York, pp. 181–91.

70. Serruys, P.W., Hooghoudt, T.E.H., Reiber, J.H.C., Slager, C., Brower, R.W. and Hugenholtz, P.G. (1983) Influence of intracoronary nifedipine on left ventricular function, coronary vasomotility, and myocardial oxygen consumption, *Br. Heart J.*, **49**, 427–41.

71. Church, J. and Zsoter, T.T. (1980) Calcium antagonist drugs. Mechanism of action. *Can. J. Physiol. Pharmacol.*, **58**, 254–64.

72. Subramanian, V.B., Lahiri, A., Paramasivan, R. and Raftery, E.B. (1980) Verapamil in chronic stable angina. A controlled study with computerised multistage treadmill exercise. *Lancet*, **i**, 841–4.

73. Mehta, J., Pepine, C.J., Day, M., Guererd, J.R. and Conti, C.R. (1981) Short-term efficacy of oral verapamil in rest angina. A double-blind placebo controlled trial in CCU patients. *Am. J. Med.*, **71**, 977–82.

74. Betriu, A., Chaitman, B.R., Bourassa, M.G., Brevers, G., Scholl, J.-M., Bruneau, P., Gagne, P. and Chabot, M. (1983) Beneficial effects of intravenous diltiazem in the acute management of paroxysmal supraventricular tachyarrhythmias. *Circulation*, **67**, 88–94.

75. Johnson, S.M., Mauritson, D.R., Willerson, J.T. and Hillis, L.D. (1981) A controlled trial of verapamil for Prinzmetal's variant angina. *N. Engl. J. Med.*, **304**, 862–6.

76. Danish Study Group on Verapamil in Myocardial Infarction (1984) Verapamil in acute myocardial infarction. *Eur. Heart J.*, **5**, 516–28.

77. de Ponti, C., Mauri, F., Ciliberto, G.R. and Caru, B. (1979) Comparative

effects of nifedipine, verapamil, isosorbide dinitrate and propranolol on exercise-induced angina pectoris. *Eur. J. Cardiol.*, **10**, 47–58.

78. Kaltenbach, M., Schulz, W. and Kober, G. (1979) Effects of nifedipine after intravenous and intracoronary administration. *Am. J. Cardiol.*, **44**, 832–8.

79. Schanzenbaecher, P., Liebau, G., Deeg, P. and Kochsiek, K. (1983) Effect of intravenous and intracoronary nifedipine on coronary blood flow and myocardial oxygen consumption. *Am. J. Cardiol.*, **51**, 712–17.

80. Muller, J.E., Turi, Z.G., Pearle, D.L., Schneider, J.F., Serfas, D.H., Morrison, J., Stone, P.H., Rude, R.E., Rosner, B., Sobel, B.E., Tate, C., Scheiner, E., Roberts, R., Hennekens, C.H. and Braunwald, E. (1984) Nifedipine and conventional therapy for unstable angina pectoris: a randomized, double blind comparison. *Circulation*, **69**, 728–39.

81. Feldman, R.L., Pepine, C.J., Whittle, J. and Conti, C.R. (1982) Short and long-term responses to diltiazem in patients with variant angina. *Am. J. Cardiol.*, **49**, 554–9.

82. Schroeder, J.S., Feldman, R.L., Giles, T.D., Friedman, M.J., DeMaria, A.N., Kinney, E.L., Mallon, S.M., Pitt, B., Meyer, R., Basta, L.L., Curry, R.C., Jr, Groves, B.M. and MacAlpin, R.N. (1982) Multiclinic control trial of diltiazem for Prinzmetal's angina. *Am. J. Med.*, **72**, 227–32.

83. Hossack, K.F., Pool, P.E., Steel, P., Crawford, M.H., DeMaria, A.N., Cohen, L.S. and Ports, T.A. (1982) Efficacy of diltiazem in angina of effort. A multicenter trial. *Am. J. Cardiol.*, **49**, 567–72.

84. Strauss, W.E., McIntyre, K.M., Parisi, A.F. and Shapiro, W. (1982) Safety and efficacy of diltiazem hydrochloride for the treatment of stable angina pectoris: Report of a cooperative clinical trial. *Am. J. Cardiol.*, **49**, 560–6.

85. Hung, J., Lamb, I., Connolly, S.J., Jutzy, K.R., Goris, M.L. and Schroeder, J.S. (1983) The effect of diltiazem and propranolol, alone and in combination, on exercise performance and left ventricular function in patients with stable effort angina. *Circulation*, **68**, 560–7.

86. Shapiro, W., DiBianco, R. and Thadani, U. (1985) Comparative efficacy of 200, 300 and 400 mg of bepridil HCl in chronic, stable angina pectoris. *Am. J. Cardiol.*, **55**, 366–426.

87. Opie, L.H., White, D., Jee, L. and Lubbe, W.F. (1982) Alternatives to beta-blockade in therapy of hypertension with angina pectoris: Role of nifedipine or of labetolol. *Br. J. Clin. Pharmacol.*, **13**, Suppl., 115S–122S.

88. Opie, L.H. (1984) Drugs and the heart four years on. *Lancet*, **i**, 495–500.

89. Opie, L.H. (1984) Calcium antagonists. Mechanisms, therapeutic indications and reservations: A Review. *Q. J. Med.*, **53**, 1–16.

90. Bassan, M.M., Weiler-Ravell, D. and Shalev, O. (1983) Comparison of the antianginal effectiveness of nifedipine, verapamil and isosorbide dinitrate in patients receiving propranolol: a double-blind study. *Circulation*, **68**, 568–75.

91. Chaitman, B.R., Wagniart, P., Paslone, A., Drevos, G., Scholl, J.-H., Lan, J., Methe, M., Fergusson, R.J. and Bourassa, M.G. (1984) Improved exercise tolerance after propranolol, diltiazem or nifedipine in angina pectoris. Comparsion at 1, 3 and 5 hours and correlation with plasma drug concentration evaluation. *Amer. J. Cardiol.*, **53**, 1–9.

92. Tolins, M., Weir, E.K. Chesler, E. and Pierpont, G.L. (1984) 'Maximal' drug therapy is not necessarily optimal in chronic angina pectoris. *J. Am. Coll. Cardiol.*, **3**, 1051–7.

93. Herling, I.M. (1984) Intravenous nitroglycerin: Clinical pharmacology and therapeutic considerations. *Am. Heart J.*, **108**, 141–9.

94. Muller, J.E., Morrison, J., Stone, P.H., Rude, R.E., Rosner, B., Roberts, R., Pearle, D.L., Turi, Z.G., Schneider, J.F., Serfas, D.H., Tate, C., Scheiner, E., Sobel, B.E., Hennekens, C.H. and Braunwald, E. (1984) Nifedipine therapy for patients with threatened and acute myocardial infarction: a randomized, double-blind, placebo-controlled comparison. *Circulation*, **69**, 740–7.

95. Abrams, J. (1985) Nitrate tolerance in angina pectoris. In *Mononitrates* (eds J.N. Cohn & R. Rittinghausen), SpringerVerlag, Berlin, pp. 154–70.

96. Torresi, J., Horowitz, J.D. & Dusting, G.J. (1985) Potentiation and reversal of tolerance to nitroglycerine with *N*-acetyl cysteine. *J. Cardiovasc. Pharmacol.*, **7**, 777–83.

97. Kukowitz, W.R. and Holzmann, S. (1985) Mechanisms of vasodilatation by molsidomine. *Am. Heart J.*, **109**, 637–40.

98. Thadani, U. and Opie, L.H. (1987) Nitrates in *Drugs for the Heart*, 2nd expanded edition (ed. L.H. Opie) Grune and Stratton Inc., Orlando. In press.

5 *Digitalis: the present position*

ROGER HAYWARD

5.1 Introduction

In dealing with a drug with a two hundred year track record, the intention has been to discuss recent developments and controversy, not to produce an encyclopaedic account. Some brief historical perspectives have been mentioned in order to set the scene. Contentious phraseology has been avoided when possible, and the term digitalis has been used to cover all related cardioactive steroidal drugs rather than solely those of *Digitalis* (foxglove plant) origin.

5.2 Digitalis actions at a cellular level

The price of progress towards an understanding of digitalis actions at a cellular level has been an acknowledgement of their complexity. Experimental conditions including electrolyte concentrations, tissue origin and method of extraction, and stimulation frequency combine to exert powerful effects upon results and require to be controlled. Dealing with isolated cardiac muscle preparations it is important to take account of indirect effects upon local release and uptake of neurotransmitter substances since these may substantially modify the direct actions of digitalis. In relation to transmembrane ionic balance and effects upon intracellular electrolyte concentrations, attention is currently being diverted from digitalis effects upon the sodium pump mechanism in cardiac and other cells towards effects upon calcium ion control in sites close to the cell membrane.

5.2.1 THE SODIUM LAG HYPOTHESIS

The theory that the cardiac effects of digitalis derive from inhibition of the sodium pump enzyme system located in the myocardial cell membrane

145

has a long history [1]. Studies undertaken some three decades ago demonstrated inhibition by digitalis of transmembrane sodium and potassium ion transport in the red blood cell. The transport enzyme responsible for maintaining sodium and potassium ion concentration gradients across the cell membrane was described soon afterwards; it is termed sodium and potassium dependent adenosine triphosphatase (Na,K-ATPase). Specific binding of digitalis glycosides to this enzyme complex on the cardiac cell membrane (sarcolemma) has been convincingly demonstrated [2]. Binding is reversible, and is directly associated both with enzyme inhibition and with modified behaviour of the cell preparation; the process has accordingly been categorized as a pharmacological drug–receptor interaction [2, 3].

The sodium lag hypothesis [4] provides an explanation of digitalis effects on the cardiac cell, starting with Na,K-ATPase binding. Inhibition of the transmembrane cation pump causes reduced extrusion of sodium from the cell, and diminished uptake of potassium.

A range of studies conducted over five decades has demonstrated increased intracellular sodium ion concentration and decreased potassium following glycoside exposure, consistent with pump inhibition. The next step in the argument involves the action of a membrane located sodium-calcium ion counter transport system. Described by Glitsch and colleagues [5] and by Reuter [6], the system provides for extrusion of calcium ions against the massive transmembrane calcium gradient, energized by sodium ion influx down the sodium concentration gradient. The magnitude of the transmembrane sodium gradient thus determines calcium ion expulsion. Raised intracellular sodium, by reducing the sodium gradient, decreases calcium exchange towards the exterior, and intracellular calcium accumulates. Electrolyte shifts in keeping with this sequence have been observed after digitalis. Sodium–calcium exchange using this mechanism is not directly energy consuming, being fuelled by the sodium gradient, though the latter process is maintained by energy derived from hydrolysis of ATP by the sodium pump ATPase system. Cardiac glycosides do not directly affect the sodium–calcium exchange mechanism. The exchange is electrogenic since three monovalent sodium ions are exchanged for one divalent calcium ion, and is accordingly affected by the state of cell membrane polarization. In addition the magnitude and direction of exchange may be manipulated, for example by altering the sodium ion gradient, and the system consistently functions to expel calcium ions in a direction opposite to that of the electrochemical sodium gradient. In the contracting heart therefore the exchange operates to expel calcium during membrane repolarization and to take in calcium during depolarization resulting from sodium ingress during phase 0 [8]. This is one of several mechanisms regulating myocardial intracellular free calcium levels to deal with calcium ingress via slow channels during phase two of depolarization, as well as with calcium liberated from intracellular stores. Regulation of ionized calcium levels in the myocardial cytoplasm (cytosol) is also supported by an ATP-dependent cell membrane located calcium pump taking calcium out across the sarcolemma, and by a similar enzyme system on the membrane of the sarcoplasmic reticulum which sequesters high concentrations of calcium in intracellular sites pending release during the next systole [9]. Provided cytosolic calcium does not accumulate to overload levels [10], an increased level of free intracellular ionized calcium represents the key step in the sequence of events by which digitalis augments contractile function through sodium pump inhibition. Levels of free calcium ion at the time of excitation contraction coupling, by acting on the troponin-tropomyosin regulatory protein complex, determine the amount of actin-myosin interaction and fibre shortening. The regulatory system described above maintains cytosolic free calcium ion concentration during diastole at 10^{-7} mol/l; against an extracellular concentration of 10^{-3} mol/l. Ingress of calcium during depolarization stimulates release from intracellular stores, so that cytosolic levels increase transiently to 10^{-5} mol/l. Demonstration of increased cytosolic free calcium levels has proved difficult in the absence of high glycoside exposure, reflecting the complex nature of intracellular calcium homeostasis. In addition interactions between sodium pump ATPase binding and effects on calcium control not directly concerning the sodium calcium exchange system have been described [11]. These have displaced the sodium lag hypothesis to a position in which a permanently elevated cytosolic sodium and calcium level during all phases of the cardiac cycle, including diastole, is considered to characterize the toxic condition. The result may be development of increased diastolic tension, leading ultimately to onset of contracture. There are parallels between this description of glycoside effects and events initiated by increased heart rate. The progressive increase in contraction velocity which results from decreasing cycle length (Bowditch effect) probably represents a sodium lag phenomenon caused by increased loading on the sodium pump [4, 12].

5.2.2 SARCOLEMMAL NA, K-ATPASE

Effects of digitalis compounds on the sodium pump ATPase enzyme system of the myocardial cell membrane are central to many of the cardiac actions of digitalis [3], though inhibition of this enzyme system is unlikely itself to explain all these effects [13]. The enzyme is orientated across the cell membrane, with an internal site stimulated by sodium ions, an external site stimulated by potassium ions, and uses energy derived from

Digitalis: the present position

ATP hydrolysis to maintain the transmembrane sodium and potassium ion gradients, moving sodium outward against a 120 mmol/l concentration gradient ($[Na^+]i/c$: 30 mmol/l; $[Na^+]$ E/C: 150 mmol/l), and potassium ions into the cell against a similar gradient ($[K^+]$ i/c: 150 mmol/l; $[K^+]$ E/C: 5 mmol/l). The enzyme carries an ATP binding site on the cell membrane interior. The sequence of events following ATP binding also requires binding of sodium and magnesium ions. ATP is hydrolysed, providing energy needed to produce a conformational change in the enzyme which results in sodium ion extrusion and inward potassium ion movement.

Enzyme activity is dependent upon availability of ATP and magnesium ions. Activity is enhanced by increased intracellular sodium, and by increased extracellular potassium so that homeostasis is maintained. Digitalis binding to the exterior of the enzyme is specific, saturable, and obeys the major criteria required to designate the process a true ligand–receptor interaction [3]. In general the result of glycoside binding is enzyme inhibition. The enzyme binding site shows high affinity for digitalis, is readily distinguishable from non-specific lipid absorption onto cell membranes, and involves a single site on a 96 000 molecular weight polypeptide α-subunit of the isolated enzyme [14]. Further molecular subfragments are needed for sodium pump activity. Binding is reversible, and glycoside may be displaced by cardioactive analogues, though not by inactive congeners. A variety of conditions modulate binding. The conformational state of the enzyme complex is important. Binding occurs to the form involved in sodium extrusion, rather than to the form associated with potassium uptake. Thus increased extracellular potassium opposes and increased extracellular sodium levels enhance digitalis binding. Similarly increased extracellular calcium levels increase digitalis receptor affinity, a likely mechanism for the synergistic relationship between calcium and digitalis. Glycoside structural requirements for binding include an unsaturated lactone ring which is probably involved via a two point attachment [15]. Binding may be facilitated by certain ring structures which enhance resonance, particularly a positive charge at C-20, and a negatively charged carbonyl group [15, 16]. Binding occurs chiefly via the side chain attached at C-17 (the lactone ring in digoxin), which is probably accommodated in a cleft in the receptor surface. The steroid ring and sugar groups at C-3 contribute slightly [15].

A degree of non-specific, non-receptor glycoside uptake onto lipid membrane constituents also occurs. Studies of binding kinetics may be complicated therefore, particularly with relatively non-polar lipophilic glycosides such as digitoxin and to a lesser extent digoxin. Binding of ouabain (polar) is highly specific, and has been favoured for kinetic studies. In man, rapid but transient myocardial uptake has been demonstrated using relatively lipid-soluble methyldigoxin, antedating effects on contractile function and considered to represent intracardiac lipid sequestration [17].

Receptor density studies provide valuable insights into ways in which disease processes and other factors may modify the response to digitalis. Hyperthyroidism is associated with clinical digitalis resistance; both increased Na,K-ATPase activity and glycoside receptor density have been described in this condition [18]. Cultured heart cell studies have linked conditions in which intracellular sodium concentrations are chronically raised, including growth in the presence of ouabain, with increased receptor site density [19]. Using the red cell membrane sodium pump ATPase system as a model or analogue of that in the heart, Ford and colleagues [20] in a series of reports have shown that chronic glycoside exposure leads to production of red cells with increased digitalis binding sites. They suggest that a similar process may take place in the myocardium, an adaptation that if confirmed might explain a progressive loss of digitalis effects on the heart in the long-term.

5.2.3 DIGITALIS BINDING SITE MULTIPLICITY

Kinetic studies mentioned previously have confirmed the presence of a high affinity, high specificity glycoside binding site on the sarcolemmal ATPase complex. It has, however, become evident that digitalis binding sites are not uniform in respect of their affinity for cardiac glycosides. Two forms of brain tissue ATPase enzyme with individual affinities for digitalis have been identified by Sweadner [21]. Godfraind and colleagues [16] have developed the view that this applies also to cardiac tissues, in that high and low affinity binding sites can be distinguished. Depending on the species and on the tissue, the relative preponderance of each receptor type varies, as does extent to which their glycoside affinities differ. In animal species showing relative digitalis insensitivity (e.g. guinea pig, rat), these workers have found two receptors with widely differing affinities, low affinity sites predominating. In sensitive species (human, cat and bovine tissues), the ratios are different and the discrepancy between affinities much reduced. Others have found similar results in insensitive tissues, but have not discerned evidence for receptor duality in human preparations [14]. When two ATPase receptors have been differentiated, however, it has been possible to link high affinity site binding to increased contractile function, and probably also to pump stimulation, while low affinity binding has correlated with pump inhibition, intracellular sodium accumulation, cell depolarization and toxic manifestations. Findings such as these open up the prospect of being able to tailor a glycoside analogue to activate the high affinity site selectively and to avoid excessive effects on intracellular sodium which may lead to

149

toxicity. Clues also come from work using dihydro ouabain (ouabain with a saturated lactone ring structure), a relatively cardioinactive derivative, which appears to bind to high affinity receptors though without causing stimulation. Attempts to alter molecular structure to stimulate only high affinity receptors, so widening the therapeutic ratio, are in progress [11].

5.2.4 PHYSIOLOGICAL ROLE OF DIGITALIS RECEPTORS

Digitalis binding to Na,K-ATPase so closely resembles a ligand–receptor interaction [2, 3] that two related questions inevitably arise. For what purpose is man, in common with many other species, equipped with receptors for which the only known ligands appear to be of extraneous plant origin? Is it not probable that endogenous materials with selective affinity for the digitalis receptor, possibly with cation pump regulatory functions, await identification?

Widely dispersed throughout mammalian tissues, the trace metal vanadium was at one time considered in this role. Vanadium is relatively concentrated in the heart (10^{-7} molar concentration) and powerfully inhibits Na,K-ATPase. The time-course of contractile enhancement with vanadium is similar to that caused by ouabain. As presently perceived, it seems to be involved in regulation of the effects of local electrolytes upon membrane Na, K-ATPase activity, rather than direct control of the cation pump [2].

Accumulating evidence indicates that one or more circulating materials may function as endogenous digitalis. A factor which reacts like digoxin in a range of highly specific digoxin radioimmunoassay systems has been described in serum from patients with renal failure [22, 23]. Though not itself shown to inhibit Na,K-ATPase, one or more materials with this capability are present in uraemic blood. No such substance has been identified in samples from subjects with normal renal function [22]. Information from a very different source is of interest. Several species of toad secrete bufagins, a cardioactive class of digoxin-like substances, in their venom. (Similar compounds are present in the traditional Chinese medicine Ch'an Su derived from skins of the toad *Bufo asiaticus*.) The serum of *Bufo marinus* is now known to contain a digoxin-like substance in substantial concentrations. It competes with ouabain for Na, K-ATPase binding sites and appropriately stimulates myocardial contractile function [2]. Although far removed from man, the toad appears therefore to have developed an endogenous digitalis substance with an undisclosed biological function. Godfraind and colleagues [24] have discerned in guinea pig and other mammalian hearts a material which competes with digitalis for ATPase receptor sites. Though its function remains unknown they suggest that exposure to low concentrations of added glycoside may displace this substance, termed 'cardiodigin', from ATPase binding sites. The result might be pump 'derepression', a possible explanation for transient pump stimulation seen after glycoside administration. Schwartz [2] favours the term 'endodigin' to describe endogenous ouabain-like activity in toad serum, others refer to 'endoxin'.

Links between cardiodigin or endodigin and material in uraemic serum which interacts with digoxin radioimmunoassays and may have Na,K-ATPase inhibitory activity would be premature [23]. Similarly attractive but unsubstantiated theories connect the uraemic substance with a long-sought natriuretic hormone. Possibly secreted by the brain in response to intravascular volume expansion, natriuretic hormone, though not yet isolated, is credited with Na,K-ATPase inhibitor effectiveness in numerous sites including the renal tubule, where its action would be to reduce sodium reabsorption. This substance appears to have a molecular weight in the 400–500 range [25]. It is possibly responsible for the widespread depression of ouabain-sensitive sodium pump activity characteristically seen in essential hypertension [26]. The role of natriuretic hormone in hypertension, in renal failure, and conceivably as a physiological cation pump regulator remains to be established [23].

Both endodigin/cardiodigin and natriuretic hormone, though still conjectural materials, are clearly separable from the recently described group of peptides termed atrial natriuretic factor (ANF) [26]. Released from granules in atrial but not ventricular myocardium these peptides prevent renal sodium reabsorption and cause natriuresis. Candidature for consideration as an endodigin is demolished since they do not inhibit Na,K-ATPase [26]; they also possess vasodilator activity contrasting with the vasoconstrictor effects of Na,K-ATPase inhibitors such as the digitalis compounds.

For the present, therefore, demonstration of a physiological role for an endogenous local or systemic digitalis hormone remains to be achieved. Successful identification of the endorphins as endogenous occupants of morphine receptors in the brain is an encouraging precedent [23].

5.2.5 SARCOLEMMAL ATPase AS THE DIGITALIS RECEPTOR

A range of pharmacokinetic studies strongly support the conclusion that sarcolemmal Na,K-ATPase behaves as a true receptor for digitalis actions. Arguments owe much to Paul Ehrlich's axiom (1909) 'corpora non agunt nisi fixata', i.e. that in order to exert a biological effect a compound must achieve binding to a receptor. The process of receptor binding is classically by reversible absorption, in which equilibrium between bound and unbound fractions obeys the law of mass action. Binding of the specific active material (the ligand) to the receptor may cause stimulation, as with catecholamines and adenylate cyclase, or exert an inhibitory action as with digitalis and ATPase. Kinetic studies in which rates of association and dissociation of a radio ligand (e.g. tritium-labelled ouabain) have been measured in preparations of human cardiac cell membrane have confirmed that absorption is by predicted zero order or saturation kinetics [18]. These workers were able to correlate binding with pump inhibition and with effects on contractile function. Digitalis binding kinetics in human ventricular tissues provided these workers with evidence for only one digitalis receptor. They identified the dissociation constant as 2 mol/l (i.e. approximately 1.5 ng/ml). This is the free drug concentration at which 50% of the receptors are occupied, a result which closely matches the accepted therapeutic plasma glycoside concentration in clinical practice. The dissociation constant was found to differ with each glycoside tested, while the total binding capacity of the preparation, a measure of the number of receptors present and of receptor density, was constant. These results have been interpreted as indicating that human cardiac tissues carry one type of digitalis receptor, having variable affinities for diverse glycosides depending on their precise structures. In addition digitalis binding was shown to be appropriately sensitive to conditions such as ionic concentrations, pH, temperature and presence of drugs such as epanutin. Accordingly these kinetic studies provide evidence linking specific binding to ATPase with contractile effects, in support of the ATPase receptor theory. Digitalis receptor binding is further discussed below.

There is a mass of evidence from a wide range of sources offering further support [3, 27], though ultimate proof is elusive and most evidence is circumstantial.

Non-digitalis compounds with a common ability to inihibit myocardial ATPase activity also increase cardiac contractile performance; in some instances parallelism exists between effects of these materials and of digitalis on ATPase and on myocardial function. Examples of compounds shown to behave in this way include n-ethylmaleimide, the erythrophleum alkaloids [3], and monovalent cations such as rubidium and thallium [15].

Manipulation of cardiac transmembrane ionic gradients also reveals common features linking digitalis effects on cardiac muscle function with ATPase inhibition. Increased extracellular potassium ion concentrations oppose the contractile stimulatory and ATPase inhibiting effects of cardiac glycosides, and reduce the amount and the rate of digitalis binding to ATPase. Decreased extracellular potassium levels inihibit ATPase activity and exert a stimulatory effect on contractile performance. There is in addition an approximate correlation between the potency with which the many structurally different forms of cardioactive digitalis-like steroids inihibit sarcolemmal ATPase activity, and their effectiveness as myocardial stimulants.

Recent elegant studies undertaken in dogs have combined measurement of cardiac contractile function in the intact animal receiving therapeutic (i.e. non-toxic) concentrations of ouabain [28] and later digoxin [29] together with sodium pump activity in ventricular muscle obtained by serial endomyocardial biopsy during the study. These workers were able to correlate approximately 25% sodium pump inhibition (assessed by uptake of labelled rubidium) with some 20% left ventricular contractile function enhancement (measured as the maximum rate of rise of pressure), in the absence of evidence of toxicity. With onset of toxic arrhythmias, over 50% sodium pump inhibition was observed. These impressive results have been criticized [13] on the ground that they do not exclude the possibility (discussed subsequently) that digitalis may transiently stimulate the sodium pump prior to causing inhibition, since the study environment included a relatively low potassium concentration which may have prevented expression of such an effect.

5.2.6 PROBLEMS WITH THE NA,K-ATPase INHIBITION THEORY

Although it has been repeatedly possible to demonstrate a correlation between Na,K-ATPase inhibition by digitalis and positive effects upon contractile function, such a correlation does not prove causation. Conversely a small number of studies which demonstrate no correlation may be enough to disprove a causal link.

A number of early reports, such as those from Ghysel-Burton and Godfraind [30] and from Blood and Noble [31], showed *in vitro* stimulation of sodium pump activity by low ouabain concentrations (less than 10^{-8} mol/l), running counter to the theories previously outlined. Rhee and co-workers [32] further showed a positive contractile response in animals receiving an ouabain infusion at a time when cardiac tissue derived by endomyocardial biopsy showed no evidence of sodium pump inhibition as measured by *in vitro* ATPase activity. This was true with ouabain concentrations of 10^{-8} mol/l, below those required to elicit signs of intoxication. Evidence of sodium pump inhibition did however emerge with increased ouabain concentrations, as did manifestations of toxicity.

It must be emphasized that in clinical use the therapeutic plasma concentration for ouabain lies in the region 7–10×10^{-10} mol/l [33]. For digoxin the figure is 1–2 nmol/l, i.e. in the 10^{-9} molar range. There is a significant gap therefore between concentrations capable in the intact animal or human heart of enhancing contractile function, and those regarded as able to generate a similar response *in vitro*. Cellular changes caused by isolation techniques may be responsible [34] though alternative possibilities exist.

153

Digitalis: the present position

The major area of difficulty which has impeded acceptance of the Na,K-ATPase digitalis receptor theory concerns effects of low glycoside concentrations, at which it has been possible to dissociate enzyme inhibition from contractile stimulation. Complementary to these difficulties have been reports concerning washout studies such as those of Okita and colleagues [35] and of Blood and Noble [31], demonstrating marked differences in the decay rates with the contractile effect declining more rapidly than enzyme inhibition. Increasingly strong evidence currently indicates that under specific conditions exhibition of a cardioactive glycoside in low concentrations (10^{-9} mol/l) may increase sodium pump activity while leaving cardiac contractile function unaltered, or causing a slight stimulant effect [36,37]. The implication is clearly that pump inhibition is not a prerequisite of effects on cardiac contraction.

Hart and co-workers [37] discerned a contractile stimulant effect in sheep ventricular tissue using relatively low glycoside concentrations (less than 10^{-7} mol/l), together with evidence based on current-voltage recordings suggesting stimulation of the pump enzyme. Recent work using canine Purkinje fibres supports this [38]. Rhee and colleagues [32] studied ATPase activity in cardiac biopsy material from animals receiving an infusion of ouabain. With non-toxic plasma levels, a stimulant effect on contractile function occurred without any measurable sodium pump enzyme effect. Enzyme inhibition emerged early as levels became toxic. This conflicts with results from similar studies by Hougen and colleagues [29] referred to earlier, and tissue isolation procedures and/or electrolyte conditions may have been involved.

By suitable adjustment of study conditions using isolated tissues it is possible to delineate a biphasic glycoside effect on the sodium pump. As an example, one may cite the rate at which a muscle preparation is driven. At low driving frequencies, contractile stimulant effects can be produced without significant change in transmembrane sodium and potassium currents. At higher frequencies, transmembrane gradients of these ions are reduced, although a contractile response may emerge first. It is suggested therefore that at slow rates pump inhibition by digitalis may be insufficient to affect transmembrane gradients. With the stress of increased rate, pump requirements are increased and inhibition becomes apparent, with increasing intracellular sodium and consequent calcium accumulation. Effects are analogous to those involved in the treppe or force-staircase response (Bowditch effect) developed by the myocardium in response to reduced cycle length [4, 12]. Since at low rates transmembrane gradients are either unaltered or slightly increased, the fraction of sodium pump sites on the membrane remaining unblocked may be in a state of increased activity consistent with glycoside-mediated stimulation [13].

The extracellular potassium ion concentration can also be manipulated to separate digitalis effects on the sarcolemmal sodium pump from those on contractile function, and to elicit biphasic responses. With high extracellular potassium and low ouabain concentrations, positive effects on contractile function may accompany a decreased intracellular sodium content. With greater ouabain exposure this is converted into a progressively increasing sodium content [39]. By increasing external potassium levels from low to high concentrations, an inhibitory glycoside effect on sodium pumping can be converted into stimulation. Noble [13] proposes that digitalis in low concentrations may occupy and inhibit a minority of pump binding sites. The remainder may then be more active because of stimulation either directly by the glycoside or by the tendency for the transmembrane cation gradient to fall. Conversion into a net inhibitory action occurs when digitalis concentrations are increased, with occupation of more binding sites. Possible additional contributions to an inhibitory effect may arise because of enhanced binding secondary to decreased extracellular potassium, or again because remaining unblocked pump sites become overloaded as a result of increased stimulation frequency. These factors clearly exert a major influence on the point of balance in the biphasic sequence of digitalis effects on pump activity, and support the possibility of initial pump stimulation by digitalis despite contractile stimulation.

5.2.7 NEUROTRANSMITTER INVOLVEMENT

The effects of low concentrations of digitalis upon the sarcolemmal cation pump are complicated by the ability of cardiac glycosides to alter concentrations of autonomic neurotransmitter substances both in the intact heart and in isolated muscle preparations. Local release of acetylcholine causes a decrease in contractile function and may occur in isolated myocardium following digitalis exposure [40]. Poole-Wilson and colleagues studying the perfused rabbit interventricular septum [34], observed a transient initial fall in developed tension with ouabain, and suggested that local acetylcholine release may have been involved. In their study progressive sodium pump inhibition was demonstrated with relatively high-dose ouabain without initial stimulation, emphasizing the apparent reduction in glycoside sensitivity characteristic of studies on isolated preparations. Grupp and colleagues [41] suggest that an Na,K-ATPase isoenzyme carried by nerve endings present in cardiac muscle may bind digitalis glycosides in low concentrations, and so affect neurotransmitter release and/or uptake.

Neurotransmitter involvement has been studied in depth by Hougen and co-workers [42]. Low ouabain concentrations (10^{-8} M) stimulated

155

monovalent cation transport (assessed by ^{86}Rb$^+$ uptake) in quiescent atrial muscle strips; stimulation could be blocked by β-adrenergic blockade or prior catecholamine depletion. Lechat and colleagues [43] similarly showed pump stimulation with very low ouabain concentrations (10^{-9} M), which could be prevented by β-blockade They were able to demonstrate no accompanying effect on contractile function, but having blocked any effect of local acetylcholine release with prior atropine a small contractile effect emerged, unaccompanied by pump changes. As these workers point out, glycoside effects on the pump and on contractile performance may be differently mediated at differing concentrations. Concentrations of 10^{-7} M ouabain as expected consistently caused pump inhibition and contractile stimulation.

Protagonists of the theory that digitalis effects on the sodium pump ATPase amount are not simply inhibitory, whose arguments have been marshalled by Noble [13] and by Hart and colleagues [37], would probably accept that local interactions with both sympathetic and parasympathetic neurotransmitter substances have a role in the balance of low dose glycoside actions. They would however argue that transient initial pump stimulation may occur with positive glycoside effects on contractile function as a direct result of glycoside activity.

Langer [12] and others have concluded in favour of an attractive scheme in which the sodium lag hypothesis as outlined above accounts for the medium-to-high dose glycoside effects and occurs at the cardiac sarcolemma, while low dose effects are caused by digitalis binding to Na,K-ATPase sites on the membranes of neuronal cells dispersed throughout the myocardium. Consequent neuronal enzyme inhibition is considered to diminish catecholamine uptake so that local levels rise, indirectly promoting contractile function to a relatively small extent in the presence of very low digitalis concentration. Inhibition of myocardial catecholamine uptake has been demonstrated in human myocardium with 10^{-8} M ouabain [44].

The cell is enclosed in a phospholipid bilayer – the cell membrane. Immediately exterior to this is the glycocalyx, which forms a superficial outer covering to the cell, and extends into the cell in continuity with internal projections of the cell membrane (the transverse tubular system). Making up the glycocalyx are glycoprotein chains extending outward from the phospholipid bilayer, together with glycolipids and a dense matrix of oligosaccharides; materials initmately involved in the control of transmembrane cation flux, particularly of ionized calcium. Unlike skeletal muscle, myocardial cells need a constant supply of 'activator calcium' from the exterior. Digitalis glycosides exert substantial effects on the quantity of calcium present at the cell surface, and on the flux of calcium into the cell. Partly discussed earlier was the involvement of locally released catecholamines following digitalis exposure on calcium influx, mediated via adenylate cyclase activation, increased cyclic AMP production and consequently increased activity of slow calcium channels conveying calcium to the interior. Glycoside enhancement of slow calcium current activity has been discerned in several studies [45, 46]. There is also good evidence that digitalis increases the amount of calcium stored as an extracellular pool within the glycocalyx, and available for translocation into the cell to enhance contractile element activation. The means by which digitalis affects extracellular calcium stores are unclear. In one possible mechanism, a consequence of digitalis binding to sarcolemmal ATPase is a reduction in the level of affinity for calcium shown by phospholipids in the close vicinity of the ATPase complex [13]. This causes a local rise in the availability of activator calcium in the glycocalyx, making more calcium available for movement into the cell during the plateau (phase 2) of the cardiac action potential.

5.2.8 CONCLUSION

Though a consensus has not yet been achieved it is attractive to suggest that important low dose but therapeutic digitalis effects involve alterations in membrane-located calcium ion availability and transport probably due to a combination of direct and neurotransmitter-mediated effects. Any alterations in intracellular sodium at this stage are transient, i.e. coincident with depolarization only. After further exposure, persistent intracellular sodium and calcium accumulation develops with blockade of a high proportion of sodium pump sites, and toxicity may ensue.

5.3 Digitalis actions on cardiovascular haemodynamics with particular reference to heart failure

The place of digitalis as a remedy for heart failure has been controversial since the studies by William Withering published two hundred years ago [47]. In making the vital connection between the diuretic effects of digitalis extract in congestive cardiac failure and improvements in cardiac motion, Withering was not in a position to differentiate between patients with and without cardiac arrhythmias. Bouillaud [48] described digitalis in 1835 as a 'great moderator and sort of opium of the heart', emphasizing that its action was to help with a fast and irregular pulse. Dominant British authorities of the early part of the present century, including Mackenzie [49] and Lewis [50], took the same line, advocating digitalis for the control of heart failure only when accompanied by atrial fibrillation. Appearing between 1919 and 1944, a number of reports [51–55] from both sides of the Atlantic subsequently described beneficial results with digitalis in heart failure with sinus rhythm. Sir Thomas Lewis' views reflected these developments. Writing in 1919 he emphasizes the negative chronotropic effect in atrial fibrillation, stating 'to the heart, foxglove is not tonic but powerfully hypnotic' [50]. In 1946, it seems after personally benefiting from digitalis, he comments 'evidence that digitalis is useful in failure with congestion presenting normal rhythm has been slower in coming . . . it is now generally recognized that digitalis is valuable in these cases . . . ' [56]. McMichael has recently described these transitional times [57]. Improvements in investigative techniques have placed beyond doubt the ability of digitalis preparations to stimulate contractile function of cardiac muscle. As described in many reviews [57–63], this effect has been shown over the years using measurements of contractile behaviour in isolated myocardium, animal models and in both the normal and failing human heart.

There is no doubt that most patients with cardiac failure and atrial fibrillation benefit from digoxin and deteriorate without it [64]. Patients with a heightened degree of pre-existent atrioventricular block in whom further control of the ventricular rate is unnecessary are an exception since further slowing by digitalis will not be helpful. Studies encompassing elderly fibrillators may not have shown clear-cut deterioration on digoxin withdrawal for this reason [65, 66]. For the present, the value of digitalis in heart failure with atrial fibrillation is relatively secure while controversy surrounds its use with sinus rhythm. As Starr and Luchi [67] observed, 'easily demonstrated in atrial fibrillation, the cardiac action of digitalis glycosides is so much less conspicuous in patients with normal rhythm that some distinguished clinicians have doubted that there was any cardiac effect at all.'

Problems that arise in considering the difficulty can be segregated into four groupings.

(1) Why has it been difficult to show that recognized short-term gains in myocardial contractile function are expressed in clinically significant improvements in cardiac performance such as in cardiac output and/or ventricular filling pressure?

(2) If significant short-term improvements in these important functions can be achieved, in which sub-groups of patient with heart failure and sinus rhythm may they be predicted?

(3) Are any short-term benefits sustained; alternatively are they soon dissipated because of myocardial adaptation or due to reduced activity of inbuilt compensatory mechanisms coping with heart failure?

(4) If long-term improvements in myocardial function can be attained in one or more sub-groups of patients with heart failure and sinus rhythm,

might this not be more safely and effectively secured by other means, for example by diuretics and/or vasodilators, so that additional driving of the weakened myocardium could be avoided?

These questions have been addressed in a number of studies, in some cases the answers are beginning to emerge.

With regard to the clinical expression of digitalis-induced changes in myocardial contractile condition, there is an evident separation between consistent and significant enhancement of myocardial pump function based upon muscle measurements [68, 69] on one hand, and on the other hand the generally inconsistent, weak and occasionally undetectable effects of digitalis on expression of overall cardiac function which would impress the clinician, such as reduced left atrial pressure or increased cardiac output.

Short-term measurements in man of myocardial developed tension [68] and of force–velocity relationships [69] have clearly demonstrated enhanced contractile function. In the latter study dealing with the non-failing human heart, Sonnenblick and colleagues [69] showed clearly how augmented left ventricular contractile function might be expressed as increased speed of myocardial shortening, and upward displacement of the force–velocity relationship, without changes in cardiac output. They point out that cardiac output in the normal heart is predominantly dependent upon heart rate, preload and afterload, while in advanced myocardial disease, contractile function becomes a major determinant.

In an early study dealing with heart failure, McMichael and Sharpey-Schafer [55] observed increased cardiac output and lowered right atrial pressure within thirty minutes of a high dose intravenous digoxin infusion in a heterogeneous group of patients, some with atrial fibrillation, who appear to have been previously untreated. Results of subsequent investigations were not uniformly so good, though increasingly the effects of concomitant therapy may be considered to have blunted the response. One-third of the patients in sinus rhythm with latent heart failure given digoxin after careful diuretic therapy by Selzer and Malmburg [70] failed to respond with increased cardiac output or decreased venous pressure. Yankopoulos and colleagues [71] summarized the problem in twenty heart failure subjects with sinus rhythm. Increased left ventricular performance was consistently expressed as an increased rate of rise of left ventricular pressure (dP/dt) after ouabain, but clinically significant improvements in cardiac output and filling pressure were observed in only twelve.

Explanations for observed failure to translate improved muscle performance into enhanced overall function have been sought in several directions. The degree to which contractile behaviour determines heart function varies with the nature and severity of heart failure [69].

Discrimination between digitalis-responsive and unresponsive varieties of heart failure on clinical or pathological grounds has not been successful. As a different approach, explanations for the inconsistent results of digitalization have been sought in connection with molecular structural dissimilarities, since these have been considered to determine speed and emphasis of cardiovascular activity. Studies reported by Lee and colleagues [72] using a range of digitalis-like substances with markedly different lipid solubility characteristics failed to distinguish differences between time to onset of activity in isolated cat papillary muscle. These workers were forced to attribute differences in timing of effects in man to variation in tissue distribution, protein binding and possibly in metabolism.

Peripheral vascular effects of digitalis compounds offer the best explanations for problems in discerning consistent haemodynamic benefit with these drugs in heart failure. First, the pre-treatment state of peripheral vascular tone is unlikely to be uniform between patient groups or individuals. Secondly, the molecular characteristics, particularly the polarity of the glycoside used for study, may determine the balance between indirect, neurally mediated activity which is responsible for the majority of vasomotor actions, and direct myocardial effects [73]. Homeostatic responses to heart failure, mediated by sympathetic hyperactivity and parasympathetic withdrawal, include venoconstriction and arterioconstriction, increased noradrenaline release from sympathetic nerve terminals in the myocardium causing increased contractile activity, and tachycardia. Without heart failure, digitalis exerts direct and indirect venous constrictor actions [68, 74]. When sympathetic overactivity has developed in response to cardiac failure, short-term studies have credited digitalis with dilator activity [74], owing to partial withdrawal of sympathetic drive in response to improved cardiac function which over-rides the venoconstrictor action. Digitalis venodilatation seems the likely explanation for striking falls in central venous pressure in the presence of severe heart failure which so impressed early investigators [55], and led to suggestions of a hepatic vein constrictor effect.

Under some conditions the vasoconstrictor effects of digitalis are however readily discernible in cardiac failure. Of the eight patients with moderately severe heart failure studied by Cohn and associates [75], haemodynamic deterioration developed in four some thirty minutes after an intravenous bolus of digoxin, an adverse effect attributed to a sharp increase in systemic vascular resistance. As shown by DeMots and colleagues [76] using ouabain, the speed with which the glycoside is given is a determinant of the peripheral vascular response. A mean 24% increase in systemic resistance seen in their subjects without heart failure after a ten second bolus injection was entirely avoided using a slow infusion over twenty minutes. Evidence from longer-term studies does not support the postulate that increased peripheral resistance may develop with sustained digitalis usage, so counteracting beneficial effects on the myocardium. The four hour haemodynamic study described by Cohn and associates [75] indicated that systemic constrictor activity was transient. The important long-term digoxin withdrawal and reintroduction study of Arnold and co-workers [77], discussed further below, revealed no change in systemic resistance over the several weeks of study.

5.3.1 SUB-GROUPS WHO MAY BENEFIT FROM DIGITALIS

The possibility that some forms of heart disease, certain degrees of severity, or particular conditions of the homeostatic response to heart failure may determine the net response to digitalis, is central to the search for factors which may predict the outcome.

In the presence of segmental or localised myocardial dysfunction, exemplified by localized myocardial fibrous replacement following myocardial infarction, or by regional infiltrative disease, it is possible that increased paradoxical movement or dyskinesia of the abnormal segment may dissipate the effects of contractile stimulation elsewhere [78]. As a result of ischaemia, long-chain fatty acids with digitalis receptor blocking actions may be released [79]. Potassium ion concentrations may increase in the vicinity of anoxic myocardium, and oppose digitalis binding in adjacent myocardium. Information is lacking concerning digitalis receptor density and Na,K-ATPase activity in a range of cardiac disease, which may modulate digoxin responsiveness. The nature of any diastolic as well as systolic ventricular abnormalities may be of decisive importance. Katz [80] has coined the term 'lusitropic' to describe effects upon diastolic ventricular relaxation. Toxic digitalis concentrations are negatively lusitropic, since they adversely affect myocardial relaxation as described above, by increasing diastolic intracellular sodium and calcium concentrations. Effects of therapeutic levels upon sequestration of cytosolic ionized calcium at end-systole are complex but not generally salutary [81], and relaxation is not improved by digitalis, in contrast with for example the catecholamines. Where raised filling pressures reflect diastolic rather than systolic functional problems they may not fall as a direct result of digitalis activity; this limits the potential of digitalis to show benefit in studies which include compliance problems, notably hypertrophic and infiltrative disorders.

Volume-Overloaded Heart Failure : Some of the best evidence supporting the use of digitalis in sinus rhythm heart failure comes from patients with a third heart sound. This clinical marker of volume overloaded ventricular dysfunction has emerged as a predictor of beneficial digitalis response with a degree of consistency. Gheorghiade and Beller [82], studying digoxin withdrawal in a group of patients with ischaemic left ventricular disease in whom cardiac failure was well compensated with diuretic and/or vasodilator therapy, observed slight deterioration following digoxin withdrawal in only two of 24 patients. Both had third sounds; while in only three of the majority who did not deteriorate was this sign present. Patients shown by Arnold and co-workers [77] to benefit from digitalis also had third sounds. By applying multivariate analysis to a scoring system for heart failure during their randomized, double-blind placebo-controlled digoxin introduction study, Lee and colleagues [83] identified the third sound as the strongest correlate of a favourable response. Of their 25 patients in sinus rhythm, 14 showed digoxin-related improvement. All 14 had third sounds, while only one of the non-responders had this sign. Since responses were noted over a period of weeks, the study dealt with medium-term changes and supports the value of digitalis in this group of subjects. Because of subsequent arguments, the care taken by these workers to stabilize patients on prior diuretic therapy needs emphasis. Benefit was most evident in the worst cases of failure, a finding reported by some previous observers [71, 77], though not by all [75]. Such a gradation in responsiveness would fit with simple extrapolation from effects upon a depressed Starling curve of drugs with myocardial stimulant properties, but the severity of failure has not generally emerged as an indicator of a favourable response.

Sub-groups of patients unlikely to benefit from digitalis therapy have been sought. Absence of desirable digitalis lusitropic activity [80] implies that patients suffering primarily from impaired diastolic ventricular compliance should not be regarded as likely responders. Infiltrative disorders such as cardiac amyloid typify this problem. (In addition there is an increased liability to arrhythmia in cardiac amyloid, conceivably caused by locally high digitalis concentrations due to avid binding by amyloid fibrils [84].) In hypertrophic cardiomyopathy, Braunwald and colleagues [85] showed early on that digitalis not only increases the left ventricular outflow tract gradient, but also causes an increase in the already abnormal diastolic pressure. Although tolerable results are achievable [86], digitalis remains contraindicated in hypertrophic myopathy. This alters if, as part of the advanced disease process, atrial fibrillation develops, usually with substantial ill-effect on function, when digitalis can assist by improving ventricular filling as the rate slows [87].

Patients with right heart failure secondary to lung disease (cor pulmonale) have long been established as digitalis-unresponsive [57].

5.3.2 LONG-TERM ACTIVITY OF DIGITALIS

Though a useful short-term response to digitalis in heart failure with sinus rhythm cannot be reliably predicted, there is little doubt that improved ventricular function can be achieved with judicious digitalis administration in an appreciable number of patients with heart failure. Disappointing attempts to prove that benefit could be sustained in the long term (i.e. weeks and months after digitalization) led one reviewer [88] to conclude 'in most patients in sinus rhythm digoxin has no long-term stimulatory action on the heart', but subsequent developments make it doubtful that such a clear statement could now be made. Contributions to the debate have come from two sources. Information has been provided from studies in which a sequence of assessments has been made before and after digitalization in suitable heart failure patients. To this can be added the results of digitalis withdrawal studies, some of which have included observations during subsequent restitution of digitalis treatment. Selzer [89] noted partial loss of digitalis activity three weeks after starting therapy. Davidson and Gibson [90], measuring displacement of the ball in the Starr–Edwards aortic prosthetic valve, found the small increment initially achieved on starting digoxin to be lost at ten days despite adequate plasma levels. Six of their ten patients were possibly not in heart failure, and all had left ventricular hypertrophy, so that substantial benefit might not have been anticipated. Using invasive measurements, Cohn and associates [75] observed loss of initial improvement in impaired left ventricular function over a brief (four hour) period, despite two doses of digoxin during this time. In addition four of their eight patients briefly deteriorated, probably because of raised ventricular afterload due to the systemic vasoconstrictor effect of digoxin. Mechanisms possibly responsible for loss of digitalis effectiveness over such a short period do not include digitalis receptor adaptations, though these may contribute in the longer term [20]. Vasoconstrictor digitalis actions may be involved [75], despite the evidence for initial withdrawal of constrictor activity in heart failure [74, 91]; in addition compensatory sympathetic drive may be partially withdrawn [90]. Myocardial disease may impair glycoside uptake, contributing to initial variability [75]. Longer-term loss of effectiveness has been studied in one patient over four months by Ford and associates [20]. They correlated loss of initial digoxin effects on systolic time intervals with similar loss of effects upon the patient's own red cell sodium pump after four months. Similar loss of effect was noted in the red cells of 46 patients on long-term digoxin; implying that an unknown compensatory mechanism is able to overcome Na,K-ATPase inhibition in the red cell and possibly also in the myocardium, and so to reduce myocardial changes. For the reasons discussed

Table 5.1 Synopsis of digitalis withdrawal studies in patients with heart failure and sinus rhythm

Ref.	Authors	Patients	Investigations	Blind Study?	Results on withdrawal (%) Im-proved	Un-changed	Worse	Comment
67	Starr & Luchi, 1969	12 geriatric women	Clinical and ballistocardiogram	Yes	25%	50%	25%	Probably not all had heart disease
93	Dall, 1970	12 of 53 geriatrics	Clinical	No	67%		33%	41 of 53 patients had no need for digitalis
94	Fonrose et al., 1974	31 elderly patients	Clinical	No	48%		52%	Patients with heart failure excluded. Over half developed failure on withdrawal
95	Hull & Mackintosh, 1977	14 general practice patients	Clinical	No	100%		0	Other therapy increased or started in 50%
65	Dobbs et al., 1977	46 hospital out-patients	Clinical	Yes	65%		35%	Included patients with AF
96	Liverpool Therapeutics Group, 1978	89 general practice patients	Clinical	No	0	100%	0	Only withdrawn if plasma digoxin level sub-therapeutic
97	Krakauer, 1978	22 geriatrics	Clinical and radiological	No	73%		27%	How many had underlying heart failure?

98	McHaffie et al., 1978	5 patients on diuretics	Exercise capacity	No	100%	0	One extra patient excluded having deteriorated
99	Johnston & McDevitt, 1979	22 fully digitalized patients	Systolic time intervals and clinical	No	68%	32%	33 of another 34 under-digitalized patients remained unchanged
77	Arnold et al., 1980	9 patients with moderate failure	Invasive and non-invasive tests	No	0–22%	78–100%	Third heart sounds present, readministration restored haemodynamics
66	Bomann et al., 1981	134 geriatrics	Clinical	No	81%	19%	'Digitalis-dependent' group excluded, some had AF
100	Griffiths et al., 1982	11 patients, 4 with coronary disease	Echocardiogram and systolic time intervals	No	0	100%	Only one patient deteriorated clinically
101	Fleg et al., 1982	80 elderly patients	Echo, exercise	Yes	Objectively slightly worse, no clinical change		Heart failure clinically unaffected in 3 months
82	Gheorgiade & Beller, 1983	24 patients with prior infarctions	Clinical and radionuclide	No	8%	84%	Most were on vasodilators. Deteriorators had third sounds
102	Taggart et al, 1983	22 heart failure patients	Clinical and systolic time intervals	Yes	13%	64%	3 improved on digitalization

earlier, it is not always necessary to achieve overt and persistent pump inhibition in order to generate a myocardial effect [13]. Similarly the nature of any adaptation is unclear, though Ford and associates [20] suggest that new generations of red cells produced under the influence of digitalis carry increased numbers of available sodium pump sites. A similar mechanism is difficult to visualize in the heart.

Sequential studies following digitalis introduction may be complicated by a number of additional considerations, such as the speed of digitalis administration, the state of peripheral vascular tone, coexistant treatment and evolution of heart disease. An alternative study design though also criticized on several grounds [92] involves measurement of the consequences of digitalis withdrawal, and has been deemed ethically acceptable in view of persistent doubts about the treatment's worth.

Results of fifteen digitalis withdrawal studies dealing wholly or partly with patients in heart failure and sinus rhythm are summarized in Table 5.1. Despite the tendency to use these results in discussion concerning digitalis long-term efficacy, the prime object of a number of these studies [93–97] was to focus attention upon indiscriminate and over enthusiastic digitalis prescribing, rather than to look for maintained compensation in cardiac failure. Indeed the investigators' faith in digitalis sometimes compelled them to exclude from study patients with a background of heart failure. A review detailing problems with a similar selection of reports has recently appeared [92]. Johnson and McDevitt [99], measuring systolic time intervals, observed deterioration in seven of 22 previously well-digitalized patients (17 on diuretic treatment) while 33 of 34 patients in whom plasma digoxin levels were sub-therapeutic showed no detriment after withdrawal. Of the deteriorators, only two straightforwardly developed heart failure. Two others developed failure while lapsing into atrial fibrillation; the remainder were deemed to have worsened having developed well-tolerated atrial fibrillation off digixin, bringing into question the significance of any underlying myocardial dysfunction. Ultimately therefore digoxin withdrawal was followed by indisputable heart failure in only two of their 22 patients; in these individuals digoxin dependency was confirmed by improvements on reintroduction.

The adequacy of methodological sensitivity for detection of subtle myocardial alterations has been questioned by Griffiths and colleagues [100]. In their series of eleven patients, four on diuretics, studied before and for six weeks after digoxin withdrawal, only one developed overt pulmonary oedema, while the group as a whole showed echocardiographic evidence of left ventricular dilation, together with diminished contractile function as determined by systolic time intervals. Fleg and colleagues [101] likewise noted no clinical change on withdrawal, despite detectable ventricular dilatation on echocardiography. Gheorghiade and Beller [82] prospectively studied a series of 24 patients with impaired left ventricular function due to prior myocardial infarction, of whom 21 were taking vasodilators and/or diuretics, making clinical, radionuclide and exercise measurements during and one month after stopping digoxin therapy. On the basis of their scoring system most patients were unaffected. Two deteriorated slightly, but two improved. Both deteriorators had third sounds, in line with arguments discussed concerning subgroups with volume overload. Taggart and colleagues [102] similarly found no clear clinical change on placebo, but systolic time-interval measurements indicated slight worsening at this stage.

These studies did little to help the pro-digitalis lobby, since they confirm the suspicion that though the early effects of digitalis may be clinically detectable, subsequent adaptations are usually enough to obscure any clinical benefit, though it may be present if looked for using sensitive equipment. It is not yet possible to say whether such a subtle effect is of importance. The authoritative report of Arnold and co-workers [77] has added helpful new information. These investigators carefully documented a range of resting and exercise haemodynamics in nine patients with heart failure and sinus rhythm, before and after digoxin withdrawal, and again after reintroduction. Cardiac function worsened without digoxin both at rest and on exercise with increased heart rates; matters were restored by restarting therapy. All their patients were on diuretics, with nitrates in two cases, third sounds were present at the outset, and the mean pre-treatment wedge pressure was high, indicating persistent volume overload. Even so, beneficial effects were consistently expressed in clinically important terms, with a fall in cardiac index from mean 2.4 ± 0.7 to 2.0 ± 0.6, and wedge presure elevated from 21 ± 8 to 29 ± 10 mmHg after withdrawal. Although the age range was relatively low (mean 51) and filling pressures were clearly relatively high at the outset, these results provide the strongest argument yet for digitalis efficacy.

Against this kind of information, some opponents have fallen back to a retrenched position, arguing that any deterioration off digoxin can be contained if necessary by adjustments to other therapy, particularly diuretics [59], essentially putting the fourth question asked at the outset. This was the policy adopted by Hull and Mackintosh [95]. In their study recurrent failure on digoxin withdrawal was avoided in all 14 of their heart failure patients, and in three with other pathology, although they needed to introduce or increase other therapy in half. It is argued that patients who benefit from digitalis are simply volume overloaded, and benefit could better be achieved by pushing diuretics more vigorously. The argument does not deny that digitalis is helpful; it remains possible that further benefit may accrue if optimum digitalization is added to well-adjusted alternative therapy including diuretics. McHaffie and colleagues [98] concluded against digoxin, finding no improvement in clinical symptoms or exercise capacity in five patients in whom oral frusemide had been used to produce an optimum 'dry' weight. Those patients shown to benefit from digoxin by Arnold and colleagues [77] were however on a diuretic, and it is doubtful if more could have been achieved by further dehydration. In addition the patient pays a price for attainment of maximal dehydration with potent diuretics, as with other therapy; renin release may follow, leading to angiotensin mediated vasoconstriction, and to counter-productive secondary hyperaldosteronism [103]. Drug combinations comprising a vasodilator and a myocardial stimulant have been shown capable of exerting synergistic effects in short-term heart failure therapy, in that effects are more than the sum of their individual actions. Short-term co-administration of digoxin and nifedipine, the latter chosen for its arteriodilator properties, acts synergistically in this way [104]. In an interesting nine month study using a 'step-care' design [105], patients with heart failure were given diuretics for three months, digoxin was added for the next three months, and in the final phase hydralazine was also brought in as an arteriodilator. Modest improvements occurred in each of the first two periods, seen as stepwise falls in left ventricular filling pressure, cardiac output rose only during the final phase of triple therapy. Benefits extended to exercise measurements. Rigid adherence to monotherapy, for example using diuretics [59], therefore seems out of place. Attenuation of long-term benefits with vasodilator therapy (e.g. prazosin, hyrdalazine) is also well recognized owing to the development of tolerance (tachyphylaxis or desensitization). Results of contractile stimulation using beta-adrenergic agonist drugs may also diminish with time because of possibly protective myocardial adaptations. These may involve either reductions in receptor numbers (down-regulation), or uncoupling of the receptor–agonist interaction from the response normally elicited by binding which leads to an effect on contractile function. Clearly any tendency of digitalis gradually to lose effectiveness in heart failure, whether or not due to receptor adaptations involving development of new sites [20], cannot be considered unique to these drugs.

Also to be included in the equation are adverse effects of digitalis compounds, particularly in patients in sinus rhythm, in whom slowing of the ventricular rate is useless as an indicator of excess digitalis effect [60]. The need for care in managing digitalis therapy is obvious, but arguments in favour of a slight yet significant beneficial long-term haemodynamic effect remain viable. Attention has been diverted from the haemodynamics towards consideration of the myocardium during long-term treatment with stimulant drugs. Katz [106] has questioned the validity of any attempt to drive the failing myocardium using stimulant drugs. He warns that a price may ultimately be paid for bolstering the failing ventricular performance, comprising accelerating disease progression and shortened survival. It is interesting that the role of digitalis was earlier visualized as being to rest the heart [48, 50]; modern thought certainly does not view it in this light [106]. Any value of beta-blockade in long-term heart failure management may derive from interactions with down-regulated beta receptors to prevent excess endogenous catecholamine drive upon the diseased myocardium. Growing interest in vasodilator therapy reflects concerns over long-term myocardial stimulation, as well as an appreciation of the counter-productive effects of the homeostatic responses to declining cardiac output.

5.3.3 DIGITALIS IN CHILDREN

The upper limit of the therapeutic plasma glycoside concentration is higher in paediatric than in adult practice, and standard paediatric doses are between twice and three times those used in adults as a function of body weight [107]. Convention holds that the response to digoxin shown by children in heart failure is greater and more consistent than in adults, so that supplementary treatment with diuretics is often not needed. Counter to the popular view that relatively high sensitivity of the infantile myocardium is the key to these differences, a degree of myocardial resistance has recently been described in the infant heart in volume overloaded failure due to ventricular septal defect (VSD) [108]. In this condition the myocardium can sometimes be shown to be performing well despite clinical heart failure, so that further increments in contractile function may be difficult to achieve. Modest and non-uniform improvements described recently in children [108] have encouraged some to adopt the 'null hypothesis' that digitalis may be unhelpful even in young children [109]. Higher digoxin concentrations found recently in the neonatal human myocardium in comparison with children and adults have been attributed to the relative inability of the immature kidney to clear digoxin [110]. Differences in digitalis binding, always an attractive explanation for age-related contrasts, have been partially confirmed in animal studies. Glycoside binding alters with age in digitalis-sensitive species such as the dog, while in less-sensitive species (e.g. sheep) no differences have been found in either contractile responsiveness or in myocardial Na,K-ATPase inhibition.

Explanations for the long-established clinical observation of favourable digitalis effects in childhood failure may rest with peripheral vascular activity. Of the 21 infants with VSDs studied by Berman and colleagues [108], twelve responded well to digoxin. Of the twelve, six showed no improvements in myocardial function measured by echocardiography, strongly implicating peripheral activity as the key. Sympathetic drive may be very substantial in paediatric heart failure, and sympathetic withdrawal may have particularly beneficial effects on ventricular after-load. Further differences characterize paediatric digitalis therapy; the toxic threshold of infantile myocardial Purkinje fibres and the central nervous system appears relatively high, so that higher plasma levels can be tolerated.

5.3.4 DIGITALIS AND MYOCARDIAL INFARCTION

Doubts over its value in heart failure, coupled with worries about toxicity, make it perhaps surprising that digitalis continues to receive authoritative endorsement in treatment of cardiac failure following myocardial infarction [78]. Patients with this type of heart failure are well represented in both short and long-term studies dealing with digitalis efficacy [77, 82, 98, 101]; cautious acceptance of a beneficial haemodynamic result extends therefore to such patients. To treat cardiac failure in the coronary care unit phase of management, a short-term effect is of paramount importance, and evidence for digitalis is perhaps strongest in this area.

To evaluate the actions of digitalis in myocardial infarction, a number of facts can be marshalled.

(1) Despite animal data to the contrary, studies in man have not demonstrated enhanced sensitivity to the toxic, pro-arrhythmic effects of digitalis after infarction [111, 112].

(2) Contractile stimulant effectiveness is not lost in patients with post-infarction heart failure, since high filling pressures can be reduced and contractile indices of left ventricular function improved after digitalis although cardiac output may not increase [113]. Stimulant effects are expressed upon remaining normal and partially ischaemic heart muscle. Animal data suggest that myocardium subtended by a totally occluded vessel rapidly becomes unresponsive to digitalis while ischaemic territory receiving some supply retains 40–50% responsiveness.

(3) A number of animal studies confirm that overall myocardial oxygen requirements are increased after digitalis, an effect attributed to the oxygen-demanding effects of enhanced ventricular contractile velocity and wall tension. Cardiac glycosides also exert coronary vasoconstrictor actions, mainly indirectly via α-adrenergic stimulation but also by a direct effect. Acting on a dilated ventricule these undesired actions are more than counter-balanced by the oxygen sparing results of reduced ventricular volumes and lessened wall tension. Canine studes [114] suggest

that digitalis may increase ischaemic damage after coronary artery occlusion in the small, non-failing heart, but may limit infarction size where there is ventricular dilatation.

Results consistent with these animal data have been reported by Morrison and colleagues [115]. In their impressive study, evidence in favour of digitalis usage was obtained in patients with large myocardial infarctions and consequent cardiac failure. Regional left ventricular wall motion defects were determined by blood pool scintigraphic imaging (the radionuclide being conventional technetium – 99m incorporated into red cells), the magnitude of the perfusion defect caused by the infarction was assessed by thallium scintigraphy; serial creatine kinase MB isoenzyme measurement also provided infarction size information. When compared against nine control subjects, fourteen digoxin recipients studied on or about days one and five showed no evidence of increased infarction size during this period, nor did they show more ventricular ectopic activity. On the positive side, left ventricular ejection function signifcantly increased during this time in the digitalized group (from mean 0.29 ± 0.09 to 0.33 ± 0.11) while the control group showed a slight but insignificant fall (from mean 0.33 ± 0.12 to 0.3 ± 0.08).

Memories of early unfavourable experiences with digoxin in the coronary care unit treatment of heart failure are exemplified by the report from Balcon and co-workers [116] who noted cardiac output reductions and one case of angina precipitation following bolus digoxin injection. The need to use a slow infusion to avoid a marked systemic constrictor response has been emphasized [76]. Though the infusion protocol is not described by Morrison and associates [115], a twenty minute infusion of 0.5mg digoxin has recently been found beneficial in 25 elderly patients in heart failure post-infarction [117], on the basis of clinically significant criteria such as cardiac index (increased by mean 18%). In this study improvements were best seen in patients with moderate failure, less evident with extreme degrees of ventricular dysfunction. Likewise this, cardiac glycosides emerged without credit when tested by Cohn and colleagues in cardiogenic shock [118]. Evidence for a positive effect on myocardial function was obtained measuring left ventricular dP/dt but there was no impact on depressed cardiac output. In addition systemic vascular resistance rose, initially causing worsened left ventricular function. On the basis of subsequent work [76] this might have been avoided using a slow infusion.

The general thrust of these reports supporting the cautious use of digitalis does not deny that alternative drugs such as dobutamine and the vasodilators may be preferable in the coronary care unit. There are two additional points of concern. Firstly, increased contractile function in

Digitalis: the present position

myocardium adjacent to an infarcted segment may dispose to aneurysmal bulging and/or progressive post-infarction wall thinning. Animal studies have shown no evidence of this undesirable effect [119]; direct measurements over some five days in man suggest this is unlikely [115]. Secondly Katz [106] has warned that the long-term consequence of myocardial stimulation in heart failure may be a counter-productive acceleration in the rate of decline, and shortened patient survival.

These theoretical worries gained credence from two investigations [120, 121] in which increased mortality was linked with digitalis usage in survivors of acute myocardial infarction. Retrospective analysis of 972 survivors of acute infarction [120] indicated a four month mortality of 11% in those on digitalis compared with 3% in the remainder. After a series of adjustments for 'non-digitalis variables' between the two groups, digitalis appeared to convey an approximate doubling of overall mortality, with a five-fold increase in a subset of particularly at-risk patients, those with congestive heart failure and complex ventricular premature depolarizations. Extensive data manipulations were required to deal with the recognized problem that digitalis therapy was itself a marker of the severity of underlying cardiac disease, being used in those with the least favourable prognosis. In a further 490 post-infarction patients followed for one year by Bigger and associates [121], mortality on digitalis was 22%, against 6% in the remainder. Again digitalization reflected the extent of underlying disease, but its use emerged as a significant contributor using multiple regression analysis. The impressive numerical weight of the coronary artery surgery study (CASS) registry has now been brought to bear on this problem [122] with revealing results. Of 14, 547 CASS patients receiving medical treatment for coronary arterial disease, the 45 year cumulative mortality in 2600 digitalized entrants was 18%, against 5% for 11 947 non-digitalized subjects. Subsequent analysis attributed this superficially striking difference to a range of prognostic variables, in particular left ventricular function impairment and number of diseased coronary arteries. Use of digitalis, though clearly a marker of severe heart disease, failed to emerge as relevant to mortality. It seems that the depth and quality of information available in relation to CASS registry entrants allowed successfully filtering out of a wider range of variables relevant to the severity of underlying disease in this [122] study. In the prior studies described [120, 121] digitalis usage may not have been successfully dissociated from uncontrolled prognostic indicators, since angiographic data in particular were unavailable. Prospective studies may provide unequivocal answers, but the CASS registry results are reassuring in regard to digitalis. Accordingly at the present stage of development digitalis is acceptable with heart failure and recent myocardial infarction, though the requirement for slow and

172

cautious introduction is clear. There is little doubt that alternative supportive treatment in the acute stage may be preferable both for control of heart failure and of supraventricular arrhythmias.

5.4 Electrophysiological effects of digitalis

Results of digitalis administration upon a specific cardiac arrhythmia are determined by the arrhythmia substrate and mechanism and by electrolyte environment, heart rate, presence of cardiac disease and additional cardioactive drugs. Digitalis effects upon the atrioventricular junction tend to assist in arrythmia control or termination (antiarrhymic actions), those expressed in the ventricles generally favour emergence and maintenance (pro-arrhythmic actions), while in the atria effects in both directions can be identified.

In studies of the electrophysiological actions of digitalis at a cellular level, the behaviour of His-Purkinje fibres is usually considered representative of effects throughout the heart. Two subtle changes in cellular electrophysiology develop with increased contractile function in the presence of low digitalis concentrations [123, 124]. Phase 2 of the action potential (the plateau phase, associated with calcium influx via slow channels and with excitation–contraction coupling) is prolonged, with similarly increased total action potential duration. In addition, threshold potential declines slightly, indicating increased membrane excitability. His-Purkinje fibre studies in the intact dog heart show slightly increased effective refractoriness, in agreement with these effects [125]. Mechanisms at this stage do not include cation transport inhibition via Na,K-ATPase. Passive resistance of the sarcolemma to current flow is increased; decreased potassium ion permeability reduces outward background potassium current and may be involved in these early effects [123]. Action potential prolongation at this stage does not protect against arrhythmias [126] and cannot be considered as a Class III antiarrhythmic effect [127].

More prolonged, non-toxic exposure accelerates repolarization, reducing action potential duration and refractoriness [126]. This has been confirmed directly in human atrium [127] and ventricular myocardium [128]. Na, K-APTase inhibition and decreased transmembrane cation gradients may now play a part probably explaining accompanying partial cell depolarization and lowered resting membrane potential. Changes in diastolic membrane function (phase 4 of the action potential) also emerge at this stage. Spontaneous diastolic depolarization (upwardly sloping phase 4), characteristic of Purkinje fibres and other cells with pacemaker capability, results from the combination of a steady background inward sodium current and a gradually diminishing outward potassium flow. By further

173

inhibiting potassium efflux and by other means, digitalis increases the rate of phase 4 depolarization, so that the intrinsic discharge rate of subsidiary potential pacemaker foci is increased. This effect is additionally pro-arrhythmic, together with previously described effects on refractoriness and on excitability, although these effects precede overt digitalis toxicity.

Toxic exposure causes substantial Na,K-ATPase inhibition. While mechanisms responsible for contractile effects and low-dose electrophysiological actions may be uncertain, cation pump inhibition is clearly central to development of toxicity. Cation gradients and resting membrane potential are decreased, and the cell becomes progressively depolarized. The rate of action potential upstroke (phase 0 depolarization), conduction velocity and action potential duration are all depressed. Two further abnormalities associated with digitalis toxicity have been observed during phase 4 of the action potential. Spontaneous depolarization is accelerated, particularly with low extracellular potassium levels, owing to a direct inhibitory effect of digitalis upon potassium ion permeability [129]. This increases the discharge rate of ectopic pacemaker foci sited in the specialized ventricular conducting system, facilitating emergence of toxic ventricular arrhythmias. As a second pro-arrhythmic mechanism in diastole, spontaneous membrane potential oscillations develop in phase 4, termed delayed after-potentials [130] or low amplitude potentials [131]. They occur soon after repolarization. After-potential amplitude increases with advancing toxicity and salvoes may develop, attaining threshold and initiating a train of extrasystolic depolarizations. Abnormal transient increased sodium currents are probably responsible, but the calcium channel blocking agent verapamil counteracts after-depolarizations in digitalis toxicity [131], probably because abnormal sodium currents reflect increased membrane permeability caused primarily by abnormal fluctuations in free calcium levels near the sarcolemma [132, 133] which are moderated by verapamil. Increasingly malignant ventricular arrhythmias and paroxysmal atrial tachycardias seen in digitalis toxicity may have this basis, though ventricular arrhythmias also owe much to sympathetic nervous system interactions [134, 135].

Digitalis actions upon physiologically discrete cardiac components are summarized in Table 5.2. Indirect effects of digitalis generally outweigh direct actions on the heart. Acetylcholine-mediated parasympathetic effects are paramount at atrial and atrioventricular junctional levels. Noradrenaline-mediated sympathetic actions predominate below this level, particularly in the presence of toxicity. Acetylcholine sensitivity is retained in the ventricles; lack of parasympathetic digitalis activity here reflects the paucity of vagal innervation below the proximal interventri-

174

Table 5.2 Cardiac electrophysiological effects of digitalis

	Direct effect	Indirect effect	Total effect
Sinoatrial node	Variable depression[157]	Slight vagal slowing	Minimally slowed conduction time and discharge rate[158]
Atrium	Variable ERP prolongation[145]	Dominant ERP reduction, but biphasic [40,127,145]	Reduced ERP, CV increased
Atrioventricular junction	Minimal slowing[145]	Significant ERP prolongation, CV increased[145]	Major increase in ERP and CV[145]
Accessory atrioventricular pathway	Probably reduced ERP	Probably vagal ERP reduction [128], but undefined	Variable, ERP often dangerously reduced[152]
His–Purkinje system	Slight ERP increase, CV unchanged[125]	Minimal effect without toxicity	Slight ERP prolongation[125]
Ventricular myocardium	Slight ERP prolongation	Vagal ERP reduction at base [128] (Sympathetic ERP reduction with toxicity)	Slight overall ERP lengthening[126]

(Key: ERP = Effective refractory period;   CV = Conduction velocity)

cular septum, although some has been discerned in the right ventricular outflow tract [128].

The dominance of parasympathetically mediated effects on supraventricular structures is achieved by digitalis actions at multiple levels in the vagal control system. Carotid, aortic and cardiopulmonary baroreceptors supplying afferent innervation are sensitized by digitalis [136], central vagal nuclei are stimulated [134], vagal efferent traffic is increased [137], there is enhanced supraventricular cardiac sensitivity to vagal stimulation [138], and acetylcholine is released from local stores in the atrial myocardium [40]. Studies in the cat show that interactions with parasympathetic innervation outside the brain are more important than effects upon vagal control centres [134].

Digitalis: the present position

Digitalis increases sympathetic drive in the heart. In experimental animal studies, sympathetic hyperactivity appears minimal until toxicity at which point hyperactivity develops in parallel with toxic ventricular arrhythmias. Removal of cardiac sympathetic innervation by spinal cord transection greatly increases the threshold to toxicity [134]. Though digitalis in sub-toxic doses does not increase sympathetic drive in the cat, part of the vasoconstrictor response to intravenous digitalis seen in normal human subjects [68, 74] reflects increased sympathetic drive, although substantial contributions come from direct stimulation of vascular α- receptors and from vasoconstriction caused by inhibition of vascular smooth muscle Na,K-ATPase. (Direct glycoside access to the central nervous system may also provoke vasoconstriction by sympathetic stimulation of renal β-receptors, provoking renin release and increased angiotensin II activity [139].) Penetration of the central nervous system is rapid after intravenous digitalis. The studies by Somberg and colleagues identify a small portion of the medulla (the area postrema) as the centre from which increased efferent sympathetic activity generates toxic ventricular arrhythmias [135] and widespread vasoconstriction [140].

Involvement of central sympathetic control centres in digitalis toxic ventricular arrhythmias has been confirmed by direct injection into the cerebral ventricles of the rat. Resultant cardiac arrhythmias were opposed by prior sympathetic ganglion blockade [141]. Predictably therefore, β-blocking drugs have proved valuable in treatment of digitalis-toxic arrhythmias [142], although alternative treatments may be preferable since β-blockers may increase digitalis-induced atrioventricular block.

Central sympathetic effects of digitalis are modified by peripheral actions. Sensitization of peripheral baroreceptor and chemoreceptor activity by sub-toxic digitalis doses tends to diminish sympathetic activity, and high dose direct digitalis effects can decrease senstivity to catecholamines shown by sinoatrial and atrioventricular nodes.

5.4.1 ATRIAL EFFECTS OF DIGITALIS

Vagal hypertonia substantially reduces action potential duration in the atrium. Repolarization is accelerated [40], conduction velocity is increased, refractory periods decreased [143] and the results may be onset of atrial fibrillation [144]. The basis of these effects is increased potassium ion permeability with acetylcholine, causing hyperpolarization, increased action potential amplitude and more rapid phase 0 depolarization [126]. Atrial effects of digitalis exposure in man very closely replicate these changes [40]. Direct effects on the atrium include slight refractory period prolongation on the basis of animal data, and are submerged by opposing indirect effects [145] until toxic conditions are attained, when

176

direct actions depress membrane potential and increase phase 4 automaticity [40]. Conflicting accounts of atrial effects of digitalis [146] and of vagal hyperactivity [147] may stem in part from two additional considerations. Firstly the initial atrial response to digitalis administration may be biphasic, particularly when the heart rate is slow, in close agreement with effects upon isolated His-Purkinje tissues described above. Action potential duration may be initially prolonged, shortening only after 15–20 minutes [40, 127]. As mentioned, atrial action potential prolongation is not antiarrhythmic, possibly because regional non-uniformity of repolarization is increased at this stage [127]. Atropine opposes both phases. Local release of acetylcholine is involved as well as increased vagal tone [40].

Secondly, inhomogeneous distribution of action potential changes [127], probably reflecting non-uniform dispersal of vagal innervation [144], may complicate results. The later effect, with action potential shortening and increased conduction velocity, underlies the well-recognized tendency to convert atrial flutter into atrial fibrillation [127, 148]. Effects on the atrioventricular junction are not involved. [148].

5.4.2 ATRIOVENTRICULAR JUNCTION EFFECTS OF DIGITALIS

Effects on and around the atrioventricular node are of cardinal importance in slowing transmission of atrial tachyarrhythmias to the ventricles. Shortened atrial refractoriness in atrial fibrillation means that partial antegrade penetration of the upper atrioventricular node, and impulse collision in the atrial approaches to the node, are increased. Simultaneously, increased junctional acetylcholine activity greatly increases nodal refractoriness and retards conduction. Digitalis also decreases sensitivity to catecholamines at this site. Studies in man after cardiac transplantation confirm the predominance of indirect vagal effects on the atrioventricular junction; the contribution from direct activity was insignificant in the denervated heart [145].

Digoxin remains the first-line treatment for ventricular rate control in atrial fibrillation. Effectiveness in controlling exercise heart rate in atrial fibrillation can be sub-optimum despite good control at rest [149]. Supplementary drugs such as beta-blocking agents or verapamil may be needed [149]. Verapamil in doses of 240–480 mg daily may be required to gain optimum exercise control in digitalized patients, and appears safe [150], despite its ability to reduce digoxin elimination [151].

Digitalis is potentially dangerous in conditions with an accessory pathway between atrium and ventricle. Approximately one third of the 21 patients with Wolff–Parkinson–White syndrome studied by Sellers and associates [152] developed faster bypass transmission to the ventricles in atrial fibrillation after digoxin, and increased liability to development of lethal atrioventricular fibrillation was confirmed. Prediction of safety or otherwise is difficult, but a patient with an accessory pathway antegrade refractory period of less than 300 ms is considered an unacceptable risk for digoxin treatment in atrial fibrillation. Most patients with re-entrant nodal tachycardia predictability benefit from the nodal actions of digitalis [153].

Prophylactic digitalization is used to reduce the incidence of supraventricular tachycardia in the perioperative phase of cardiac surgery. Striking success has recently been achieved, with apparent reduction in tachyarrhythmia incidence from 72% to 5% [154].

Digitalis may be effective against supraventricular arrhythmias in the mitral prolapse syndrome [155]. Digoxin has no place in management of ventricular rhythm disturbances. In a recent Holter monitoring study, digoxin had no impact on complex ventricular arrhythmias against placebo in patients with heart failure or with normal ventricular functions, although a slight and questionably important reduction in ectopic beat frequency occurred in those with normal function [156]. The slight increase in effective refractoriness of the His-Purkinje system noted in dogs after digitalis may be relevant [125], though worries over the indirect, sympathetically mediated pro-arrhythmic effects of high dose exposure counteract any tendency to use digitalis for ventricular arrhythmia protection.

5.5 Clinical pharmacology of digitalis

5.5.1 BIOLOGICAL AVAILABILITY

Digitalis absorption from the gastrointestinal tract involves first-order kinetics, in which absorption proceeds by passive diffusion. Intrinsic lipid solubility of the molecule is therefore influential in determining the fraction of the oral dose which is absorbed so as to exert its pharmacological effect, that is the biological availability [158, 159]. Non-lipophilic digoxin, with a relatively polar molecule, is approximately 65% absorbed from tablets which fulfil current formulation standards, lanatoside C is closely similar. Less polar β-acetyldigoxin is approximately 80/ absorbed; substantial loss of the acetyl group during absorption means this side chain acts solely as a facilitator of absorption. Lipophilic digitoxin and newer β-methyl digoxin [160] achieve near-complete absorption. The relationship between lipophilic properties and biological availability is frequently obscured by further determinants of gastrointestinal absorption. The particle size of the active drug present in the tablet has emerged as a major influence [159] since it governs the readiness of the drug to enter solution in the gut. Digoxin is nearly insoluble in water, but dissolves better in organic solvents; absorption can be improved by giving it orally as a solution. A weak solution of 0.05% digoxin with 10% alcohol (digoxin elixir) provides improved absorption (70–85%). Capsules are now available containing a relatively high concentration of digoxin, dissolved in ethanol plus polyethylene glycol and propylene glycol. Nearly complete (90–100%) absorption is claimed using these capsules, indicating that prior complete dissolution overcomes any inherent limitations on absorption caused by molecular polarity. Using this oral formulation the initial plasma level peak is high. Though this in unlikely to reflect levels in the myocardium [17, 161], centres in the medulla mediating the nausea and vomiting reaction may be provoked. There is no evidence that this concern extends to the adjacent control centres in sympathetic cardiac and vasomotor responses. Complete absorption is usually equated with predictable and constant absorption. Variations in serum digoxin levels between and within patients should be minimized using new digoxin formulations with enhanced absorption characteristics.

Certain malabsorption syndromes, scleroderma and post-irradiation damage decrease digoxin absorption, but partial gastrectomy (Bilroth types I and II), and jenunoileal bypass operations do not. Most absorption takes place in the jejunum; provided that the proximal twelve inches is intact, uptake is satisfactorily preserved, though there is a correlation between digoxin absorption and the length of jejunum remaining after resection [162].

Co-administered drugs exert significant effects. Interference with uptake may occur through physical adsorption of digoxin in the gut by anti-diarrhoea preparations based on kaolin–pectin, by charcoal, and by bile acid binding resins including cholestyramine and colestipol – advantage can be taken of this phenomenon in treating toxicity. A similar though milder effect occurs with high-fibre foods. Interference with digoxin absorption can be simply pre-empted by giving it not less than fifteen minutes before these materials [163]. Drugs which increase gut motility and reduce transit time (metoclopramide) decrease absorption; those which decrease motility (propantheline, diphenoxylate) promote uptake. Liquid antacids decrease absorption (magnesium hydroxide, magnesium trisilicate, aluminium hydroxide). Anti-cancer chemotherapeutic agents decrease absorption [164], probably due to gut epithelial damage. (Adriamycin interacts with digitalis in the myocardium. Digitalis was considered protective against adriamycin cardiotoxicity; more recently adriamycin has been shown to oppose ouabain-toxic delayed after depolarizations.) Neomycin and sulphasalazine reduce digoxin absorption by a mechanism which is undefined but dissimilar from effects on metabolism of other antibiotics discussed below. Absorption remains unimpaired with cardiac and renal failure.

Enterohepatic recycling of digitalis glycosides is important in man, and is sufficient with β-methyl digoxin [160] and digitoxin [165] to generate secondary plasma level peaks after initial gastrointestinal uptake. Biliary intubation and external drainage accelerate digitoxin clearance.

5.5.2 DRUG INTERACTIONS WITH DIGITALIS

Since the quinidine–digoxin interaction was recognized an increasing number have come to light, with implications for therapy. Quinidine increases the rate though possibly not the total amount of digoxin absorbed from the gut. Digoxin elimination by renal and non-renal routes declines, and the apparent volume of distribution is reduced. Serum digoxin concentrations may increase by 50 to 200% within a few days of starting quinidine, particularly if renal impairment is present [166]. It has been suggested that the cardiac effect of this rise may be less than expected since quinidine displaces digoxin from Na,K-ATPase receptors [166, 167]; not all studies confirm this. Digoxin doses should in general be halved if quinidine is to be introduced. Quinine now appears to exert similar effects. Other local anaesthetic antiarrhythmic agents such as procainamide, disopyramide and mexiletine do not generate this problem. Quinidine affects digitoxin elimination in the same way, though the total effect is less than with digoxin, since the volume of distribution is unaffected.

Verapamil similarly increases serum digoxin concentrations by reducing distribution volume, and elimination by renal and non-renal routes [151, 166]. Its effect may diminish with time, unless there is renal disease. High dose verapamil has been successfully used with digoxin [150] but caution is needed [151], and digoxin levels may increase by some 40%. Incomplete or conflicting data are available on other calcium antagonist drugs. Nifedipine and diltiazem probably have minimal effects in this direction. Amiodarone may precipitate digoxin toxicity, and significantly increases serum digoxin levels [168]. The trend towards multiple antiarrhythmic drug regimes increases the probability of three-way interactions.

Vasodilator drugs do not affect digoxin absorption, but hydralazine may increase renal tubular secretion and reduce serum digoxin concentrations. Drugs which alter serum protein binding affect free levels of digitoxin (95% protein bound), though not digoxin (20–30% protein bound). Of a number tested, only tolbutamide and clofibrate increased free digitoxin levels; warfarin did not [169]. Enzyme-inducing drugs such as rifampicin, phenobarbitone and epanutin increase metabolic inactivation of digitoxin [169] though there is no discernable effect on digoxin.

Epanutin also opposes digitalis binding to Na,K-ATPase as discussed in the preceding text.

5.5.3 DIGOXIN METABOLISM

Though there is substantial variation between individuals, usually more than 75% of digoxin absorbed into the body is eliminated unchanged, whereas over 90% of digitoxin is eliminated as metabolites. Digoxin metabolism however takes place in several directions. Digitoxose sugars are serially hydrolysed, producing in turn cardioactive and increasingly lipophilic digoxigenin bis- and mono-digitoxoside, and ultimately digoxigenin. The genin is some 50% less cardioactive than digoxin though it readily penetrates the central nervous system and may thus elicit side effects. The mono-digitoxide is probably 50% more cardioactive; studies in the cat (like man, a digitalis sensitive species) suggest it has a wider therapeutic ratio than digoxin, in line with concepts of digitalis receptor duality [16] discussed above. Most hydrolosis occurs in the liver; some in the stomach if the pH is very low. A fraction of these metabolites undergoes hepatic conjugation with sulphate or glucuronate radicals, and is inactivated. Secreted into the bile, some is reabsorbed from the gut to appear in the urine. Epi- and keto-derivatives are also formed.

First observed in 1968 [170], a new pathway of digoxin metabolism has been the subject of increasing interest. In that year digoxin resistance in a man with atrial fibrillation was attributed to conversion of digoxin into dihydrodigoxin, a cardioinactive metabolite in which the lactone ring at C-17 is fully saturated. (As described, this structure is of key importance in achieving successful binding to Na,K-ATPase [15, 16].) The capacity of the individual to metabolize digoxin to dihydrodigoxin and other di-hydrometabolites of the products of sugar hydrolysis (collectively termed digoxin reduced products, DRPs) varies enormously. Watson and colleagues [171] identified up to 39% of total digoxin and methylene chloride extractable metabolites as DRPS. Greenwood and co-workers [172] used mass spectroscopy to identify an average of 16% urinary digoxin-related compounds as dihydrodigoxin in unselected long-term digoxin takers. Having developed a specific radioimmunoassay for DRPs, Lindenbaum, Butler and associates have extensively researched this phenomenon [173]. The DRP source is in the gut, probably in the colon. The lactone ring reduction step is performed by a number of strains of *Eubacterium lentum*, a Gram-negative non-spore forming anaerobic rod with a very limited metabolic repertoire. Possession of this organism and hence of DRP forming capacity is unpredictable. It is absent in the very young, and more prevalent in some ethnic groups, but in general age, sex, renal function and serum digoxin concentrations have no bearing on DRP production. Some rare individuals produce 40% DRPs in their urine (expressed as a function of total digoxin-like material); DRPs may be detected in the serum in such cases. The organism can be eradicated by antibiotics, particularly erythromycin and tetracycline. Deletion of this diversionary pathway by erythromycin may result in digoxin toxicity in substantial DRP producers.

Intravenous digoxin administration does not circumvent DRP formation, since enterohepatic recycling and possibly intestinal secretion of digoxin provide substrate for the organism in the lower bowel. Production of DRPs is lessened during oral digoxin treatment if preparations with high biological availability are used, on the grounds that near-complete upper bowel absorption reduces the substrate supply. This may be valuable in patients in whom apparent digoxin resistance turns out to be due to substantial DRP formation. Avoidance of DRP formation using well-absorbed preparations represents a further indication for their use, adding to familiar arguments concerning variability of absorption with the less biologically available formulations. Between one in three and one in ten of digoxin recipients have been found to produce significant quantities of DRPs (more than 5% of the total digoxin elimination) in the urine [173].

5.5.4 DIGITALIS TOXICITY

A number of factors contribute to toxicity in digitalized patients, found in up to 35% of recipients in past years. The therapeutic ratio of traditional glycosides remains strikingly low, though this may be improved in the future [11, 16]. The therapeutic: toxic ratio has been calculated as 1 : 4. Renal impairment increases digoxin levels; drug interactions (preceding section) are increasingly recognized. Patients with impaired atrioventricular conduction may progress to complete block. Those with atrial fibrillation and a ventricular rate of 60 or less should not receive digitalis. Hypokalaemia, often diuretic-induced, potentiates digitalis efects on Na,K-ATPase (as discussed), and adds to toxictiy. Hypercalcaemia and hypomagnesaemia act similarly. Hyperthyroidism causes digoxin insensitivity [18] and increased digoxin elimination; digitalis sensitivity is increased in myxoedema. Amyloid infiltration may cause local digoxin toxicity in the myocardium [84]. Sensitivity is increased with high sympathetic drive or exogenous catecholamines and with chronic lung disease. Diagnosis may be difficult in borderline cases with plasma digoxin concentrations between 1.3 and 2.5 nmol/l, and is more likely if the simultaneously measured serum potassium is low [174].

Digitalis removal, potassium correction and toxic arrhythmia control are the corner-stones of toxicity management. Ventricular tachyarrhythmias require epanutin 100 mg i.v, with repeated doses at intervals (favoured since it opposes digitalis binding, and may improve atrioventricular conduction), or lignocaine. If cardioversion is needed, energy levels must be low, and toxic arrhythmias may re-emerge. Correction of low serum potassium is important, giving 20–40 mmol/h by slow infusion [174]; this will reduce digitalis binding to Na,K-ATPase. Extreme overdosage with attempted suicidal digoxin ingestion may present with hyperkalaemia due to intracellular potassium efflux so that potassium is contraindicated. Atropine is helpful for atrioventricular block owing to the heavy vagal involvement.

Digoxin absorption from the gut can be reduced with cholestyramine. Removal is not achieved with dialysis. The steroidal aldosterone antagonist canrenoate opposes digitalis arrhythmias, but not by preventing binding. A dramatic reduction in the usual two thirds mortality of extreme digitalis toxicity accompanying massive overdose (with serum concentrations in the range 6–20+ nmol/l) has been achieved using digoxin antibody to inactivate circulatory digoxin (or digitoxin [174, 175]. Sheep antidigoxin antibody is cleaved into three fragments using papain. The 50 000 dalton molecular weight Fab fragment carries specific digoxin binding sites and rapidly picks up digoxin on a molecule for molecule basis. The serum is quickly cleared, and the conjugate is eliminated via the kidneys. Anaphylaxis is a source of concern, but has not been a problem. Preliminary intradermal testing is necessary. Some digoxin radioimmunoassays may be invalidated after Fab fragment infusion [176]. The material is available from regional poisons units, the dose is calculated on the basis of the digoxin load, using plasma digoxin concentration and body weight. In addition to the present encouraging results, the principle involved has potential for other toxic conditions.

References

1. Repke, K.R.H., Herrman, J., Kunze, R., Portius, H.J., Schön, R. and Schönield, W. (1973) Mechanism of digitalis action. In *Digitalis* (eds O. Storstein, S. Nitter-Hauge & L. Storstein), Gyldendal Norsk Forlag, Oslo, pp. 143–51.
2. Schwartz, A. and Adams, R.J. (1980) Studies on the digitalis receptor. *Circ. Res.*, **46** (Suppl. 1), 1-154–60.
3. Akera, T. (1977) Membrane adenosine triphosphatase: A digitalis receptor? *Science*, **198**, 569–74.
4. Langer, G.A., (1983) The sodium pump lag revisited. *J. Mol. Cell. Cardiol.*, **15**, 647–51.
5. Glitsch, H.G., Reuter, H. and Scholz, H. (1970) The effect of the internal sodium concentration on sodium fluxes in isolated guinea-pig auricles. *J. Physiol.*, **209**, 25–43.
6. Reuter, H. (1974) Exchange of calcium ions in the mammalian myocardium. Mechanisms and physiological significance. *Circ. Res.* **34**, 599–605.
7. Langar, G.A. and Serena, S.D. (1970) Effects of strophanthidin upon

contraction and ionic exchange in rabbit ventricular myocardium: relation to control of the active state. *J. Mol. Cell. Cardiol.*, 1, 65–90.

8. Carafoli, E. (1984) How calcium crosses plasma membranes including the sarcomere. In *Calcium Antagonists and Cardiovascular Disease* (ed. L.H. Opie), Raven Press, New York, pp. 29–41.

9. Katz, A.M. (1984) Calcium fluxes across the sarcoplasmic reticulum. in *Calcium Antagonists and Cardiovascular Disease* (ed. L.H. Opie), Raven Press, New York, pp. 53–66.

10. Vassalle, M. and Lin, C.I. (1979) Effect of calcium on strophanthidin-induced electrical and mechanical toxicity in cardiac Purkinje fibres. *Am. J. Physiol.*, 236, H689.

11. Lüllmann, H., Peters, T. and Preuner, J. (1982) Mechanism of action of digitalis glycosides in the light of new experimental observations. *Eur. Heart J.*, 3 (Suppl. D) 45–51.

12. Langer, G.A. (1968) Ion fluxes in cardiac excitation and contraction and their relation to myocardial contractility. *Physiol. Rev.*, 48, 708–57.

13. Noble, D. (1980) Mechanism of action of therapeutic levels of cardiac glycosides. *Cardiovasc. Res.*, 14, 495–514.

14. Erdmann, E. and Brown, L. (1984) The cardiac glycoside-receptor system in the human heart. *Eur. Heart J.*, 5 (Suppl. A), 61–5.

15. Thomas, R., Brown, L., Boutagy, J, and Gelbart, A. (1980) The digitalis receptor. Inferences from structure–activity relationship studies. *Circ. Res.*, 46, (Suppl 1), 1-167–72.

16. Godfraind, T. (1984) Subclassification of cardiac glycoside receptors. In *Cardiac Glycoside Receptors and Positive Inotropy. Evidence for more than one receptor?* (ed. E. Erdmann), Supplement to *Basic Research in Cardiology*, Vol. 79, Steinkopff Verlag, Darmstadt, pp. 27–34.

17. Hayward, R., Greenwood, H., Stephens, J., and Hamer, J. (1983) Relationship between myocardial uptake and actions in heart failure of methy-digoxin. *Br. J. Clin. Pharmacol.*, 15, 41–8.

18. Erdmann, E. and Brown, L. (1983) The cardiac glycoside-receptor system in the human heart. *Eur. Heart J.*, 4 (Suppl A), 61–5.

19. Smith, T.W., Kim, D. and Barry, W.H. (1984) Studies of the inotropic mechanisms of cardiac glycosides in cultured heart cells. In *Cardiac Glycoside Receptors and Positive Inotropy* (ed. E. Erdmann), supplement to *Basic Research in Cardiology* Vol. 79, Steinkopff Verlag, Darmstadt, pp 140–6.

20. Ford, A.R., Aronsen, J.K., Grahame-Smith, D.G. and Carver, J.G. (1979) The acute changes seen in cardiac glycoside receptor sites, [86]rubidium uptake and intracellular sodium concentrations in the erythrocytes of patients during the early phases of digoxin therapy are not found during chronic therapy: pharmacological and therapeutic complications for chronic digoxin therapy. *Br. J. Clin. Pharmacol.*, 8, 135–42.

21. Sweadner, K.J. (1979) Two molecular forms of $(Na^+ + K^+)$ -stimulated ATPase in brain. *J. Biol. Chem.*, 254, 6060–70.

22. Graves, S.W., Brown, B. and Valdes, R. (1983) An endogenous digoxin-like substance in patients with renal impairment. *Ann. Intern. Med.*, 99, 604–8.

23. Lancet (Editorial) (1983) Endogenous foxglove. *Lancet*, ii, 1463–4.

24. Godfraind, T., De Pover, A., Castaneda, H. and Fagoo, M. (1982) Cardiodigin endogenous digitalis like material from mammalian heart. *Arch. Int.*

Pharmacodyn. Ther., **258**, 165–7.

25. De Wardener, H.E. and Clarkson, E.M. (1982) The natriuretic hormone: recent developments. *Clin. Sci.*, **63**, 415–20.
26. Thibault, G., Garcia, R., Contin, M. and Genest, J. (1983) Atrial natriuretic factor, characterization and partial purification. *Hypertension*, **5**, 1-75–80.
27. Langer, G.A. (1981) Mechanism of action of the cardiac glycosides on the heart. *Biochem. Pharmacol.*, **30**, 3261–4.
28. Hougen, T.J. and Smith, T.W. (1978) Inhibition of myocardial monovalent cation active transport by subtoxic doses of ouabain in the dog. *Circ. Res.*, **42**, 856–63.
29. Hougen, T.J., Lloyd, B.L. and Smith, T.W. (1979) Effects of inotropic and arrhythmogenic digoxin doses and of digoxin specific antibody on myocardial monovalent cation transport in the dog. *Circ. Res.*, **44**, 23–31.
30. Ghysel-Burton, J. and Godfraind, T. (1977) Importance of the lactone ring for the action of therapeutic doses of ouabain in guinea pig atria. *J. Physiol.*, **266**, 75–6P.
31. Blood, B.E. and Noble, D. (1978) Two mechanisms for the inotropic action of ouabain on sheep cardiac Purkinje fibre contractility. In *Biophysical Aspects of Cardiac Muscle* (ed. Morad), Academic Press, New York, pp. 369–78.
32. Rhee, H.M., Dutta, S. and Marks, B.H. (1976) Cardiac Na^+ -K^+, ATPase activity during positive inoptropic and toxic actions of ouabain. *Eur. J. Pharm.*, **37**, 141–53.
33. Selden, R. and Smith, T.W. (1972) Ouabain pharmacokinetics in dog and man: determination by radioimmunoassay. *Circulation*, **45**, 1176–82.
34. Poole-Wilson, P.A., Galindez, E. and Fry, C.H. (1979) Effect of ouabain in therapeutic concentrations on K^+ exchange and contraction of human and rabbit myocardium. *Clin. Sci.*, **57**, 415–20.
35. Okita, G.T., Richardson, F. and Roth-Schechter, B.F. (1973) Dissociation of the positive inotropic action of digitalis from inhibition of sodium- and potassium-activated adenosine triphosphatase. *J. Pharm. Exp. Ther.*, **185**, 1–11.
36. Gadsby, D.C. (1980) Activation of electrogenic Na^+/K^+ exchange by extracellular K^+ in canine cardiac Purkinje fibres. *J. Gen. Physiol.*, **65**, 345–65.
37. Hart, G., Noble, D. and Shimoni, Y. (1983) The effects of low concentrations of cardiotonic steroids on membrane currents and tension in sheep Purkinje fibres. *J. Physiol.*, **334**, 103–31.
38. Bernabei, R. and Vassalle, M. (1984) The inotropic effects of strophanthidin in Purkinje fibres and the sodium pump. *Circulation*, **69**, 618–31.
39. Ghysel-Burton, J. and Godfraind, T. (1979) Stimulation and inhibition of the sodium pump by cardioactive steriods in relation to their binding sites and their inotropic effect on guinea-pig isolated atria. *Br. J. Pharmacol.*, **66**, 175–84.
40. Hordof, A.J., Spotnitz, A., Mary-Rabine, L., Edie, R.N. and Rosen, M. R. (1978) The cellular electrophysiologic effects of digitalis on human atrial fibres. *Circulation*, **57**, 223–9.
41. Grupp, G., Grupp, I., Ghysel-Burton, J., Godfraind, T. and Schwartz, A. (1982) Effects of very low concentrations of ouabain on contractile force of isolated guinea-pig, rabbit and rat atria and right ventricular papillary muscles: an interinstitutional study. *J. Pharmacol. Exp. Ther.*, **220**, 145–51.

42. Hougen T.J., Spicer, N. and Smith, T.W. (1981) Stimulation of monovalent cation active transport by low concentrations of cardiac glycosides. Role of catecholamines. *J. Clin. Invest.*, **68**, 1207–14.
43. Lechat, P., Malloy, C.R. and Smith, T.W. (1983) Active transport and inotropic state in guinea-pig left atrium. *Circ. Res.* **52**, 411–22.
44. Petch, M.C. and Nayler, W.G. (1979) Concentration of catecholamines by human cardiac muscle in-vitro. *Br. Heart. J.*, **41**, 336–9.
45. Weingart, R., Kass, R.S. and Tsien, R.W. (1978) Is digitalis inotropy associated with enhanced slow inward calcium current? *Nature*, **273**, 389–91.
46. Marban, E. and Tsien, R.W. (1979) Oubain increases the slow inward calcium current in ventricular muscle. *J. Physiol.*, **292**, 72–3P.
47. Withering, W. (1785) An account of the foxglove, and some of its medical uses: with practical remarks on dropsy, and other diseases. In *Cardiac Classics* (eds F.A. Willius & T.E. Keys), H Kimpton, London, 1941 pp. 231–52.
48. Bouillaud, J. (1835) *Traité Clinique des Maladies du Coeur.* Paris.
49. Mackenzie, J. (1911) Digitalis, *Heart*, **2**, 273–386.
50. Lewis T. (1919) On cardinal principles in cardiological practice. *Br. Med. J.*, **2**, 621–5.
51. Christian, H.A. (1919) Digitalis therapy: satisfactory effects in cardiac cases with regular pulse-rate. *Am. J. Med. Sci.*, **157**, 593–603.
52. Harrison, T.R., Calhoun, L.A. and Turley, F.C. (1931) Congestive heart failure. XI. The effect of digitalis on the dyspnoea and on the ventilation of ambulatory patients with regular cardiac rhythm. *Arch. Int. Med.*, **48**, 1203–16.
53. Gavey, C.J. and Parkinson, J. (1939) Digitalis in heart failure with normal rhythm. *Br. Heart J.*, **1**, 27–44.
54. Wood, P. (1940) The action of digitalis in heart failure with normal rhythm. *Br. Heart J.*, **2**, 132–40.
55. McMichael, J. and Sharpey-Schafer, E.P. (1944) The action of intravenous digoxin in man. *Q. J. Med. (NS)* **13**, 123–35.
56. Lewis, T. (1946). *Diseases of the Heart*, 4th edn, MacMillan, London.
57. McMichael, Sir J. (1982) Digitalis in the last half century. *Eur. Heart J.*, **3** (Suppl D), 3–4.
58. Smith, T.W. and Haber, E. (1973) Digitalis (Second of four parts). *N. Engl. J. Med.*, **289**, 1010–5.
59. Guz, A. and McHaffie, D. (1978) The use of digitalis glycosides in sinus rhythm. *Clin. Sci. Mol. Med.*, **55**, 417–21.
60. Hamer, J. (1979) The paradox of the lack of the efficacy of digitalis in congestive heart failure with sinus rhythm. *Br. J. Clin. Pharmacol.*, **8**, 109–13.
61. Hayward, R. and Hamer, J. (1979) Digitalis. In *Drugs for Heart Disease* (ed. J. Hamer), 1st edn, Chapman and Hall, London, pp. 244–317.
62. Storstein, L. (1982) Clinical and circulatory aspects of digitalis in heart failure. *Eur. Heart J.*, **3** (Suppl. D), 59–64.
63. Wilkins, M.R., Kendall, M.J. and Wade, O.L. (1985) William Withering and digitalis, 1785–1985. *Br. Med. J.* **290**, 7–8.
64. Rogen, A.S. (1943) Maintenance treatment with digitalis. *Br. Med. J.*, **1**, 694–5.
65. Dobbs, S.M., Kenyon, W.I and Dobbs, R.J. (1977) Maintenance digoxin after

an episode of heart failure: placebo-controlled trial in outpatients. *Br. Med. J.*, **1**, 749–52.

66. Bomann, K., Allgulander, S. and Skoglund, M. (1981) Is maintenance digoxin necessary in geriatric patients? *Acta Med. Scand.*, **210**, 493–5.

67. Starr, I. and Luchi, R.J. (1969) Blind study on the action of digitalis on elderly women. *Am. Heart J.*, **78**, 740–51.

68. Braunwald, E., Bloodwell, R.D., Goldberg, L.I. and Morrow, A.G. (1961) Studies on digitalis. IV. Observations in man on the effect of digitalis preparations on the contractility of the non-failing heart and on total vascular resistance. *J. Clin. Invest.*, **40**, 52–9.

69. Sonnenblick, E.H., Williams, J.F. Jr, Glick, G., Mason, D.T. and Braunwald, E. (1966) Studies on digitalis. XV. Effects of cardiac glycosides on myocardial force-velocity relations in the non-failing human heart. *Circulation*, **34**, 532–8.

70. Selzer, A. and Malmborg, R.O. (1962) Hemodynamic effects of digoxin in latent cardiac failure. *Circulation*, **25**, 695–702.

71. Yankopoulos, N.A., Kawai, C., Federici, E.E., Adler, L.N. and Abelmann, W.H. (1968) The hemodynamic effects of ouabain upon the diseased left ventricle. *Am. Heart J.*, **76**, 466–80.

72. Lee, G., Peng, C.L., Mason D.T., Amsterdam, E.A., Massumi, R.A. and Zelis, R. (1972) Similarity of the inotropic time course of differing digitalis preparations in isolated cardiac muscle. *Circulation*, **46**, (Suppl. II), 31 (abstract).

73. Runge, T.M. (1977) Clinical implications of differences in pharmacodynamic action of polar and nonpolar cardiac glycosides. *Am. Heart J.*, **93**, 248–55.

74. Mason, D.T. and Braunwald, E. (1964) Studies on digitalis. X. Effect of ouabain on forearm vascular resistance and venous tone in normal subjects and in patients with heart failure. *J. Clin. Invest.*, **43**, 532–43.

75. Cohn, K., Selzer, A., Kersh, E.S. Karpman, L.S. and Goldschlager, N. (1975) Variability of hemodynamic responses to acute digitalisation in chronic cardiac failure due to cardiomyopathy and coronary artery disease. *Am. J. Cardiol.*, **35**, 461–8.

76. DeMots, H., Rahimtoola, S.H., McAnulty, J.H. and Porter, G.E. (1978) Effects of ouabain on coronary and systemic vascular resistance and myocardial oxygen consumption in patients without heart failure. *Am. J. Cardiol.*, **41**, 88–93.

77. Arnold, S.B., Byrd, R.C., Meister, W., Melmon, K., Cheitlin, M.D., Bristow, J.D., Parmley, W.W. and Chatterjee, K. (1980) Long-term digitalis therapy improves left ventricular function in heart failure. *N. Eng.*, **303**, 1443–8.

78. Marcus, F.I. (1980) Editorial: Use of digitalis in acute myocardial infarction. *Circulation*, **62**, 17–19.

79. Adams, R.J., Pitts, B.J.R., Wood, J.M., Gende, O.A., Wallick, E.T. and Schwartz, A. (1979) Effect of palmityl carnitine on ouabain binding to Na, K-ATPase. *J. Mol. Cell Cardiol.*, **11**, 941–59.

80. Katz, A.M. and Smith, V.E. (1982) Regulation of myocardial function in the normal and diseased heart. *Eur. Heart J.*, **3** (Suppl. D) 11–18.

81. Nayler, W.G. and Williams, A. (1978) Relaxation in heart muscle: some morphological and biochemical considerations. *Eur. J. Cardiol.*, **7** (Suppl) 35–50.

82. Gheorghiade, M. and Beller, G.A. (1983) Effects of discontinuing maintenance digoxin therapy in patients with ischaemic heart disease and congestive heart failure in sinus rhythm. *Am. J. Cardiol*, **51**, 1243–50.

83. Lee, D.C.S., Johnson, R.A., Bingham, J.B., Leahy, M., Dinsmore, R.E., Goroll, A.H., Newell, J.B., Strauss, W. and Haber, E. (1982) Heart failure in outpatients. A randomised trial of digoxin versus placebo. *New. Engl. J. Med*, **306**, 699–705.

84. Rubinow, A., Skinner, M. and Cohen, A.S. (1981) Digoxin sensitivity in amyloid cardiomyopathy. *Circulation*, **63**, 1285–8.

85. Braunwald, E., Brockenbrough, E.C., and Frye, R.L. (1962) Studies on digitalis. V. Comparison of the effect of ouabain on left ventricular dynamics in valvular aortic stenosis and hypertrophic subaortic stenosis. *Circulation*, **26**, 166–73.

86. Storstein, L. and Amlie, J.P. (1981) The effect of practolol, propranolol and strophanthin compared with placebo on exercise tolerance and a postural test in patients with hypertrophic cardiomegaly. *Eur. Heart J.*, **2**, 289–96.

87. Glancy, D.L., O'Brien, K.P., Gold, H.K., Epstein, S.E. (1970) Atrial fibrillation in patients with idiopathic hypertrophic subaortic stenosis. *Br. Heart J.*, **32**, 652–9.

88. Anonymous (1979) Digoxin in sinus rhythm. *Br. Med. J.*, **1**, 1103–4.

89. Selzer, A. (1960) Comparative studies of acute and chronic effects of digitalis in cardiac failure. *Circulation*, **22**, 807 (abstract).

90. Davidson, C. and Gibson, D. (1973) Clinical significance of positive inotropic action of digoxin in patients with left ventricular disease. *Br. Heart J.*, **35**, 970–6.

91. Mason, D.T. and Braunwald, E. (1963) Studies on digitalis. IX. Effects of ouabain on the non-failing human heart. *J. Clin. Invest.*, **42**, 1105–11.

92. Mulrow, C.D. (1984) Re-evaluation of digitalis efficacy. New light on an old leaf. *Ann. Int. Med.*, **101**, 113–7.

93. Dall, J. (1970) Maintenance digoxin in elderly patients. *Br. Med. J.* **2**, 705–6.

94. Fonrose, H.A., Ahlbaum, N., Bugatch, E., Cohen, M., Genovese, C. and Kelly, J. (1974) The efficacy of digitalis withdrawal in an institutional aged population. *J. Am. Geriatric Soc.*, **22**, 208–11.

95. Hull, S.M. and Mackintosh, A. (1977) Discontinuation of maintenance digoxin therapy in general practice. *Lancet*, **ii**, 1054–5.

96. Liverpool Therapeutics Group (1978) Use of digitalis in general practice. *Br. Med. J.*, **2**, 673–5.

97. Krakauer, R. (1978) Use of digitalis in general practice. *Br. Med. J.*, **2**, 1019–20.

98. McHaffie, D., Purcell, H., Mitchell-Heggs, P. and Guz, A. (1978) The clinical value of digoxin in patients with heart failure and sinus rhythm. *Q. J. Med.*, **47**, 401–19.

99. Johnston, G.D. and McDevitt, D.G. (1979) Is maintenance digoxin necessary in patients with sinus rhythm? *Lancet*, **i**, 567–70.

100. Griffiths, B.E., Penny, W.J., Lewis, M.J. and Henderson, A.H. (1982) Maintenance of the inotropic effect of digoxin on long-term treatment. *Br. Med. J.*, **284**, 1819–22.

101. Fleg, J.L. Gottlieb, S.H. and Lakatta, E.G. (1982) Is digoxin really important in treatment of compensated heart failure? *Am. J. Med.*, **73**, 244–50.

102. Taggart, A.J., Johnston, G.D. and McDevitt, D.G. (1983) Digoxin withdrawal after cardiac failure in patients with sinus rhythm. *J. Cardiovasc. Pharmacol.*, **5**, 229–34.
103. Knight, R.K., Miall, P.A., Hawkins, L.A., Dacombe, J., Edwards, C.R.W. and Hamer, J. (1979) Relationship of plasma aldosterone concentrations to diuretic treatment in patients with severe heart disease. *Br. Heart J.*, **42**, 316–25.
104. Cantelli, I., Pavesi, P.C., Parchi, C., Naccarella, F. and Bracchetti, D. (1983) Acute hemodynamic effects of combined therapy with digoxin and nifedipine in patients with chronic heart failure. *Am. Heart J.*, **106**, 308–15.
105. Taylor, S.H., Silke, B. and Nelson, G.I.C. (1982) Principles of treatment of left ventricular failure. *Eur. Heart J.*, **3**, (Suppl. D), 19–43.
106. Katz, A.M. (1973) Biochemical 'defect' in the hypertrophied and failing heart. Deleterious or compensatory? *Circulation*, **47**, 1076–9.
107. Soyka, L.F. (1981) Pediatric clinical pharmacology of digoxin. *Pediat. Clin. North Am.*, **28**, 203–16.
108. Berman, W. Jr, Yabek, S.M., Dillon, T., Niland, C., Corlew, S. and Christensen, D. (1983) Effects of digoxin in infants with a congested circulatory state due to a ventricular septal defect. *N. Engl. J. Med.*, **308**, 363–6.
109. LeBlanc, M.H. (1983) Digoxin in infants with a congestive circulatory state. *N. Engl. J. Med.*, **309**, 279.
110. Hastreiter, A.R. and Van der Horst, R.L. (1983) Post mortem digoxin tissue concentration and oxygen content in infancy and childhood. *Am. J. Cardiol.*, **52**, 330–5.
111. Lown, B., Klein, M.D., Barr, I, Hagemeijer, F., Kosowski, B.D. and Garrison, H. (1982) Sensitivity to digitalis drugs in acute myocardial infarction. *Am. J. Cardiol*, **30**, 388–95.
112. Reicansky, I, Conradson, T.B., Holmberg, S., Rydén, L., Waldenström, A. and Wennerbolom, B. (1976) The effect of intravenous digoxin on the occurrence of ventricular tachyarrhythmias in acute myocardial infarction in man. *Am. Heart J.*, **91**, 705–11.
113. Rahimtoola, S.H., Sinno, M.R., Chuquimia, R., Loeb, H.S., Rosen, K.M. and Gunnar, R.M. (1972) Effect of ouabain on impaired left ventricular function in acute myocardial infarction. *N. Engl. J. Med.*, **287**, 527–31.
114. Maroko, P.R. and Braunwald, E. (1973) Modification of myocardial infarction size after coronary occlusion. *Ann. Intern. Med.*, **79**, 720–33.
115. Morrison, J., Coromilas, J., Robbins, M., Oug, L., Eisenberg, S., Stechel, R., Zema, M., Reiser, P. and Scherr, L. (1980) Digitalis and myocardial infarction in man. *Circulation*, **62**, 8–16.
116. Balcon, R., Hoy, J. and Sowton, E. (1968) Haemodynamic effects of rapid digitalisation following acute myocardial infarction. *Br. Heart. J.*, **30**, 373–6.
117. Marchionni, N., Vannucci, A., Pini, R., Greppi, B., Conti, A., Di Bari, M. and Bertini, G. (1980) Hemodynamic effects of digoxin in acute myocardial infarction. *Eur. Heart J.*, **1**, 319–26.
118. Cohn, J.N., Tristani, F.E. and Khatri, I.M. (1969) Cardiac and peripheral vascular effects of digitalis in clinical cardiogenic shock. *Am. Heart J.*, **78**, 318–30.
119. Banka, V.S., Chadda, K.D., Bodenheimer, M.M. and Helfant, R.H. (1975)

Digitalis: the present position

Digitalis in experimental acute myocardial infarction. *Am. J. Cardiol.*, **35**, 801–18.

120. Moss, A.J., Davis, H.T., Conard, D.L., DeCamilla, J.J. and Odoroff, C.L. (1981) Digitalis associated cardiac mortality after myocardial infarction. *Circulation*, **64**, 1150–6.

121. Bigger, J.T., Weld, F.M, Rohitzky, L.M. and Fenick, K.J. (1981) Is digitalis treatment harmful in the year after acute myocardial infarction? *Circulation*, **64** (Suppl. IV) IV-83.

122. Ryan, T.J., Bailey, K.R., McCabe, C.H., Luk, S., Fisher, L.D., Mock, M.B. and Killip, T. (1983) The effects of digitalis on survival in high-risk patients with coronary artery disease. *Circulation*, **67**, 735–42.

123. Kassebaum, D.C. (1963) Electrophysiological effects of strophanthin on the heart. *J. Pharmacol. Exp. Ther.*, **140**, 329–38.

124. Rosen, M.R., Gelband, H. and Hoffman, B.F. (1973) Correlation between effects of ouabain on the canine electrocardiogram and transmembrane potentials of isolated Purkinje fibres. *Circulation*, **47**, 65–72.

125. Gomes, J.A.C., Damato, A.N., Bobb, G.A. and Lau, S.H. (1978) The effect of digitalis on refractoriness of the intact canine His-Purkinje system. *Circulation*, **58**, 284–94.

126. Rosen, M.R., Wit, A.L. and Hoffman, B.F. (1975) Electrophysiology and pharmacology of cardiac arrhythmias. IV. Cardiac antiarrhythmic and toxic effects of digitalis. *Am. Heart J.*, **89**, 391–9.

127. Hayward, R., Hamar, J., Taggart, P. and Emanuel, R. (1983) Observations on the biphasic nature of digitalis electrophysiological actions in the human right atrium. *Cardiovasc. Res.*, **18**, 533–46.

128. Edvardsson, N., Hirsch, I. and Olsson, S.B. (1984) Acute effects of lignocaine, procainamide, metoprolol, digoxin and atropine on human myocardial refractoriness. *Cardiovasc. Res.*, **18**, 463–70.

129. Aronson, R.S. and Gelles, J.H. (1977) The effect of ouabain, dinitrophenol and lithium on the pacemaker current in sheep cardiac Purkinje fibres. *Circ. Res.*, **40**, 517–24.

130. Ferrier, G.R. (1977) Digitalis arrhythmias: role of oscillatory after-potentials. *Prog. Cardiovasc. Dis.*, **19**, 459–74.

131. Rosen, M.R., Ilvento, J., Gelband, H. and Merker, C. (1974) Effects of verapamil on electrophysiologic properties of canine cardiac Purkinje fibres. *J. Pharmacol. Exp. Ther.*, **189**, 414–22.

132. Kass, R.S., Lederer, W.J., Tsien, R.W. and Weingart, R. (1978) Role of calcium ions in transient inward currents and after contractions induced by strophanthidin in cardiac Purkinje fibres. *J. Physiol.*, **281**, 187–208.

133. Kass, R.S., Tsien, R.W. and Weingart, R. (1978) Ionic basis of transient inward current induced by strophanthidin in cardiac Purkinje fibers. *J. Physiol.*, **281**, 209–26.

134. Pace, D.G. and Gillis, R.A. (1976) Neuroexcitatory effects of digoxin in the cat. *J. Pharmacol. Exp. Ther.*, **199**, 583–600.

135. Somberg, J.C. and Smith, T.W. (1979) Localization of the neurally mediated arrhythmogenic properties of digitalis. *Science*, **204**, 321–3.

136. Imamura, T., Takeshita, A., Ashihara, T., Yamamoto, K., Hoka S. and Nakamura, M. (1985) Digitalis-induced augmentation of cardiopulmonary baroreflex control of forearm vascular resistance. *Circulation*, **71**, 11–16.

137. Gillis, R.A., Raines, A., Sohn, Y.J., Levitt, B. and Standaert, G. (1972) Neuroexcitatory effects of digitalis and their role in the development of cardiac arrhythmias. *J. Pharmacol. Exp. Ther.*, **183**, 154–68.
138. Greenspan, K. and Lord, T.J. (1973) Digitalis and vagal stimulation during atrial fibrillation: effects on atrioventricular conduction and ventricular arrhythmias. *Cardiovasc. Res.*, **7**, 241–6.
139. Caldwell, R.W., Songu-Mize, E. and Bealer, S.L. (1985) The vasopresser response to centrally administered ouabain. *Circ. Res.*, **55**, 773–9.
140. Somberg, J.C., Kuhlman, J.E. and Smith, T.W. (1981) Localization of the neurally mediated coronary vasoconstrictor properties in the cat. *Circ. Res.*, **49**, 226–33.
141. Puryear, S.K., Nash, C.B. and Caldwell, R.W. (1981) Effect of cardiac β-adrenergic blockade or denervation on cardiotoxicity of digoxin and on aminosugar cardenolide. *J. Cardiovasc. Pharmacol.*, **3**, 113–27.
142. Gibson, D. and Sowton, E. (1969) The use of beta-adrenergic receptor blocking drugs in dysrhythmias. *Prog. Cardiovasc. Dis.*, **12**, 16–39.
143. Prystowsky, E.N., Naccarelli, G.V., Jackman, W.M., Rinkenberger, R.L., Heger, J.T., and Zipes, D.P. (1983) Enhanced parasympathetic tone shortens atrial refractoriness in man. *Am. J. Cardiol*, **51**, 96–100.
144. Alessi, R., Nusynowitz, M., Abildskov, J.A. and Moe, G.K. (1958) Non uniform distribution of vagal effects on the atrial refractory period. *Am. J. Physiol.*, **194**, 406–410.
145. Goodman, D.J., Rossen, R.M., Cannom, D.S., Rider, A.K. and Harrison, D.C. (1975) Effect of digoxin on atrioventricular conduction. Studies in p t-ients with and without cardiac autonomic innervation. *Circulation*, **151**, 251–6.
146. Engel, T.R. and Gonzalez, A.D.C. (1978) Effects of digitalis on atrial vulnerability. *Am. J. Cardiol*, **421**, 570–6.
147. Dhingra, R.C., Amat-y-Leon, F., Wyndham, C., Denes, P., Wu, D., Pouget, J.M. and Rosen, K.M. (1976) Electrophysiologic effects of atropine on human sinus node and atrium. *Am. J. Cardiol*, **38**, 429–34.
148. Weiner, P., Bassan, M.M., Jarchovsky, J., Lusim, S. and Plavnick, L. (1983) Clinical course of acute atrial fibrillation treated with rapid digitalization. *Am. Heart J.*, **105**, 223–7.
149. Beasley, R., Smith, D.A. and McHaffie, D.J. (1985) Exercise heart rates at different serum digoxin concentrations in patients with atrial fibrillation. *Br. Med. J.*, **290**, 9–11.
150. Panidis, I.P., Morganroth, J. and Baessler, C. (1983) Effectiveness and safety of oral verapamil to control exercise-induced tachycardia in patients with atrial fibrillation receiving digitalis. *Am. J. Cardiol.*, **52**, 1197–201.
151. Klein, H.O., Lang, R., Weiss, E., DiSegni, E., Libhaber, C., Guerrero, J. and Kaplinsky, E. (1982) The influence of verapamil on serum digoxin concentration. *Circulation*, **65**, 998–1003.
152. Sellers, T.D. Jr, Bashore, T.M. and Gallagher, J.J. (1977) Digitalis in the preexcitation syndrome: analysis during atrial fibrillation. *Circulation*, **56**, 260–70.
153. Wu, D., Wyndham, C., Amat-y-Leon, F., Denes, P., Dhingra, R.C. and Rosen, K.M. (1975) The effects of ouabain on induction of atrioventricular nodal re-entrant paroxysmal supraventricular tachycardia. *Circulation*, **52**, 201–7.

154. Chee, T.P., Prakash, N.S., Desser, K.B. and Benchimol, A. (1982) Post-operative supraventricular arrhythmias and the role of prophylactic digoxin in cardiac surgery. *Am. Heart J.*, **104**, 974–7.

155. Saltissi, S., Crowther, A., Bryne, C., Clarke, S., Jenkins, B.S. and Webb-Peploe, M.M. (1983) The effects of oral digoxin therapy in primary mitral leaflet prolapse. *Eur. Heart J.*, **4**, 828–37.

156. Gradman, A.H., Cunningham, M., Harbison, M.A., Berger, H.J. and Zaret, B.L. (1983) Effects of oral digoxin on ventricular ectopy and its relation to left ventricular function. *Am. J. Cardiol*, **51**, 765–9.

157. Goodman, D.J., Rossen, R.M., Ingham, R., Rider, A.K, and Harrison, D.C. (1975) Sinus node function in the denervated human heart. Effect of digitalis. *Br. Heart J.*, **37**, 612–8.

158. Dhingra, R.C., Amat-y-Leon, F., Wyndham, C., Wu, D., Denes, P. and Rosen, K.M. (1975) The electrophysiological effects of ouabain on sinus node and atrium in man. *J. Clin. Invest.*, **56**, 555–62.

159. Shaw, T.R.D. (1981) Bioavailability of cardiac glycosides. In *Cardiac glycosides. Handbook of experimental pharmacology* (ed. K. Greef), Springer Verlag Berlin, **56** (11), 169–87.

160. Hayward, R.P., Greenwood, H. and Hamer, J. (1978) Comparison of digoxin and medigoxin in normal subjects. *Br. J. Clin. Pharmacol.*, **6**, 81–6.

161. Kelman, A.W:, Sumner, D.J., Lonsdale, M., Lawrence, J.R. and Whiting, B. (1980) Comparative pharmacokinetics and pharmacodynamics of cardiac glycosides. *Br. J. Clin. Pharmacol.*, **10**, 135–43.

162. Gerson, D.G., Lowe, E.H. and Lindenbaum, J. (1980) Bioavailability of digoxin tablets in patients with gastrointestinal dysfunction. *Am. J. Med.*, **69**, 43–9.

163. Woods, M.N. and Ingelfinger, J.A. (1979) Lack of effect of bran on digoxin absorption. *Clin. Pharmacol. Ther.*, **26**, 21–3.

164. Kuhlmann, J., Zilly, W., and Wilke, J. (1981) Effects of cytostatic drugs on plasma level and renal excretion of beta-acetyldigoxin. *Clin. Pharmacol. Ther.*, **30**, 518–27.

165. Storstein, L. (1975) Studies on digitalis, III. Biliary excretion and extrahepatic circulation of digitoxin and its cardioactive metabolites. *Clin. Pharmacol. Ther.*, **17**, 313–20.

166. Bussey, H.I. (1984) Update on the influence of quinidine and other agents on digitalis glycosides. *Am. Heart J.*, **107**, 143–6.

167. Warner, N.J., Barnard, J.T., Leahey, E.B. Jr, Hougen, T.J., Bigger, J.T. Jr and Smith, T.W. (1984) Myocardial monovalent cation transport during the quinidine–digoxin interaction in dogs. *Circ. Res.*, **54**, 453–60.

168. Moysey, J.O., Jaggarao, N.S.V., Grundy, E.N. and Chamberlain, D.A. (1981) Amiodarone increases plasma digoxin concentrations. *Br. Med. J.*, **282**, 272.

169. Peters, U. (1982) Pharmacokinetic review of digitalis glycosides. *Eur. Heart J.*, **3**, (Suppl D), 65–78.

170. Luchi, R.J. and Gruber, J.W. (1968) Unusually large digitalis requirements. *Am.J. Med.*, **45**, 322–8.

171. Watson, E., Clark, D.R. and Kalman, S.M. (1973) Identification by gas chromatography–mass spectroscopy of dihydrodigoxin – a metabolite of digoxin in man. *J. Pharmacol. Exp. Ther.*, **184**, 424–31.

172. Greenwood, H., Snedden, W., Hayward, R.P. and Landon, J. (1975) The measurement of urinary digoxin and dihydrodigoxin by radioimmunoassay and by mass spectroscopy. *Clin. Chim. Acta*, **62**, 213–24.
173. Dobkin, J.F., Saha, J.R., Butler, V.P. Jr, Neu, H.C. and Lindenbaum, J. (1983) Inactivation of digoxin by *Eubacterium lentum*, an anaerobe of the human gut flora. *Trans. Assoc. Am. Physicians*, **95**, 22–9.
174. George, C.F. (1983) Digitalis intoxication: a new approach to an old problem. *Br. Med. J.*, **286**, 1533–4.
175. Smith, T.W., Butler, V.P. Jr, Haber, E., Fozzard, H., Marcus, F., Bremner, F., Schulman, I. and Phillips, A. (1982) Treatment of life-threatening digitalis intoxication with digoxin specific Fab antibody fragments. *N. Engl. J. Med.*, **307**, 1357–62.
176. Gibb, I., Adams, P.C., Parnham, A.J. and Jennings, K. (1983) Plasma digoxin: assay anomalies in Fab-treated patients. *Br. J. Clin. Pharmacol.*, **16**, 445–7.

6 Positive inotropic drugs for treating heart failure

LEON RESNEKOV

6.1 Introduction

A failing ventricle adapts poorly to changes in outflow resistance. In heart failure resistance to ventricular outflow greatly increases, stroke-volume falls and a reduction in cardiac output follows. In an effort to maintain peripheral perfusion further vasoconstriction comes about that eventually will depress ventricular function even further.

At the cellular level myocardial contractility is regulated by myosin isonzymes, activator Ca^{2+} for binding to troponin C, and calmodulin. An additional important regulating mechanism improves ventricular relaxation that is impaired in the energy-deprived heart. In the presence of heart failure, there is both a lack of energy as well as a reduction in ventricular compliance, a result of progressive fibrosis.

In early heart failure compensatory mechanisms have a significant effect that progressively lessens in importance as failure becomes advanced. Three such reflex mechanisms come into play. The first is the Frank Starling principle. This effect becomes greatly blunted when the heart is dilated and failing. Stimulation of the sympathetic nervous system is the second mechanism, the effect being produced by releasing noradrenaline from sympathetic nerve terminals. Not only does this increase contractility but also heart rate is augmented. Cardiac output is maintained and peripheral blood flow redistributed. In the third compensatory mechanism retention of sodium stimulates renin secretion and the release of aldosterone.

It is the aim of positive inotropic therapy to enhance myocardial contraction. In addition, treatment with arterial dilators to reduce excess afterload, venodilators to reduce preload and diuretics to lessen salt and water retention are important [1, 2]. The overall effect therefore is not only to improve systolic contraction function but to lessen diastolic stiffness and to redistribute blood flow to appropriate vascular beds.

In this chapter the use of inotropic agents for managing heart failure will be considered.

195

Positive inotropic drugs for treating heart failure

6.2 Positive inotropic drugs

Until very recently, only digitalis glycosides have been readily available as oral positive inotropic drugs. During the last decade, however, many new positive inotropic drugs have been introduced although in the main, still on an experimental basis.

Most of these agents fall into two general categories: (1) sympathomimetics; (2) non-glycoside, non-sympathomimetics.

6.2.1 DIGITALIS GLYCOSIDES

Introduced into medicine in 1785, digitalis glycosides have admirably stood the test of time. It should be recognized, however, that as first used it was a diuretic effect that was being sought. It took almost 50 years before it was recognized that additional important effects were slowing

Table 6.1 Positive inotropic drugs

Digitalis Glycosides	
β-*Adrenergic Agonists*	– Norepinephrine, Epinephrine, Isoproterenol, Dopamine, Dobutamine
β₂ Selective	– Terbutaline, Salbutamol, Pirbuterol
β₁ Selective	– Prenalterol, ICI-118587, Butopamine
Dop agonists	– Levodopa, Ibopamine, Propylbutyldopamine
α-*Adrenergic agonists*	– Cause increase in contractility without heart rate increase
	Combine with peripheral vasodilator
Forskolin	
(endogenous diterpene)	– Stimulates adenylate cyclase increasing cAMP production, Ca^{2+} flux, contractility, heart rate
Cyclic nucleotides	– Dibutryl-cAMP, increases contractility and causes peripheral vasodilation
Phosphodiesterase inhibitors	– Inhibit cAMP breakdown, Theophylline
Non-glycoside	
Non-sympathomimetic agents	– Inhibit phosphodiesterase F-111 (cardiac)
	– Amrinone, Milrinone, MDL-17043 MDL-19205, RO-13-6438, ARL-115-BS (Sulmazol, Vardax)
	Berberine
	Benzimidazole derivatives, UD-CG-212, UD-CG-115
	Carbazeran

an inappropriately rapid heart rate and even regularizing abnormal heart rhythms. Digitalis has a direct inotropic effect, increasing force and velocity of myocardial contraction. How this is achieved has been an area of considerable investigation and not a little controversy. It is now recognized that inhibition of Na, K-ATPase is not the sole receptor mechanism that causes both contractility and electrophysiological effects of the drug. Calcium-magnesium-ATPase is also important [3].

Curiously, digitalis compounds will stimulate the sodium–potassium pump at low concentrations, wheras at high concentrations inhibition occurs. Although a negative inotropic effect is difficult to demonstrate in man further study may help formulate a digitalis-like drug that would have little such inhibition and therefore be safer to use.

Despite recent questions regarding the efficacy of digitalis glycosides there is little doubt that reviewing invasive and non-invasive carefully controlled studies demonstrates a positive inotropic effect that is long lasting [4]. In consequence, digitalis remains a first-line drug in the treatment of heart failure.

Digoxin is excreted mainly through the kidneys; digitoxin is extensively metabolized by the liver and about 55% excreted by the kidneys. Thus, in the presence of renal dysfunction the digoxin dosage needs to be reduced; digitoxin can often be used without modification of dosage in renal failure.

Possible drug interactions need to be considered, particularly quinidine. In addition, similar interactions occur with verapamil, amiodarone, spironolactone and triamterene. When used with digoxin an appropriate reduction in digoxin dosage is needed to avoid increases in plasma digoxin levels.

6.2.2 SYMPATHOMIMETIC AGENTS (see Table 6.1)

The adrenergic nervous system influences the state of contractility of the myocardium by interacting endogenous catecholamines with beta-adrenergic receptors of the myocardium and also to alpha-adrenergic receptors [5].

In the presence of severe heart failure the myocardial catecholamine stores become depressed and the role of circulating catecholamines becomes even more important. It can be shown that a persistent increase in circulating epinephrine and norepinephrine levels parallels the severity of heart failure.

(a) Beta-adrenergic agonists

Norepinephrine, epinephrine and isoproterenol, although efficiently stimulating beta-adrenergic receptors of the heart are limited clinically because of an associated increase in heart rate, exacerbation of ventricular dysrhythmias and concomitant constriction of the peripheral vasculature. Dopamine, a precursor of noradrenaline synthesis is a beta$_1$-adrenergic agonist releasing noradrenaline from sympathetic nerve endings [6]. It is also unusual in activating dopamine vascular receptors to produce dilation of renal, coronary, cerebral and mesenteric vascular beds. In higher dosage, dopamine is a powerful constrictor of arteries and veins.

(i) Dobutamine
Selectively increases contraction without any significant effect on heart rate or peripheral vascular resistance. This synthetic agent is particularly useful when heart failure is associated with high filling pressures of the ventricles, low cardiac output but relative preservation of the blood pressure [7]. When the blood pressure is severely compromised, dopamine should be given. Thus the choice of these two intravenous beta-adrenergic agonist drugs will depend on the haemodynamic abnormality being treated. In point of fact, at times, a combination of both dopamine (to maintain blood pressure) and dobutamine (to help reduce filling pressures of the ventricles) can be extremely beneficial.

Unfortunately neither of these agents can be administered orally. Thus they are of use only in the short-term management of patients admitted to hospital.

A great deal of effort has been undertaken to develop sympathomimetic amines that can be taken orally and be effective over a prolonged period of time. Several are now available but it is important to recognize that their pharmacological properties vary widely.

(ii) Beta$_2$ selective agonists – terbutaline [8] salbutamol [9], pirbuterol [10–12]
These agents increase myocardial contractility and relax vascular smooth muscle. In patients with severe heart failure cardiac output and indices of ventricular contraction increase; systemic vascular resistance falls. Usually there is only a small concomitant decrease in left ventricular filling pressure. Plasma glucose rises as do plasma potassium levels (temporary). Pirbuterol maintains haemodynamic benefit over many months of oral use.

(iii) Beta$_1$ selective agonists – prenalterol, ICI-118587 [13, 14]
Prenalterol increases contractility of the heart more than its effect on heart rate. It has no alpha-adrenoceptor effects, it can be used both intrevenously and orally and appears not to be subject to tachyphylaxis.

ICI-118587 is a selective partial beta$_1$ agonist that can be considered as an alternative to isoproterenol. It has no beta$_2$ vasodilation effect, causes considerable increase in contraction of the heart but very little change in heart rate. In addition, it has little effect in precipitating ventricular rhythm disturbances. It also improves segmental contraction of the ventricle in the presence of coronary heart disease and may well be an important drug for the management of heart failure in association with ischaemic heart disease.

(iv)   Dopaminergic receptor agonists (oral) – levodopa [15]
ibopamine,
propylbutyldopamine [16,17].
The use of levodopa as an oral positive inotropic drug was first reported by Goldberg, Hsieh and Resnekov [18]. Subsequently its beneficial haemodynamic effects have been reported by Rajfer and colleagues [15]. Following ingestion, levodopa is decarboxylated to dopamine, a significant positive inotropic effect is achieved and in addition, reduction of systemic vascular resistance occurs. Following a single oral dose of 1.5 to 2.0 g these effects persist for 4–6 hours with little change in ventricular filling pressures, heart rate or mean arterial blood pressure. A plasma concentration of dopamine of about 35 ng/ml at one hour after ingestion is achieved that slowly decreases towards control values at 4 to 5 hours. Significant diuresis is associated. The haemodynamic responses are due to activation of beta$_1$-adrenergic, dopamine-1 and dopamine-2 receptors derived from the decarboxylation of levodopa. Continued long-term benefit over a three month period of haemodynamic monitoring has been shown and clinical benefit beyond that time is frequent. Side effects are few but certain patients cannot take the high oral dose needed (1.5–2.0 g each 6 hours) because of nausea. Tachyphylaxis does not appear to limit its use long-term.

Ibopamine and propylbutyldopamine [16,17] appear to produce more peripheral vasodilation (and probably less positive inotropy) than does levodopa.

(b)   Alpha-adrenergic agonists

Curiously stimulation of alpha$_1$-receptors will increase the contractile state. How this is achieved is still uncertain. The receptors are not coupled to adenylate cyclase and act through a biochemical pathway that is different from the beta-adrenergic receptors. The positive inotropic effect builds up slowly and is less marked than with other sympathomimetic amines. They do not increase heart rate nor do they enhance myocardial relaxation.

Since their dominant effect is peripheral vasoconstriction the only possible use of alpha-adrenergic agonists in heart failure would be

199

combined with a vasodilator drug to provide a selective increase in contraction with little effect on heart rate.

Tachyphylaxis

Beta-adrenergic desensitization may cause a decline of haemodynamic effectiveness over weeks or months. This unfortunate effect appears to result from both a decrease in the number of beta-adrenergic receptors and an uncoupling of the receptor from adenylate cyclase [19–21]. It can greatly decrease the initial clinical benefit when beta-adrenergic agonist drugs are used long term.

(c)   Forskolin [22]

This is an endogenous diterpene; it acts directly on adenylate cyclase increasing cardiac cAMP production, calcium ion flux and contractility. Clinical trials of it have already been completed and positive inotropy demonstrated with associated modest vasodilation. Unfortunately the drug seems to have a profound effect on heart rate causing an inappropriate tachycardia.

(d)   The cyclic nucleotides

Dibutryl-cAMP has been shown to improve heart failure in patients and to increase cardiac output and reduce ventricular filling pressures. It is still uncertain, however, whether benefit is achieved primarily as a positive inotropic intervention or through peripheral vasodilation; probably it is a combination of both.

(e)   Phosphodiesterase inhibitors

Theoretically phosphodiesterase inhibitors should increase contraction of the heart muscle since inhibiting cAMP breakdown increases its intracellular concentration. The prototype drug theophylline has been extensively studied and does have a positive inotropic effect in man, although its potency is low. In addition, undesirable side effects may emerge, particularly affecting the gastrointestinal and neurological systems. At high doses there is often an inappropriate tachycardia and emergence of ventricular rhythm disturbances.

6.2.3   NON-GLYCOSIDE, NON-SYMPATHOMIMETIC AGENTS
(see Table 6.1)

A new class of drugs with both positive inotropic and peripheral vasodilation effects has been developed and several have already been used with success for treating heart failure in man. These effects are not brought about by interfering with the sodium–potassium pump mechanism. They continue despite a reduction in endogenous catecholamine. Pre-treatment with beta-or alpha-adrenergic blockers, or with agents that specifically block prostaglandin synthesis or with drugs that block the fast inward sodium current do not decrease their effectiveness. They have therefore been called 'non-glycoside, non-sympathomimetic' drugs.

As can be seen from Table 6.1 many such agents are already available. As a group they appear selectively to inhibit phosphodiesterase F-III which is a cAMP-specific heart muscle phosphodiesterase.

(a)   Amrinone

A great deal of patient evaluation of this drug has already occurred [23–26]. It causes a powerful positive inotropic effect with associated peripheral vasodilation. Its effects are presumed to result from inhibition of cyclic nucleotide phosphodiesterase F-III that allows an increase of cardiac cAMP. The drug also causes an increased entry of calcium ion into the myocardial cell and may increase the sensitivity of troponin for calcium.

Considerable haemodynamic improvements have occurred when amrinone has been given to patients in heart failure. These include increases in cardiac output and exercise tolerance. Ventricular filling pressure and systemic vascular resistance are lowered. Only a small increase in heart rate is associated. There is still controversy regarding the relative potency of its positive inotropic effect versus its causation of peripheral vasodilation in bringing about clinical improvement.

Unfortunately when used orally serious adverse effects emerged that were common [27]. These have included dose-dependent reversible thrombocytopenia, liver dysfunction, fever and gastrointestinal upsets.

At present, therefore, the clinical use of amrinone in the USA is limited to its intravenous preparation.

(b)   Milrinone

This drug is closely related to amrinone but is much more potent. It has similar beneficial haemodynamic and pharmacological effects and its oral use is not associated with severe side effects. Haemodynamic studies have demonstrated not only peripheral vasodilation but also positive inotropy, and ventricular compliance in diastole is improved [28].

The beneficial haemodynamic and exercise tolerance effects appear to be maintained when used long term [29]. At high dosage ventricular rhythm disturbances may emerge.

The drug has a half-life of about two hours, being excreted largely by the kidneys. A smaller dose than usual should be given in the presence of renal dysfunction.

Positive inotropic drugs for treating heart failure

(c) MDL-17043 [30]; MDL-19205 [31]

These drugs are derived from imidazolone. Their effects are very similar to amrinone and milrinone. They are phosphodiesterase F-III inhibitors, increase contractility of the heart, cause peripheral vasodilation and reduce ventricular filling pressures. Little change in heart rate is associated. Improvement in ventricular compliance occurs.

The drugs may be used intravenously or orally and in their oral form continue to produce benefit long term.

(d) ARL-115 BS (sulmazol) [32]

This drug is an imidazopyridine derivative and is similar in its effects to amrinone, milrinone and the MDL drugs. Its effect is produced by phosphodiesterase F-III inhibition.

When used in patients considerable improvement in heart failure occurs, left ventricular function is enhanced and peripheral vasodilation produced. Unfortunately ARL-115BS may not be without side effects, thrombocytopenia has been reported and gastrointestinal side effects have also occurred following its use.

(e) RO13-6438

This is an imidazo-quinazolinone derivative. It is a powerful positive inotropic drug that also causes peripheral vasodilation. Following a single oral dose haemodynamic effects persist for up to 8 hours. It has not, as yet, been extensively tried in humans but animal work is encouraging.

(f) Carbazeran

Also acting as an inhibitor of phosphodiesterase F-III, the initial clinical investigations with this drug are encouraging. It provides positive inotropy and peripheral vasodilation. It has replaced the earlier introduced UK-14275 that had to be withdrawn because it prolonged QT time and could cause torsades-de-pointes.

(g) Other agents

Other compounds that have been tried and which are active by mouth include berberine, D13625 and UD-CG212, and UD-CG115. Although chemically dissimilar all these agents act as inhibitors of phosphodiesterase F-III, producing positive inotropy and peripheral dilation. Their role in the management of heart failure in humans has not, as yet, been established.

6.3 Discusssion

It is indeed remarkable how many new drugs have now been introduced, many of which show great promise for managing severe heart failure. Whereas in the not too distant past only digitalis glycosides orally and intravenous sympathomimetic amines were available, a very large number of drugs have now emerged with important positive inotropic effects as well as being powerful peripheral vasodilators. In addition, many of these new compounds reduce the abnormal stiffness of the ventricle. All these beneficial effects occur without any untoward increase in heart rate. Most of the newer agents are not subject to tachyphylaxis. With many, side effects are few.

To be clinically useful, haemodynamic benefit must occur not only at rest but also during effort. There should be no serious or frequent side effects and the drugs must be well tolerated orally. Their effects should persist during long-term administration without tolerance emerging. Continued clinical benefit should occur. Ideally longevity should be enhanced but in any event it should not be shortened by the drug. Ideally dosage schedules should be simple and relatively infrequent to improve patient compliance.

There remain many uncertainties about using these new compounds. It is unclear, for example, whether continuing a positive inotropic effect on a myocardium already subject to heart failure may not, in the long term, be detrimental. Fortunately many of the drugs improve diastolic compliance and thereby reduce myocardial oxygen requirement. Long term this could be of considerable benefit to the overall energetics of the myocardium.

The ultimate survival of the patient depends not only on improving haemodynamics in the short or long term. We still have little definite evidence to show that patients treated with the newer agents necessarily live longer, although their symptoms may be greatly alleviated, a most desirable end in itself. It seems as if such patients are still succumbing to acute cardiac rhythm disturbances and complications of thromboembolism. At least half the patients in severe heart failure eventually die suddenly.

We badly need, therefore, a better understanding of the molecular basis of cardiac contraction and the cellular causes of heart failure. Better diagnostic methods, preferably non-invasive, are required to categorize the overall cardiac status of the patient more reliably. This will permit a much better definition of the individual's ventricular dysfunction even when its clinical manifestations are few. Therapy appropriate for that

Positive inotropic drugs for treating heart failure

patient's disability can be given early to improve long-term results of treatment.

Not only do we require to treat systolic function but we need to improve diastolic function and reduce the inappropriate lack of ventricular compliance. Fortunately, many of the newer oral positive inotropic drugs succeed in reducing ventricular stiffness.

Approaching the patient in heart failure with these physiological concepts will permit individualizing therapy for each patient, tailoring the therapeutic programme to the pathophysiological and clinical requirement.

Fortunately for the patient in heart failure the therapeutic future is encouraging. We already have very powerful drugs available for heart failure managment. The newer agents should permit us to relieve the unacceptable suffering the patient in heart failure endures, and at the same time allow him to live a more normal life that hopefully will be prolonged by the newer drugs introduced.

References

1. Cohn, J.N. and Franciosa, J.A. (1977) Vasodilator therapy of cardiac failure. *N. Engl. J. Med.*, **297**, 27–31.
2. Chatterjee, K. and Parmley, W.W. (1977) The role of vasodilator therapy in heart failure. *Progr. Cardiovasc. Dis.* **19**, 301–26.
3. Akera, T. and Brody, T.M. (1977) The role of Na,$^+$, K$^+$-ATPase in the inotropic action of digitalis. *Pharmacol. Rev.*, **29**, 187–220.
4. Arnold, S.B. (1980) Long-term digitalis therapy improves left ventricular function in heart failure, *N. Engl. J. Med.*, **303**, 1443–7.
5. Colucci, W.S. and Braunwald, E. (1984) Adrenergic receptors: New concepts and implications for cardiovascular therapeutics. In *Cardiac Drug Therapy*, (ed. C.R. Conti), F.A. Davis, Philadelphia, p. 39.
6. Goldberg, L.I. (1974) Dopamine – clinical uses of an endogenous catecholamine. *N. Engl. J. Med.*, **291**, 707–10.
7. Bendersky, R., Chatterjee, K. and Parmley, W.W. (1981) Dobutamine in chronic ischemic heart failure: alterations in left ventricular function and coronary hemodynamics. *Am. J. Cardiol.*, **48**, 554–8.
8. Awan, N.A., Amsterdam, E.A., Evenson, M.K., Needham, K.E., Laslett, L.J. and Mason, D.T. (1982) Oral terbutaline: an effective cardiac stimulant for beneficial augmentation of left ventricular function in severe congestive heart failure. *Clin. Res.*, **30**, 24A.
9. Sharma, B. and Goodwin, J.F. (1978) Beneficial effect of salbutamol on cardiac function of severe congestive cardiomyopathy. *Circulation*, **58**, 449–60.
10. Selective beta$_2$-adrenergic bronchodilator. *J. Pharmacol. Exp. Ther.*, **207**, 410–14.
11. Awan, N.A., Evenson, M.K. and Needham, K.E. (1981) Hemodynamic effects of oral pirbuterol in chronic severe congestive heart failure. *Circulation.*, **63**, 96–101.

References

12. Sharma, B., Hoback, J. and Francis, G.S. (1981) Pirbuterol: a new oral sympathomimetic amine for the treatment of congestive heart failure. *Am. Heart. J.* **102**, 533–41.
13. Heedberg, A., Mattson, H. and Carlsson, E. (1980) Prenalterol, a non-selective beta-adrenoceptor ligand with absolute beta$_1$-selective partial agonist activity. *J. Pharmacol.*, **32**, 660–5.
14. Awan, N.A., Needham, K.E., Evenson, M.K., Win, A. and Mason, D.T. (1981) Hemodynamic actions of prenalterol in severe congestive heart failure due to chronic coronary disease. *Am. Heart J.* **101**, 158–61.
15. Rajfer, S.I., Anton, A.H., Rossen, J.D. and Goldberg, L.I. (1984). Beneficial hemodynamic effects of oral levodopa in heart failure. *N. Engl. J. Med.*, **310**, 1357–61.
16. Melloni, G.F., Melloni, R., Minoja, G.M., Scarazzati, G., Bruni, G.C., Loreti, P. and Bauer, R. (1981) Clinical tolerability of ibopamine hydrochloride (SB 7505). *Eur. J. Clin. Pharmacol.*, **19**, 409–11.
17. Melloni, G.F., Minoja, G.M., Scarazzati, G., Bauer, R., Brusoni, B. and Ghiradi, P. (1981) Renal effects of SB 7505: A double-blind study. *Eur. J. Clin. Pharmacol.*, **19**, 177–80.
18. Goldberg, L.I., Hsieh, Y-Y. and Resnekov, L. (1977) Newer catecholamines for treatment of heart failure and shock, an update on dopamine and first look at dobutamine. *Progr. Cardiovasc Dis.*, **19**, 327–340.
19. Unverferth, D.V., Blaunford, H., Kates, R.E. and Leier, C.V. (1980) Tolerance to dobutamine after a 72-hour continuous infusion. *Am. J. Med.*, **69**, 262–5.
20. Colucci, W.S., Alexander, R.W., Williams, G.H., Rude, R.E., Holman, B.I., Konstam, M.A., Wynn, E.J., Mudge, G.H. Jr. and Braunwald, E. (1981) Decreased lymphocyte beta-adrenergic-receptor density in patients with heart failure and tolerance to the beta-adrenergic agonist pirbuterol. *N. Engl. J. Med.*, **305**, 185–8.
21. Lefkowitz, R.J., Caron, M.G. and Stiles, G.L. (1984) Mechanisms of membrane-receptor regulation. *N. Engl. J. Med.*, **310**, 1570–9.
22. Colucci, W.S. and Wright, R.F. (1984) Positive inotropic therapy of congestive heart failure: an update. Newsletter, *Am. Heart Assoc. Council Clin. Cardiol.*, **10**, SC-84-CLC, 1–4.
23. Benotti, J.R., Grossman, W., Braunwald, E., Davolos, D.D. and Alousi, A.A. (1978) Hemodynamic assessment of amrinone. *N. Engl. J. Med.*, **299**, 1373–77.
24. LeJemtel, T.H., Keung, E. and Sonnenblick, E.H. (1979) Amrinone: a new non-glycosidic, non-adrenergic cardiotonic agent effective in the treatment of intractable myocardial failure in man. *Circulation*, **59**, 1098–104.
25. Weber, K.T., Andrews, V., Janicki, J.S., Wilson, J.R. and Fishman, A.T. (1981) Amrinone and exercise performance in patients with chronic heart failure. *Am. J. Cardiol.*, **48**, 164–9.
26. Wynne, J., Malcoff, R.F., Benotti, J.R. (1980) Oral amrinone in refractory congestive heart failure. *Am. J. Cardiol.*, **45**, 1245–9.
27. Wilmshurst, P.T. and Webb-Peploe, M.M. (1983) Side effects of amrinone therapy. *Br. Heart J.*, **49**, 447–51.
28. White, H.D., Ribeiro, J.P., Hartley, L.H., Jaski, B.E., Fiffer, M.A., Wright, R.F. and Colucci, W.S. (1984) Acute beneficial effects of milrinone on aerobic capacity, anaerobic threshold and catecholamine response in heart failure. *Clin. Res.*, **32**, 216A.

Positive inotropic drugs for treating heart failure

29. Maskin, C.S., Sinoway, L., Chadwick, B., Sonnenblick, E.H. and LeJemtel, T.H. (1983) Sustained hemodynamic and clinical effects of a new cardiotonic agent, WIN47203, in patients with severe congestive heart failure. *Circulation*, **67**, 1065–9.
30. Uretsky, B.F., Generalovich, T., Reddy, P.S., Spangenberg, R.B. and Follenberg, W.P. (1983) The acute hemodynamic effects of a new agent MDL17,043, in the treatment of congestive heart failure. *Circulation.*, **67**, 823–8.
31. Petein, M., Garberg, V., Carlyle, P., Cohn, J.N. and Levine, T.B. (1983) Acute hemodynamic and neurohumoral effects of NDL19205, a new inotropic agent in congestive heart failure. *J. Am. Coll. Cardiol.*, **1**, 675–9.
32. Hagemeijer, F., van Mechelen, R. and Schelling, (1983) Hemodynamic effects of the new inotropic agent sulmazol (AR-L115BS) administered intravenously to patients with severe heart failure. *Herz*, **8**, 41–5.

7 Diuretics

ARIEL LANT

7.1 Introduction

The history of diuretics extends back to antiquity with the knowledge that extracts of tea and coffee possessed the ability to enhance urine flow. In addition, inorganic mercury salts such as mercurous chloride (calomel) were employed in the middle ages amongst other uses, as diuretics; they continued to be held in high esteem well into the nineteenth century. In a text entitled: *The Diseases of the Heart and Aorta*, Stokes states: 'the exhibition of mercury will, as if by enchantment, remove the anasarca'. [1]. However, such treatments bore the harsh penalty of substantial toxicity [2].

It was with the development of organometallic compounds as potential chemotherapeutic agents, stimulated by the ideas of Paul Ehrlich in Germany that diuretic drugs indirectly owe their origin. In 1919, one of the most dramatic discoveries of modern medicine was made by the chance occurrence and noting of an adverse reaction to an organomercurial compound, merbaphen (Novasurol). A third-year medical student at the University of Vienna, Vogl, observed that parenteral administration of this substance to a non-oedematous young patient with congenital syphilis evoked a substantial diuresis [3, 4]. This impressive 'man-made' diuresis paved the way for the development of many scores of other less-toxic organomercurials, culminating in the production of synthetic diuretic molecules that lacked any heavy metallic ion [5]. Then, in the mid-1950s, the first orally effective sulphonamide diuretic, chlorothiazide, emerged [6], and the modern era of diuretics had begun in earnest.

Now, thirty years later, diuretics rank among the most extensively used drugs in cardiovascular practice world-wide. Estimated sales in the United States alone exceed five hundred million dollars per annum [7]. Although oral diuretics were originally introduced into medicine primarily to treat oedematous conditions, current prescribing trends indicate that the most extensive use of diuretics today is in the management of hypertension [8].

The realization that a variety of non-metallic organic chemicals could profoundly affect salt and water metabolism gave a considerable boost to the search for compounds that possessed increasing degrees of selectivity of action. Thus molecules with attractive new attributes such as anti-kaliuresis or high ceiling characteristics made their appearance. Availability of these agents offered for the first time opportunity for the molecular biologist to explore the mechanisms of membrane transport. Thus hand in hand with the dramatic transformation in the management of cardiac failure brought about by the new era of synthetic diuretic discovery, there has occurred a parallel explosion in knowledge concerning cellular transport of ions and water. Much of our current understanding of the operation of ion pumps in cell membranes not only within the nephron but in a variety of other tissues throughout the animal kingdom, owes its basis to the use of synthetic diuretics as investigative agents with which transport processes could be probed [9].

7.2 Classification of diuretics

Since much of the synthetic development of diuretics has occurred by a process of logical manipulation of molecules, it might have been thought that chemical structure would offer a useful framework upon which to classify available compounds. Unfortunately, this is not the case. For example, amongst sulphonamide diuretics, there exist compounds which, despite a common sulphamoyl radical ($- SO_2-NH_2$), display at least three different modes and characteristics of action: carbonic anhydrase inhibitors (e.g. acetazolamide); benzothiadiazines (e.g. hydrochlorothiazide) and high-ceiling sulphamoylbenzoates (e.g. frusemide). Similarly, within the 'high-ceiling' group of diuretics, we can identify at least three totally dissimilar chemical groupings as represented by each of the following agents: ethacrynic acid, frusemide and muzolimine [Fig. 7.1].

From a practical clinical standpoint, the most useful classification of diuretics is one based on the maximal amount of filtered sodium chloride that is rejected in the urine by the renal activity of the diuretic concerned. To some extent, of course, such excretory maxima are themselves determined by where a particular diuretic acts within the nephron, but the concept of single or even exclusive sites of action has had to be modified by the knowledge that many diuretics act at more than one tubular locus. In the classification set out in Table 7.1, the major site of action for each group has been emphasized.

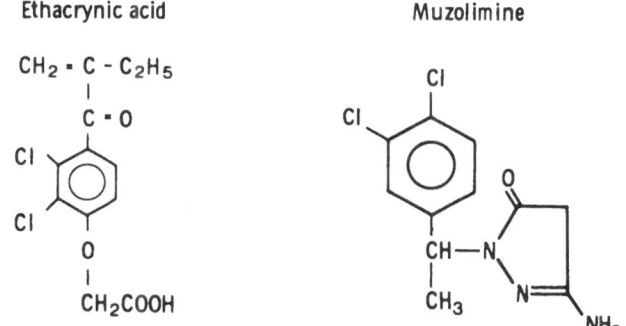

Compound	R_4	R_3	R_2
Furosemide	Cl	H	$NHCH_2$ furan
Bumetanide	$-O-$ phenyl	$NH \cdot (CH_2)_3 \cdot CH_3$	H
Piretanide	$-O-$ phenyl	$-N$ pyrrolidine	H

Ethacrynic acid

Muzolimine

Fig. 7.1 Chemical heterogeneity amongst 'loop' diuretics. In the upper half of the figure, the common sulphonamide structure that forms the basis of the sulphamoylbenzoate group of diuretics is shown. The prototype is frusemide (furosemide). Below are shown the structures of the phenoxyacetic acid derivative, ethacrynic acid, and alongside, the aminopyrazolinone, muzolimine, which is unique in being a highly basic compound.

7.3 Localization of diuretic action in the nephron

Apart from the xanthines, theobromine and theophylline, which act primarily as dilators of the afferent arterioles feeding the glomerular tufts, all available diuretics act by inhibiting electrolyte reabsorption within different tubular segments of the nephron [10]. The rejected electrolyte increases luminal osmolality, thereby depressing water reabsorption and so generates an increase in urinary flow. Extensive use of tubular

Diuretics

Table 7.1 Classification of diuretics

Group I. High efficacy (> 15%) [TAL; site II]
    SH-binders   Organomercurials
                      Ethacrynic acid

    Sulphamoylbenzoates   Frusemide (furosemide)
                            Bumetanide
                            Piretanide

    Aminopyrazolinones   Muzolimine

Group II. Medium efficacy (5–10%) [cds; site III]
    Benzothiadiazines and related heterocycles   Thiazides
                                              Hydrothiazides

    Polyvalent uricosuric saluretic agents   Indacrinone

Group III. Low Efficacy (<5%)
    Xanthines   Aminophylline   [glomerulus; site I]

    Osmotic agents   Mannitol [site I]

    Antikaliuretics: [site IV]

        Aldosterone antagonists
                Spironolactone
                Canrenoate

        Pteridines
                Triamterene

        Pyrazinecarboxamides
                Amiloride

The numbers in parentheses refer to the maximal percentage of filtered sodium chloride excreted through action of the different groups of diuretic.

The principal sites of action for each group are given. The location of individual sites is shown in Fig. 7.2

TAL = thick ascending limb of Henle's loop; cds = cortical diluting site of early distal tubule.

micropuncture and microperfusion techniques has made it possible to localize with accuracy the sites of action of different diuretics. In addition, application of clearance techniques has enabled localization studies to be carried out *in vivo*. This last method of defining sites of action is the only approach that has proved feasible thus far in man. Allowing for the difficulties in extrapolating data from animal studies to human subjects, remarkable agreement has been reached between results obtained in experimental animals and those found in man [9].

As has already been pointed out, the patterns of electrolyte excretion evoked by different diuretics reflect their sites of action within the nephron and have much more relevance to their classification and application to clinical practice than do either chemical structure or what has

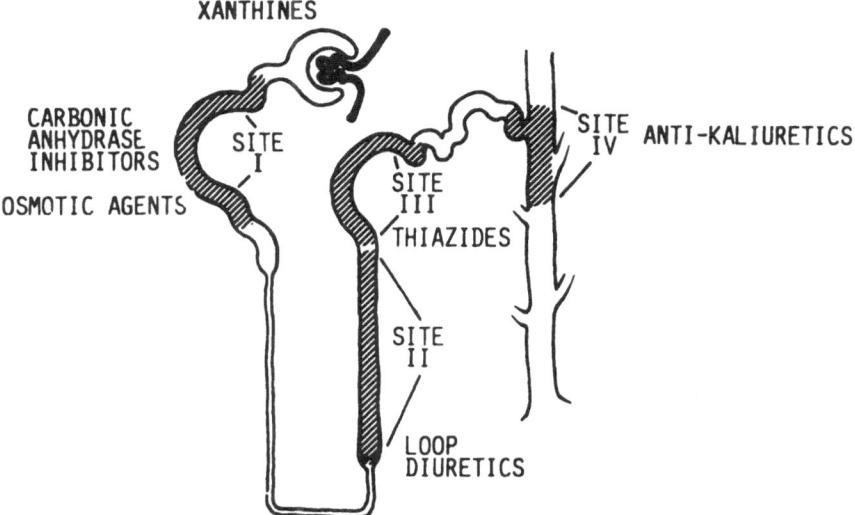

Fig. 7.2 Diagrammatic representation of the four principal tubular sites of action of diuretics in the nephron with xanthine compounds acting upon afferent arterioles at the glomerulus.

so far been elucidated about the cellular or subcellular mechanisms of action of these agents.

Four major tubular sites of diuretic action have been identified (Fig. 7.2). Within the proximal tubule (site I), approximately two-thirds of the glomerular filtrate is reabsorbed iso-osmotically. Site I also serves an important role in transporting diuretic molecules into tubular urine via the active secretory pathways that normally serve as elimination paths for most drugs and their metabolites. Since most 'loop' diuretics and the non-aldosterone antagonist antikaliuretics work from inside the tubule, secretory activity at site I is obviously an important determinant of the renal response to diuretics [11].

The substantial reabsorptive capacity of site I might suggest that this site was a particularly attractive target against which to direct inhibitory effects when designing new diuretics. Unfortunately, experience has shown that the overall effect of those diuretics working mainly at site I is relatively unimpressive as reflected in the relatively weak efficacy of osmotic agents or carbonic anhydrase inhibitors. The reason for this paradox is that although a proximally active compound may block as much as 65% of the reabsorption of the glomerular filtrate, the reabsorptive reserve of the remaining tubular segments that are still functioning normally beyond site I, notably the thick portion of the ascending limb of

211

Diuretics

Henle's loop (TAL), will overshadow the proximal salt and water rejection. The final outcome is one of little extra saluresis.

The loop of Henle absorbs approximately 25% of the glomerular filtrate and this nephron segment has been the subject of much intensive study in the last decade [12]. The TAL is virtually impermeable to water and so solute reabsorption occurs without the osmotic accompaniment of water. The net result of this is to create a milieu which helps to maintain hypertonicity of the medullary interstitium. At the same time, tubular urine becomes progressively more dilute as flow continues upwards out of the medulla back into the cortex.

Hypertonicity of the inner medulla is the result of the combined activities of the hairpin structure of the long hoops of Henle acting as counter-current multiplier systems and of their associated vasa recta acting as counter-current exchange systems. Recycling of urea between the two limbs of the vasa recta and between the loops of Henle and collecting ducts also contributes to maintaining medullary hypertonicity. In the presence of antidiuretic hormone (ADH), the collecting ducts which pass through the hypertonic medulla on their way to the renal pelvis become permeable to water. The progressive extraction of solute-free water from the collecting ducts into the medullary interstitium makes the final urine hypertonic.

Two morphologically distinct portions of the TAL can be identified – a medullary portion lined by cuboidal cells (site II) and a cortical portion, lined by flattened cells (site III). Because cortical solute reabsorption does not contribute to medullary hypertonicity and urinary concentration, site III is commonly referred to as the 'cortical diluting segment'. The process of urine dilution can thus be considered to occur at both sites II and III. During water diuresis, total urine volume can be divided into two moieties. First, there is the volume of urine needed to excrete urinary solutes at plasma tonicity, that is, the osmolal clearance (C_{osm}). Second, there is the volume of solute-free water generated at sites II and III, which can be collectively termed solute-free water clearance or C_{H_2O}. When fluid intake is restricted and hypertonic urine is formed, C_{H_2O} becomes negative and is referred to as $^TC_{H_2O}$. $^TC_{H_2O}$ reflects the reabsorption of water into the hypertonic medulla from the collecting ducts as they become permeable to water under the influence of ADH.

Study of the detailed functional characteristics of the TAL only really became possible with the introduction by Burg and his colleagues in the early 1970s of the technique of perfusion of isolated nephron segments *in vitro* [13]. By using this technique, it proved possible to show for the first time that the mechanism of NaCl reabsorption in the TAL is unique when compared to other portions of the nephron. A lumen-positive transtubular electrical potential difference is present in the TAL. Coupled reabsorption of Na^+ and Cl^- appears to be driven by the chemical gradient for Na^+, which, in turn, is sustained by the activity of the sodium pump or Na,K-ATPase, located at the basolateral membrane of each cell lining the TAL. These observations have led to the use of the term 'secondary active transport' as applied to the chloride reabsorptive process within the TAL [14]. So-called 'loop' diuretics act primarily within site II and because of their powerful action in rejecting more than 15% of the filtered load of salt together with their steep dose–response relationships, they are often referred to as 'high-ceiling' diuretics.

Clearance technology has proved particularly helpful in localizing the action of the benzothiadiazines and related compounds to the cortical diluting segment (site III). Thus, whereas these diuretics inhibit C_{H_2O} under conditions of maximal hydration, they do not interfere with $^TC_{H_2O}$ during hydropenia, distinguishing their action clearly from classical 'loop' diuretics which inhibit both C_{H_2O} and $^TC_{H_2O}$ [15]. In this manner, it has been possible to show that the two stereoisomers or the uricosuric saluretic, indacrinone, act in different portions of the TAL. (−)-indacrinone acts primarily at site II whereas (+)-indacrinone acts primarily at site III [16].

Antikaliuretic diuretics act at site IV which incorporates the late distal convoluted tubule and cortical collecting duct. It is at these nephron segments that the final regulation of potassium excretion occurs. The activity of site IV is controlled by aldosterone, plasma potassium, acid–base status and the amount of sodium that is delivered within the tubular urine reaching this part of the nephron [17]. When distal urinary flow increases with increase in salt delivery, NaCl reabsorption also increases and the lumen-negative transepithelial potential difference increases. In this way, a favourable electrical gradient is created for passive exit of potassium and hydrogen ions from cell into lumen. Since most potent diuretics act in front of site IV, and increase distal sodium delivery, urinary potassium wastage is a common accompaniment of their action. With the short-acting compounds as contrasted, for example, with the benzothiadizines, the net potassium loss tends to be less because, during the compensatory period following saluresis, delivery of sodium chloride to the distal nephron falls off markedly and thus allows a degree of potassium conservation to occur.

7.4 Molecular mechanisms of diuretic action

The sophisticated structural and functional characteristics of the mammalian kidney have made it a particularly difficult organ to study experimentally, in particular with respect to finding out how different

Diuretics

diuretics cause their effects at a cellular level. Because the renal tubules share transport characteristics with epithelia derived from other cellular systems, a number of simpler tissues have been employed to investigate the molecular mechanisms of diuretic action [9]. These have ranged from red or white cells, corneal membranes, shark rectal gland, teleost intestine to amphibian skin or bladder [18–20]. In this manner, diuretic drugs have served as remarkable chemical probes for exploring the mechanisms of solute transport across cell membranes. At the same time, in some instances, we have learnt how these drugs may be working in molecular terms, though obviously care has to be taken when extrapolating findings from isolated tissues in different species to the likely mechanisms operative within tubular cells of the intact human kidney.

The biochemical basis for the action of most diuretics still remains incomplete. In the case of the widely used benzothiadizines, it is completely obscure, despite their availability for close on thirty years. The classic studies by Pitts and his colleagues in the 1940s paved the way for the explanation of molecular action of carbonic anhydrase inhibitors such as acetozolamide [21]. The action of these compounds is to block the major fraction of HCO_3- reabsorption at site I by preventing the production of H^+ within tubular cells. Recent work has shown that these processes are not just intracellular but involve membrane-bound carbonic anhydrase that is present in high concentrations not only at luminal brush border but also at the peritubular blood membrane [22].

Localization of the action of the classic 'loop' diuretics to the luminal surface of the TAL implies interaction with an electrolyte transport system specific to this portion of the nephron. The system in question has been characterized as a Na^+ K^+ $2Cl^-$ electroneutral co-transporter and it has furthermore been suggested that the Tamin–Horsfall glycoprotein, which is concentrated within the luminal membrane of the TAL may be the diuretic receptor or a component of it [23]. However, this concept seems to hold true for only certain loop diuretics, notably the sulphamoylbenzoates, typified by frusemide. Other diuretics, such as muzolimine or indacrinone, do not necessarily work at the luminal surface or inhibit specifically the Na^+ K^+ $2Cl^-$ co-transporter [24]. In the case of indacrinone, there is evidence for high affinity binding to a membrane chloride exchange mechanism [25].

As we have seen, potassium-sparing diuretics exert their major effect in the late distal nephron and in particular within the cortical collecting tubule. The mechanisms of antikaluresis produced by these agents are not the same. Spirolactones are competitive inhibitors of aldosterone at the peritubular membrane site of the mineralocorticoid receptor; for this reason, spironolactone and canrenoate only inhibit aldosterone-mediated transport events. Triamterene and amiloride, on the other

214

hand, block conductive sodium channels on the luminal side of the tubular epithelium and, by so doing, prevent sodium from gaining access to the sodium pump or Na, K-ATPase which is located at the basolateral membrane on the peritubular surface [18]. Thus the inhibition of distal potassium and hydrogen ion secretion that occurs under the influence of these agents is in large part due to diminished passive entry of sodium into the cell and the dramatic resultant fall produced in the lumen-negative transepithelial voltage.

7.5 Extrarenal vascular effects of diuretics

Mention has been made of the widespread actions of diuretics on all manner of electrolyte transporting tissues in many species besides man. Such effects normally play a very subsidiary role in the therapeutic application of diuretic drugs, since the major goal in using diuretics to treat the syndrome of chronic heart failure is to correct the secondary salt-retaining consequences. This is achieved by utilizing the primary action of diuretics within the kidney. However, two important situations arise where the extrarenal actions of diuretics take precedence.

First, there is the use of diuretics in the management of hypertension where long-acting compounds, especially members of the benzothiadiazine family, continue to enjoy a key role [26]. This is despite recent concerns as to the potentially adverse consequences of the long-term metabolic sequelae of diuretic administration [9,27–29]. Although the initial antihypertensive effect of diuretics is due to shrinkage of the extracellular fluid and plasma volume compartments, with reduction in cardiac output, the sustained effect in lowering blood pressure relates to reduction in peripheral vascular resistance. The precise cause of the reduced resistance is uncertain [30]. Autoregulatory adjustments within tissues, so as to normalize cardiac output, may be responsible and these may involve finely balanced adjustments in the ratios of intra- to extracellular sodium and calcium [31].

The second important application of the extrarenal actions of diuretics also relates to vascular responsiveness but in the acute as opposed to the chronic setting. In acute heart failure, loop diuretics, such as frusemide, given intravenously, lower left heart filling pressure *before* a significant saluretic effect has become apparent [32]. This is usually achieved without compromising cardiac output [33]. The beneficial effect is due to increased capacitance of small veins with reduction in pulmonary capillary pressure and this, together with a degree of peripheral venodilatation, lowers cardiac preload and causes an overall improvement in left ventricular performance. These early extrarenal effects on venous capacitance appear to be prostaglandin-mediated, either by intrarenal prostaglandins liberated into the circulation or by locally released prostaglandins from vein walls [34].

7.6 'High ceiling' diuretics

The main members of this group are shown in Table 7.1. Included are a variety of chemically dissimilar compounds all capable of causing a rapid and powerful diuresis in which at least 15% of the filtered load of sodium chloride is excreted in the urine. Although rarely used today, the organo-mercurial, mersalyl, is included as it is still available (BNF, 1985). Ethacrynic is a non-mercurial phenoxyacetic acid derivative which shares chemical similarities with the first organomercurial, merbaphen (see Section 7.1) and mersalyl, but lacks any heavy metal in its structure.

Although introduced in the United States at about the same time as the first sulphonamide 'high ceiling' diuretic, frusemide, ethacrynic acid has never gained the same popularity in clinical usage as the latter drug. Phenoxyacetic acid analogues that are diuretically active react with sulphydryl containing molecules in a manner that correlates with their saluretic potential.

Introduction of a phenoxy [C_6H_5–O–) group at position 4 instead of Cl, together with substitution at position 3 of the sulphamoylbenzoate ring present in frusemide, has led to the development of bumetanide and piretanide (Fig. 7.1). The action of these compounds is similar though, on a weight basis, bumetanide is the more potent. Bioavailability of bumetanide and piretanide is considerably higher than frusemide [9, 35]. Absorption of oral frusemide may be impaired in patients with decompensated cardiac failure [36]. Clearance studies in man have shown that all the sulphamoylbenzoates have actions at tubular site I in addition to their main effect in the TAL; this is not the case with ethacrynic acid which behaves as a pure 'loop' diuretic [37]. Although the three sulphamoylbenzoates are effective in the management of chronic cardiac failure, piretanide has only been marketed as a slow-release preparation for the treatment of hypertension.

Muzolimine stands apart from the other 'high-ceiling' diuretics in having neither a sulphamoyl nor an acidic radical in its structure. It shares a dichlorobenzene ring with the phenoxyacetic acid analogues but, unlike these, it is a highly basic and lipophilic substance. It is ususual also in acting more slowly than classic 'loop' diuretics and its length of action is also protracted, probably reflecting its extensive metabolism *in vivo* [38]. Muzolimine is only available for clinical use in certain European countries.

A miscellany of other chemicals have been studied and found to display high-ceiling diuretic properties. None of these has thus far been introduced into clinical practice. Of particular interest are two compounds – ozolinone and indacrinone – which are chemically unrelated but both have asymmetric carbon atoms in their structures and each has been resolved into its respective stereo-isomers. It turns out that only one optically active isomer acts in the TAL to cause saluresis in each instance. Thus the laevorotatory isomers of ozolinone and indacrinone both behave like 'loop' diuretics, whereas the d-rotatory isomer of ozolinone is non-saluretic and that of indacrinone causes minor saluresis and prominent uricosuria [16, 39]. These findings suggest that a remarkable degree of stereospecificity exists at the target transport system for diuretics located in the TAL.

7.7 Medium efficacy diuretics

This is numerically the largest family of diuretics and it consists mainly of benzothiadiazine and related heterocyclic compounds. All possess modest diuretic activity and, at most, lead to excretion of 5–10% of the filtered load of sodium chloride. By contrast with loop diuretics, the dose–response curves for both saluretic and antihypertensive effects tend to be relatively flat [40, 41]. Some of the earlier members of the group, such as chlorothiazide, possess a degree of carbonic anhydrase inhibitory activity but nearly all of the substituted hydrofluazides derived from hydrochlorothiazide and the related heterocyclic analogues increase urinary chloride as opposed to bicarbonate output. Action is limited to the cortical diluting segment of the early distal tubule and the compounds reach their target site after passing through the probenecid-sensitive organic acid pathway in the proximal tubule.

There are currently thirteen members of this group available for prescription in the UK under the guise of 17 proprietary names: in addition, a further six preparations are combined with potassium.

Since the renal action of all these compounds is the same, there is therapeutic cross resistance in the group as a whole. A patient who has responded to maximal doses of one thiazide-like drug is unlikely to respond to another member of the same family. The only exception is metolazone which has significant sites of action in the nephron, additional to site III, and so in some respects overlaps with the 'loop' diuretics [42].

The time course of diuretic action varies among different members of the group. Whereas hydrochlorothiazide, bendrofluazide, cyclopenthiazide act for about 10–12h, the action of polythiazides, and especially chlorexolone and chlorthalidone, may persist for 48h or longer. The longer action may be advantageous in respect of low-dose use in

Diuretics

hypertension but can be the cause of troublesome nocturia when medium efficacy diuretics are used in the management of chronic cardiac failure.

7.8 Adjunct diuretics

In this group are to be found a number of different diuretics, each of which may be too weak to be effective on its own but which may possess special properties that may be useful in company with benzothiadiazine or loop diuretics.

7.8.1 XANTHINES

The main xanthine that remains in use today is theophylline. Its use in management of cardiac failure is usually reserved for cases of advanced disease where there may be disproportionate reduction in renal blood flow relative to glomerular filtration. By relaxation of the efferent arteriolar bed, theophylline may help to diminish the filtration fraction and restore responsiveness to benzothiadiazine or loop diruetics where this has lapsed due to inadequacy of the tubular solute load.

7.8.2 OSMOTIC DIURETICS

As an osmotic agent, mannitol suffers the major disadvantage of requiring intravenous administration. Its main mode of action is to block passive reabsorption of sodium chloride at site I via the paracellular shunt pathway which operates between the loose-fitting cells of this part of the nephron [43].

7.8.3 ANTI-KALIURETICS

Although potassium-sparing diuretics are only weak saluretics in their own right, their clinical usefulness mainly lies in their ability to potentiate the saluretic effects of other diuretics that act more proximally to site IV, whilst at the same time blocking urinary potassium wastage that is activated by the increased distal solute load.

Aldosterone interacts with specific receptors on the basolateral surface of the cells of the cortical collecting tubule. As a result, a signal is despatched to the cell nucleus where other receptors are activated to induce DNA-dependent RNA synthesis which codes for a specific aldosterone-induced protein that encourages sodium reabsorption. The peritubular receptor interaction is competitively blocked by aldosterone antagonists of which two are commercially available – orally active spironolactone and parenterally active potassium canrenoate. Both compounds are slow-acting and their full effect takes 3–4 days to become apparent.

Triamterene and amiloride do not possess a steroidal structure and both conserve potassium irrespective of the level of circulating aldosterone [9]. Triamterene is a pterideni and amiloride a pyrazine carboxamide derivative. Both act on the luminal surface of site IV producing an immediate block of passive sodium entry which drops the lumen-negative transepithelial voltage sharply and thereby discourages potassium and hydrogen ion secretion. The principal hazard in clinical use of anti-kaliuretics is hyperkalaemia, especially when renal function is already compromised. For this reason, no potassium-sparing diuretic should ever be used without first having undertaken a basal measurement of the plasma urea and electrolyte concentrations.

7.9 Polyvalent compounds

Under this heading comes a class of unusual diuretics that combine the properties of saluresis with uricosuria. The first to be discovered was tienilic acid which is a phenoxyacetic acid derivative, related to ethacrynic acid and possessing a thienyl heterocycle in its side-chain. The drug has been extensively studied and its saluretic properties derive from an action at site III, whereas the uricosuria emanates from interference with probenecid-sensitive urate handling at site I [44]. The limited saluretic potential of the compound places it in company with the medium efficacy benzothiadiazine group. Unfortunately, development of hepatotoxicity associated with its clinical use led to withdrawal of tienilic acid from the United States in 1980; the drug continues, however, to be used as an antihypertensive agent in France.

Indacrinone is an indanylacetic acid derivative that lacks a sulphur residue in its structure. It is a racemic mixture and, when its constituent enantiomers were separated, it emerged that each had different renal actions reflecting different sites of action in the nephron. Thus the (−) enantiomer behaves like a loop diuretic acting, as far as its saluretic potential is concerned, predominantly in site II, whereas the (+) enantiomer resembles tienilic acid and benzothiadiazines in localizing primarily to site III [16, 19]. [Fig. 7.3]. Indacrinone remains an experimental drug at the present time.

7.10 Therapeutic choice of diuretic

A number of basic principles should always guide the clinician when

219

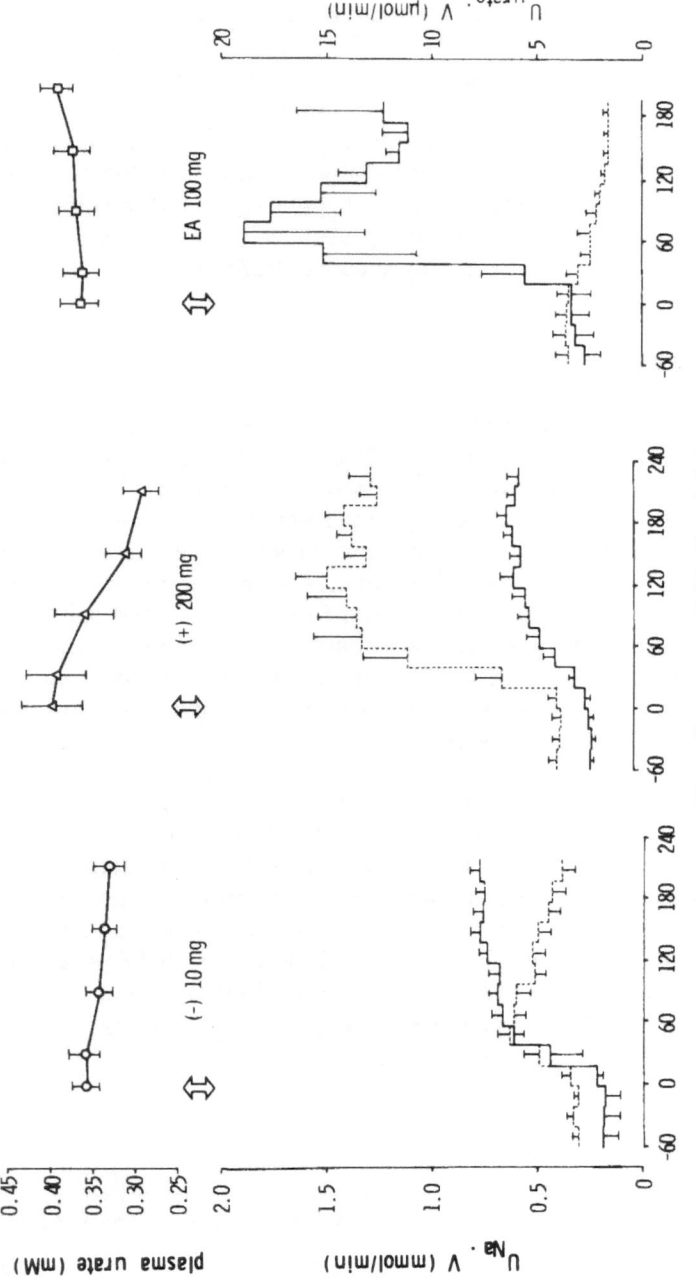

Fig. 7.3 Comparison of the sequential effects of single doses of the enantiomers of indacrinone with the effects of ethacrynic acid in normal human subjects undergoing maximal water diuresis. (−)-indacrinone causes a modest natriuresis and a small degree or uricosuria; (+)-indacrinone causes modest natriuresis with prominent uricosuria, whilst ethacrynic acid causes prominent natriuresis and a modest reduction in urinary uric acid excretion. Note also the striking fall in plasma urate produced by (+)-indacrinone and the elevation in plasma urate produced by ethacrynic acid [16].

choosing a particular diuretic in treatment. Probably the most important of these is the knowledge of the pharmacological qualities of diuretics in order to allow drug action to be appropriately matched to the pathophysiology of the disease state requiring control. One can speculate whether, had this premise been kept in mind, the widespread inappropriate use of excessively high doses of diuretics in treating hypertension might have been avoided.

7.10.1 HIGH EFFICACY VS. MEDIUM EFFICACY DIURETICS

The rapid effect of an intravenously administered loop diuretic in increasing venous capacitance and in reducing left ventricular filling pressure makes for an ideal choice in the emergency management of acute pulmonary oedema where the administration of a benzothiadiazine would be both inappropriate and clinically ineffective.

In oedematous states, generally, the main aim of adminstering a diuretic is to remove excess salt and water from the body. The potency of the diuretic must always be carefully titrated against the severity of the abnormal fluid retention. Powerful loop diuretics should be reserved for states of advanced fluid retention. Minimal oedema may need no more than bed rest, salt restriction, or digitalization if atrial fibrillation is present. In the early stages of cardiac failure, a medium-efficacy diuretic of the benzothiadiazine family or one of its congeners is the most appropriate agent. However, if this ultimately proves inadequate, it is pointless increasing the dose beyond the plateau of the rather flat dose–response curve characteristic of this group of diuretics, since little or no additional saluresis will occur [41]. If effective doses of a medium-efficacy diuretic are failing to achieve control, then *small* doses of a loop diuretic should be initiated. Unnecessarily large doses of loop diuretics given too early in the management of cardiac failure merely worsen peripheral hypoperfusion secondary to acute shrinkage of the plasma compartment. The drop in plasma volume serves to activate the renin–angiotensin–aldosterone system and the secondary aldosteronism stimulates increased renal potassium wastage.

7.10.2 ANTIKALIURETICS VS. POTASSIUM SUPPLEMENTS

The clinical use of potassium-sparing diuretics is intimately linked to the controversial issue of how important is the state of diuretic-induced hypokalaemia and what, if anything, should be done about it [45–48]. We have already discussed the mechanisms involved in successful saluresis with either a loop diuretic or a benzothiadiazine, or of both, given together. Inevitably, the induced diuresis causes an enhancement of distal nephron leakage of potassium. Diuretic-induced hypokalaemia is thus a common occurrence. About one-fifth of all patients on ben-zothiadiazine therapy develop hypokalaemia [47]. Although this does not necessarily mean that there is any associated deficit in body potassium stores, low plasma potassium can be significant in predisposing to cardiac dysrrhythmias [49]. This is specially so in high-risk patients such as the elderly, those on other drugs besides diuretics that cause renal potassium wastage (e.g. glucocorticoids, carbenoxolone), those on drugs that pro-long the QT interval (e.g. phenothiazines and tricyclic antidepressants), or where the patient is digitalized. Whether mild hypokalaemia poses a real hazard to the uncomplicated patient remains an unresolved and much debated issue [46, 50].

Once adequacy of dietary intake of potassium has been safeguarded, the choice in either trying to prevent or treat diuretic-induced hypoka-laemia lies between either giving potassium supplements or an anti-kaliuretic. Potassium chloride supplements are remarkably inefficient in preventing or correcting hypokalaemia, even when given in sizeable dosage, e.g. 64 mmol per day [51, 52]. Yet, physicians world wide have prescribed and continue to prescribe vast amounts of potassium chloride, to the tune of nearly 180 million US$ per annum in the United States alone [7]. In most instances, trivial dosage of 6–16 mmol per day is given as either a combined preparation with a benzothiadiazine a loop diuretic, or separately. The prescriber (and the patient) maintain the mistaken belief that body potassium status is being preserved and even being benefited by this gesture, especially when it can be claimed that a combined preparation has the 'built-in potassium.'

Against this widespread and illogical prescribing of ineffective doses of potassium chloride has to be weighed the cost-effectiveness, safety and convenience of antikaliuretic diuretics, qualities which, in turn, depend on the relative dosage equivalents of the drugs used. In safety terms, the key danger of antikaliuretic usage is the risk of hyperkalaemia, and for this reason, no potassium-sparing drug should ever be used before the patient's basal electrolyte and renal status has been determined. Equiva-lent potassium-sparing doses of amiloride or triamterene are of the order 20–30 mg vs 200 mg, respectively [52], and each of these dosages is equivalent to 50 mg spironolactone [51, 52]. In efficacy terms, this tends to make spironolactone the more economic contrary to popular belief. But this aldoesterone antagonist does have a number of unwanted effects that limit its long-term clinical usefulness. It can cause painful gynaecomastia in men and menstrual disturbances in women.

A number of fixed-combination preparations of an antikaliuretic with either a loop or benzothiadiazine diuretic are available in the United Kingdom [Table 7.2]. These offer convenience of administration to

Table 7.2 Fixed drug combination mixtures of potassium-sparing diuretics

Amiloride/Thiazide (mg)			Amiloride/Frusemide (mg)	
Amilco	5	50 (hydrochlorothiazide)	Frumil	
Moduret	2,5	25 (hydrochlorothiazide)	5	40
Moduretic	5	50 (hydrochlorothiazide)		

Triamterene/Thiazide (mg)			Triamterene/Frusemide (mg)	
Dyazide	50	25 (hydrochlorothiazide)	Frusene	
Dytide	50	25 (benzthiazide)	50	40
Kalspare	50	50 (chlorthalidone)		

Spironolactone/Thiazide (mg)			Spironolactone/Frusemide (mg)	
Aldactide 25	25	25	Lasilactone	
		(hydroflumethiazide)	50	20
Aldactide 50	50	50		

patients whose diuretic needs both in terms of sodium-loss and potassium-sparing requirements have been quantified and appear to be stable. The disadvantages are the obvious inability to vary independently the constituent compounds if requirements change, plus the arbitrary choice of dosages of the ingredients which may not necessarily counterbalance one another. A further difficulty relates to differences in bioequivalence between various commercial preparations as has been shown, for example, when Dyazide (50 mg triamterene; 25 mg hydrochlorothiazide) was compared with an alternative formulation, Maxzide (75 mg triamterene; 50 mg hydrochlorothiazide). Urinary recovery of triamterene after dosing with two capsules of Dyazide was about one-third of that following administration of one Maxzide tablet [53].

7.10.3 DIURETICS IN HYPERTENSION

For over twenty years, diuretics have been in the forefront of choice when initiating therapy for mild hypertension, especially in the United States [26, 45]. Diuretics have proved particularly effective in elderly and black patients. On the other hand, in Western Europe, beta-adrenoceptor blocking drugs have been the more popular first choice, especially in younger patients, and this role might have been strengthened even further had the role found for these drugs in secondary prevention of coronary artery disease also been demonstrated in primary prevention.

In the last few years, the supremacy of diuretics in the initial management of hypertension has been challenged [8, 45]. Whilst no one has

Diuretics

doubted that the sustained antihypertensive effect of diuretics reduces the incidence of stroke, cardiac and renal failure in hypertensive patients, the drug-induced elevations in plasma lipids, glucose and uric acid, together with the reductions in circulating potassium and magnesium concentrations have caused concern. The question has been raised as to whether these metabolic sequelae might be increasing the risk for cardiovascular disease [54]. Could we be merely substituting one risk factor for another? This issue was particularly highlighted by publication of the controversial MRFI trial [55].

It seems extraordinary that, just as physicians have for many years been busily prescribing routine potassium supplements at doses too low to have any useful effect, so they have misused diuretics in managing hypertension and to some considerable extent generated the problem of the unwanted metabolic sequelae of therapy. Already in 1963, Cranston *et al*. [40], showed clearly that the antihypertensive dose-response curves to three different members of the benzothiadiazine family is relatively flat and that no additional benefit is gained from using higher doses of these compounds. These observations have been confirmed more recently by other investigators in different countries. Yet, for reasons that are not clear, most of the recent large-scale studies of diuretic use in hypertension, including the MRFI trial, have used high-dosage schedules. For example, the Australian Therapeutic trial in Mild Hypertension (1980) [56] used 0.5–1.0 g chlorothiazide per day and the Medical Research Council study [57] used 10 mg bendrofluazide per day. An exception is the EWPHE study which employed a comparison of one Dyazide capsule (25 mg hydrochlorothiazide; 50 mg triamterene) with placebo [58]. Observations such as these would suggest that, in the majority of instances, there continues to be a misconception as to the relationship between dose and antihypertensive action of diuretics. It implies that continued effective diuresis is necessary to cause the maintained lowering of blood pressure. Yet this is clearly not so [30] (see also above, p. 213). The manufacturers of indapamide ingeniously fixed the maximal daily dose at 2.5 mg, so as to discourage prescribers from stepping up the dose in an attempt to increase the antihypertensive efficacy of the drug. Other manufacturers have done the opposite as for example, with xipamide, which is marketed as a 20 mg unit dose, well above doses known to produce effective lowering of blood pressure without prominent diuretic effects [59].

The lesson of all this is that when choosing a long-acting diuretic of the medium-efficacy group for use in hypertension, a much less aggressive approach is called for. The *lowest effective dose* should be the goal. If we all followed this direction, then diuretics might be reinstated to their rightful place as relatively safe, cost-effective agents of choice for starting treatment in most patients with mild hypertension. Where not effective as monotherapy, the dosage should not be increased into the saluretic zone, but, instead, a vasodilator, as for example, an ACE inhibitor, should be added with potentiation of clinical effectiveness.

7.11 Diuretic resistance

Resistance to the action of diuretics, when encountered today, is rarely due to lack of intrinsic drug potency, bearing in mind the steep dose-response characteristics of the loop diuretics. It is most commonly the result of interference at a pharmacodynamic or pharmacokinetic level with the renal mechanisms responsible for saluresis. Thus, for example, inadequate *control of salt intake* in a patient with cardiac failure may offset the saluretic potential of diuretic administration, especially if powerful salt-retaining processes involving the renin–angiotensin–aldosterone systems are already maximally stimulated.

Excessive enthusiasm in using inappropriately large doses of potent diuretics too early in the evolution of congestive cardiac failure may lead to diuretic resistance by invoking a major fall in plasma volume. This volume contraction, in turn, stimulates the renin–angiotensin–aldosterone system, and, as a result, not only is there diuretic resistance but enhanced renal potassium and magnesium wastage.

With the recent development of techniques capable of accurately detecting and quantitating the amounts of diuretic drugs and their metabolites in body fluids, it has proved possible to investigate the relevance of altered pharmacokinetics on the clinical response to diuretic therapy. It emerges that particularly for loop diuretics, the overall saluretic response is a function of the *total amount of drug* that has access to the tubular site(s) of action within the kidney. This, in turn, is dependent on the *dose administered*, the *absorption characteristics* and the *capacity of the transporting systems of the proximal renal tubule* for transferring drug from plasma to urine. It is also clear that the *time-course for drug delivery* into tubular urine is also critical [60, 61].

In decompensated as compared to compensated cardiac failure, for example, delayed absorption of frusemide has been found, even though the total absorption of drug remains unaltered [36]. Bioavailablity of frusemide is, in any event, normally only about 50–60% as compared with values of 90–100% found with other sulphamoylbenzoates such as bumetanide or piretanide. Considerations such as these explain why resistance to frusemide in severe congestive cardiac failure may be circumvented by intravenous use of the drug or by substantially raising the oral dose. With other loop diuretics having the much higher bioavailability, such modifications of route of administration or dosage may be unnecessary.

Another manoeuvre that may help to restore diuretic responsiveness is to increase renal blood flow with a xanthine such as aminophylline or an ACE inhibitor, thereby generating a more satisfactory tubular solute load as well as drug presence. Alternatively, different diuretics whose sites of tubular action do not overlap can be combined with additive, and sometimes synergistic, effects. This is the rationale for combined use of, for example, metolazone with a conventional loop diuretic or a K-sparing compound with either a benzothiadiazine or loop diuretic. In the case of combined use of thiazide or loop diuretics with an ACE inhibitor, the striking benefit in control of cardiac failure is, of course, not just due to the enhanced saluresis but also to the additional relief of afterload through perpheral vasodilatation. Where significant renal insufficiency is present, diuretic resistance reflects decreased drug delivery to the tubular site(s) of action. This is the reason that the diuretic response in the elderly to conventional doses of loop diuretics may be inadequate [62]. It is also the justification for using very large doses of loop diuretics where there is advanced renal failure; this helps to overcome both the massive fall in glomerular filtration and tubular transporting capacity. It is important to remember that in these circumstances, there is not only a global reduction in functional nephron mass but also accumulation of endogenous organic acids that are end-products of intermediary metabolism and directly interfere with the residual function of the proximal transport pathway.

Non-steroidal anti-inflammatory drugs blunt or totally negate the saluretic response to loop diuretics and are thus an important cause of diuretic resistance. The mechanisms involved have been studied extensively and the bulk of available evidence points to an interference with intrarenal haemodynamic repsonses to these diuretics rather than any major interference with the time-course of delivery of diuretic into the renal tubule [63, 64].

Thus in seeking to account for the occasional failure of diuretic therapy in different clinical situations, a therapeutic strategy has to be evolved which considers the possible participation of one or more of the processes discussed above, bearing in mind that in the seriously ill patient with heart failure, several mechanisms may be operative together.

7.12 Adverse effects

As a group of drugs which has enjoyed widespread usage throughout the world over the past thirty years, diuretics emerge with quite an impressive safety record. This is all the more remarkable when one considers that, at least as far as usage in the management of hypertension is concerned, consistent prescribing of unnecessarily large doses has highlighted and perhaps unmasked metabolic sequelae that might otherwise have gained less prominence or even been avoided. In the recent MRC trial of treatment in mild hypertension, as many as 25% of male patients and 14% of female patients stopped treatment with bendrofluazide because of unwanted effects; the daily dose used in the study was 10 mg [57]. Such problems have not featured to any significant extent in the application of diuretic therapy to the management of chronic heart failure mainly because of the much more limited patient survival as compared with mild to moderate hypertension [65].

As far as organ system disturbances directly attributable to diuretics are concerned, these are rare events overall. They include acute cholecystitis or pancreatitis, thrombocytopenia with thiazides, gynaecomastia in males and menstrual disturbances in females treated with spironolactone, and ototoxicity with high-dose loop diuretics [9]. The surprising finding of an incidence of 12.6 per 1000 patient years of observation with respect to impotence in bendrofluazide-treated patients in the MRC study [57] emphasizes the importance of asking the appropriate questions whenever investigation of the adverse reaction profile of long-term drug therapy is being undertaken.

By far, the issue that has received most attention in the literature concerning the long-term safety profile of diuretic therapy has been the continuing debate as to whether the metabolic complications that accompany diuretic treatment exert an independent unfavourable influence on known cardiovascular risk factors [9, 27, 54, 66, 67]. Maybe, if physicians had followed the guidance given on using the lowest effective dosage, there might have been no debate at all. Now that the patent protection has expired on all available thiazides, it is highly unlikely that any large-scale study will ever be mounted to provide a definitive answer as to the real benefit–risk ratio of truly low-dose thiazide therapy in hypertension.

7.12.1 HYPONATRAEMIA

In the management of chronic heart failure with diuretics, hyponatraemia can occur; usually it is mild, asymptomatic and requires no correction. It may, however, become a significant metabolic complication with nausea, headache, mental confusion and ultimately, convulsions and coma. The pathogenesis remains uncertain but clinical experience suggests that hyponatraemia occurs more commonly with long-acting members of the benzothiadiazine family of diuretics than with loop diuretics. Despite the different ways in which diuretics can cause hyponatraemia, it is also clear that patients with cardiac failure may develop a low plasma sodium concentration without ever having been given a diuretic [68]. A number of different mechanisms of diuretic-induced hyponatraemia have been implicated. Genuine sodium depletion may result associated with hypovolaemia, diminished glomerular filtration and an impaired renal ability to excrete dilute urine. More commonly, total body sodium is normal or increased, and when total body water is disproportionately increased, dilutional hypo-osmolality results. These changes may result from activation of vasoconstrictor hormones such as angiotensin and vasopressin which stimulate thirst and enhance renal water reabsorption. Another factor may relate to diuretic-induced cellular depletion of potassium which encourages a shift of sodium into the cells in order to restore osmotic equilibrium between the extra-and intracellular fluid compartments [69].

Management of severe hyponatraemia has involved a number of therapeutic approaches such as the traditional restriction of water intake, withdrawal of diuretics, administration of mannitol, hypertonic saline or corticosteroids. Yet many patients have proved resistant to one or more of these manoeuvres, and the situation has become irreversible. Recent work has supported a major causative role for the renin–angiotensin-aldosterone system, particularly when this system undergoes pronounced activation. It is upon this background that treatment of hyponatraemia with converting-enzyme inhibitors has been advocated. Hyponatraemic patients may, however, be dependent on angiotensin for support of their systemic blood pressure and thus become extremely sensitive to treatment with any drug interfering with the renin–angiotensin-aldosterone system. Careful titration of dose of ACE-inhibitor is essential and concurrent use of a loop diuretic may be necessary to reverse the hyponatraemic state [70, 71].

7.12.2 POTASSIUM AND MAGNESIUM BALANCE

The reasons for disturbance in balance of these two cations following continued diuretic therapy have been discussed at length already (p.212). Any diuretic that acts upon tubular sites in front of the distal cation exchange sites will inevitably cause an increase in urinary losses of potassium and magnesium. Hypokalaemia in young ambulant patients with uncomplicated hypertension treated with a thiazide is usually preventable by employing the lowest effective diuretic doses; if hypokalaemia occurs, it is mild, well tolerated and requires no corrective measures. On the other hand, in oedematous patients, with cardiac and/or hepatic disease, the risks of diuretic-induced hypokalaemia may be substantial [72]. This is especially so in certain groups of patient: those requiring digitalis glycosides or drugs affecting ventricular repolarization such as the tricyclic antidepressants or phenothiazines; the elderly and chronically sick in whom anorexia and deficient dietary intake are common; diabetic patients; those requiring concomitant therapy with corticosteroids, carbenoxolone or potent purgatives; and patients in the early phase after myocardial infarction.

Hypomagnesaemia frequently co-exists in patients with significant diuretic-induced hypokalaemia [49]. Failure to correct the underlying deficiency of magnesium may make it difficult or impossible to correct the intracellular depletion of potassium [73].

At the other end of the spectrum, *hyperkalaemia* is the most serious adverse effect associated with use of potassium-sparing diuretics and is a direct consequence of the pharmacological action of these agents. To avoid this occurrence, K-sparing agents should never be initiated in treatment without prior knowledge of the basal urea and electrolyte status of the patient.

7.12.3 CALCIUM BALANCE

Chronic thiazide therapy causes a reduction in urinary calcium excretion which has led to the use of these diuretics in the treatment of idiopathic hypercalciuria with recurrent renal calculi, as well as in the prevention of post-menopausal osteoporosis [74, 75]. The initial calciuria which is seen with loop diuretics may or may not be sustained in chronic therapy [76].

7.12.4 URIC ACID BALANCE

Asymptomatic hyperuricaemia is a common accompaniment of chronic diuretic therapy with loop or thiazide diuretics. The main mechanism involved in its causation is the enhanced proximal tubular reabsorption of urate secondary to diuretic-induced shrinkage of the extracellular fluid volume [77]. Hyperuricaemia, *per se*, in the absence of clinical gout, does not appear to constitute a significant cardiovascular risk factor. For patients with a predisposition to gout, the discovery of polyvalent diuretics capable of causing both uricosuria and saluresis offered a major potential advance in management. Unfortunately, the first of these compounds, tienilic acid, was only in clinical use for a few months before it was withdrawn in 1980 on account of hepatotoxicity; the drug remains in clinical use in France. The only other member of this series of diuretics, indacrinone, remains an experimental drug to date [78].

Diuretic-induced gout can be treated effectively with non-steroidal anti-inflammatory agents just as in primary gout. It must, however, be remembered that NSAI agents will blunt or negate the saluretic effects of coincidentally administered diuretics. Prophylactic lowering of plasma

Diuretics

urate in patients predisposed to gout who need continued diuretic therapy can be achieved with allopurinol.

7.12.5 IMPAIRED GLUCOSE TOLERANCE

The relative lack of significant disturbance in glucose tolerance where thiazide or loop diuretics have been used in low dosage lends support for a possible link between hypokalaemia and expression of diuretic-induced worsening of carbohydrate tolerance. There is also some evidence to suggest that loop diuretics may be less diabetogenic in long-term treatment than benzothiadiazines. However, length of therapy and dosage are important [79, 80]. Thus, not surprisingly, sporadic cases of hyperosmolar non-ketotic states have been precipitated by high-dose frusemide [81].

7.12.6 ALTERATIONS IN CIRCULATING LIPIDS

Increases in serum triglycerides and low-density lipoprotein (LDL)-cholesterol with a decrease or no change in HDL-cholesterol have been documented after long-term treatment with thiazide and loop diuretics [9]. Occurrence of such changes has, not unnaturally, focused attention on the question of whether chronic diuretic therapy has a significant atherogenic potential [82]. Subtle differences between the representatives of different diuretic groups have been noted but the mechanism of these diuretic-induced changes in lipid metabolism remains unknown. As with other metabolic effects of diuretics, the influence of dose may be critical [8, 67]. At the present time, there is no evidence that the hyperlipidaemic effect of diuretics is either a consistent phenomenon or one associated with aggravation of a major cardiovascular risk factor that might be offsetting or even negating the benefits conferred by long-term treatment with diuretics.

References

1. Stokes, W. (1854) *The Diseases of the Heart and the Aorta*, Hodges and Smith, Dublin, pp.354–5.
2. Heidenreich, O. (1969) Quecksilberhaltige diuretica. In *Handbuch der Experimentellen Pharmakologie*, Vol.24, Springer-Verlag, Berlin, pp.62–194
3. Saxl, P. and Heilig, R. (1920) Über die diuretische Wirkung von Novasurol und anderen Quecksilberinjektionen. *Wiener Klin. Wochenschr.*, 33, 943–4.
4. Vogl, A. (1950) The discovery of the organic mercurial diuretics. *Am. Heart J.*, 39, 881–3.
5. Maren, T.H., Mayer, E. and Wadsworth, B.C. (1954) Carbonic anhydrase

References

inhibition. I. The pharmacology of Diamox. 2-acteylamino-1,3,4-thiadiazole-5-sulfonamide. *Bull. Johns Hopkin Hosp.*, **95**, 199–243.

6. Novello, F.C. and Sprague, J.M. (1957) Benzothiadiazine dioxides as novel diuretics. *J. Am. Chem. Soc.*, **79**, 2028–9.

7. Hollenberg, N.K. (1984) Diuretic-induced potassium deficits: principles, opinions and practical therapeutics. *Am. J. Med.*, **77**, (5A), 1–2.

8. Gifford, R.W. (1984) The role of diuretics in the treatment of hypertension. *Am. J. Med.*, **77**, 102–6.

9. Lant, A. (1985) Diuretics: clinical pharmacology and therapeutic use. Part I. *Drugs*, **29**, 57–87; Part II, *Drugs*, **29**, 162–88.

10. Kokko, J.P. (1984) Site and mechanism of action of diuretics. *Am. J. Med.*, **77**(5A), 11–17.

11. Odlind, B. (1983) Determinants of access of diuretics to their site of action. *Fed. Proc.*, **42**, 1703–6.

12. Greger, R. (1985) Ion transport mechanisms in thick ascending limb of Henle's loop in mammalian nephron. *Physiol. Rev.*, **65**, 760–97.

13. Burg, M.G. and Green, N. (1973) Function of the thick ascending limb of Henle's loop. *Am. J. Physiol.*, **224**, 659–69.

14. Greger, R. (1981) Chloride reabsorption in the rabbit cortical thick ascending limb of the loop of Henle. A sodium-dependent process. *Pflügers Archiv.*, **390**, 38–43.

15. Lant, A.F., Baba, W.I. and Wilson, G.M. (1967) Localization of the site of action of oral diuretics in the human kidney, *Clin. Sci.*, **33**, 11–12.

16. Brooks, B.A., Lant, A.F., NcNabb, W.R. and Noormohamed, F.H. (1984) Stereospecificity of diuretic receptors in the nephron: a study of the enantiomers or indacrinone (MK-196) in man. *Renal Physiol.*, **7**, 304–10.

17. Stokes, J.B. (1981) Potassium secretion by cortical collecting tubule: relation to sodium absorption, luminal sodium concentration and transepithelial voltage. *Am. J. Physiol.*, **241**, F395–F402.

18. Benos, D.J. (1982) Amiloride: a molecular probe of sodium transport in tissues and cells. *Am. J. Physiol.*, **242**, C131–C145.

19. Brooks, B.A. and Lant, A.F. (1978) The use of the human erythrocyte as a model for studying the action of diuretics on sodium and chloride transport. *Clin. Sci.*, **54**, 679–83.

20. Frizzell, R.A., Field, M. and Schultz, S. (1979) Sodium-coupled chloride transport by epithelial tissue. *Am. J. Physiol.*, **236**, F1–F8.

21. Pitts, R.F. (1958) Some reflections on mechanisms of action of diuretics. *Am. J. Med.*, **24**, 745–56.

22. Dobyan, D.C. and Bulger, R.E. (1982) Renal carbonic anhydrase. *Am. J. Physiol.*, **243**, F311–F324.

23. Greven, J. (1982) Studies on the renal receptors of loop diuretics. *Clin. Exp. Hypertension*, **A5(2)**, 193–208.

24. Schlatter, E., Greger, R. and Weidtke, C. (1983) Effect of 'high ceiling' diuretics on active salt transport in the cortical thick ascending limb of Henle's loop of rabbit kidney. Correlation of chemical structure and inhibitory potency. *Pflügers Archiv.*, **396**, 210–17.

25. Lant, A. (1984) Red cell chloride transport in relation to the action of diuretics. In *Diuretics, Chemistry, Pharmacology and Clinical Applications* (eds J.B. Puschett & A. Greenberg), Elsevier, New York, pp.313–19.

Diuretics

26. Freis, E.D. (1984) Advantages of diuretics. *Am. J. Med.*, **77**, (4A) 107–9.
27. Grimm, R.H., Leon, A.S., Hunninghake, D.B., Lenz, K., Hannan, P. and Blackburn, I. (1981) Effects of thiazide diuretics on plasma lipids and lipoproteins in mildly hypertensive patients. A double-blind controlled trial. *Ann. Intern. Med.*, **94**, 7–11.
28. Moser, M. (1984) Clinical trials and their effect on medical therapy: The Multiple Risk Factor Intervention Trial. *Am. Heart J.*, **107**, 616–18.
29. Nicholls, M.G. (1980) Diuretic treatment of hypertension: benefits and risks. In *The Therapeutics of Hypertension*. RSM International Congress and Symposium Series, No.26, Academic Press, London, pp.13–22.
30. Shah, S., Khatri, I. and Freis, E.D. (1978) Mechanism of antihypertensive effect of thiazide diuretics. *Am. Heart J.*, **95**, 611–18.
31. Struyker-Boudier, H.A.J., Smits, J.F.M., Kleinjans, J.C.S. and van Essen, H. (1983) Haemodynamic actions of diuretic agents. *Clin. Exp. Hypertension*, **A5**, 209–23.
32. Johnston, G.D., Nicholls, D.P. and Leahey, W.J. (1984) The dose response characteristics of the acute non-diuretic peripheral vascular effects of frusemide in normal subjects. *Br. J. Clin. Pharmacol.*, **18**, 75–81.
33. Nelson, G.I.C., Ahuja, R.C., Silke, B., Okoli, R., Hussain, M. and Taylor, S.H. (1983) Haemodynamic effects of frusemide and its influence on repetitive rapid volume loading in acute myocardial infarction. *Eur. Heart J.*, **4**, 706–11.
34. Gerber, J.G. (1983) Role of prostaglandins in the hemodynamic and tubular effects of furosemide. *Fed. Proc.*, **42**, 1707–10.
35. Marcantonio, L.A., Auld, W.H.R., Murdoch, W.R., Purohit, R., Skellern, G.G. and Howes, C.A. (1983) The pharmacokinetics and pharmacodynamics of the diuretic bumetanide in hepatic and renal disease. *Br. J. Clin. Pharmacol.*, **15**, 245–52.
36. Vasko, M.R., Brown-Cartwright, D., Knochel, J.P., Nixon, J.V. and Brater, D.C. (1985) Furosemide absorption altered in decompensated congestive heart failure. *Ann. Intern. Med.*, **102**, 314–18.
37. McNabb, W.R. Noormohamed, F.H., Brooks, B.A. and Lant, A.F. (1984) Renal actions of piretanide and three other 'loop' diuretics in man. *Clin. Pharmacol. Ther.*, **35**, 328–37.
38. Gorrod, J.W., Messis, P.D. and Ritter, W. (1985) The metabolism of muzolimine. *Z. Kardiol.*, **74** (Suppl.2), 152–6.
39. Greven, J., Defrain, W., Glaser, K., Meywald, K. and Heidenreich, O. (1980) Studies with the optically active isomers of the new diuretic drug ozolinone. I. Differences in stereoselectivity of the renal target structures of ozolinone. *Pflügers Archiv.*, **384**, 57–60.
40. Cranston, W.I., Juel-Jensen, B.E., Semmence, A.M., Handfield Jones, R.P.C., Forbes, J.A. and Mutch, L.M.M. (1963) Effects of oral diuretics on raised arterial pressure. *Lancet*, **ii**, 966–70.
41. Peters, G. and Roch-Ramel, F. (1969) Thiazide diuretics and related drugs. In *Handbuch der Experimentellen Pharmakologie*, Vol.24, Springer-Verlag, Berlin, pp.257–385.
42. Puschett, J.B., Steinmuller, S.R., Rastegar, A. and Fernandez, P. (1973) Metolazone: Mechanisms and sites of action. In *Modern Diuretic Therapy in the Treatment of Cardiovascular and Renal Disease* (eds A.F. Lant, & G.M. Wilson),

Excerpta Medica, Amsterdam, pp.168–75.

43. Mathisen, O., Raeder, M. and Kiil, F. (1981) Mechanism of osmotic diuresis. *Kidney Int.*, **19**, 431–7.

44. Steele, T.H. (1979) Mechanism of the uriocosuric activity of ticrynafen. *Nephron*, **23**, 33–7.

45. Kaplan, N.M. (1983) The clinical use of diuretics in the treatment of hypertension. *Clin. Exper. Hypertension*, **A5**, 167–76.

46. Kaplan, N.M. (1984) Our appropriate concern about hypokalemia. *Am. J. Med.*, **77**, 1–4.

47. Knochel, J.P. (1984) Diuretic-induced hypokalemia. *Am. J. Med.*, **77**(5A), 18–27.

48. Seldin, D.W. (1983) Diuretic-induced potassium loss. In *Recent Advances in Diuretic Therapy* (ed V.E. Andreucci), Excerpta Medica, Amsterdam, pp.9–20.

49. Hollifield, J.W. (1984) Potassium and magnesium abnormalities: diuretics and arrhythmias in hypertension. *Am. J. Med.*, **77**(5A), 28–32.

50. Harrington, J.T., Isner, J.M. and Kassirer, J.P. (1982) Our national obsession with potassium. *Am. J. Med.*, **73**, 155–9.

51. Jackson, P.R., Ramsay, L.E. and Wakefield, V. (1982) Relative potency of spironolactone, triamterene and potassium chloride in thiazide-induced hypokalaemia. *Br. J. Clin. Pharmacol.*, **14**, 257–63.

52. Ramsey, L.E., Hettiarachichi, J. Fraser, R. and Morton, J.J. (1980) Amiloride, spironolactone and potassium chloride in thiazide treated hypertensive patients. *Clin. Pharmacol. Ther.*, **27**, 533–43.

53. Blume, C.D. and Williams, R.L. (1984) A new antihypertensive agent: maxzide (75 mg triamteren/50 mg hydrochlorothiazide). *Am. J. Med.*, **77**,(5A) 52–8.

54. Goldman, A.I., Steele, B.W., Schnaper, H.W., Fitz, A.E., Frohlich, E.D. & Perry, H.M. Jr (1980) Serum lipoprotein levels during chlorthalidone therapy. A Veterans Administration – National Heart, Lung and Blood Institute cooperative study on antihypertensive therapy: mild hypertension. *J. Am. Med. Assoc.*, **244**, 1691–5.

55. Multiple Risk Factor Intervention Trial (MRFIT) (1982) Risk factor change and mortality results. *J. Am. Med. Assoc.*, **248**, 1465–77.

56. Australian National Blood Pressure Study (1980) The Australian therapeutic trial in mild hypertension. Report by the Management Committee. *Lancet*, **i**, 1261–7.

57. Medical Research Council Working Party (1985) MRC trial of treatment of mild hypertension: principal results. *Br. Med. J.*, **291**, 97–104.

58. EWPHE Study (1985) Mortality and morbidity results from the European working party on high blood pressure in the elderly trial. *Lancet*, **i**, 1349–54.

59. MacGregor, G.A., Banks, R.A., Markandu, N.D. and Roulston, J. (1982) Xipamide and cyclopenthiazide in essential hypertension – comparative effects on blood pressure and plasma potassium. *Br. J. Clin. Pharmacol.*, **13**, 859–63.

60. Brater, D.C. (1981) Resistance to diuretics: emphasis on a pharmacological perspective. *Drugs*, **22**, 477–94.

61. Kaojarern, S., Day, B. and Brater, D.C. (1982) The time course of delivery of furosemide into urine is an independent determinant of overall response. *Kidney Int.*, **22**, 69–74.

Diuretics

62. Kerremans, A.L.M., van Baars, H., van Ginneken, C.A.M. and Gribnau, F.W.J. (1983) Furosemide kinetics and dynamics in aged patients. *Clin. Pharmacol. Ther.*, **34**, 181–9.
63. Chennavasin, P., Seiwell, R. and Brater, D.C. (1980) Pharmacokinetic–dynamic analysis of the indomethacin–furosemide interaction in man. *J. Pharmacol. Exp. Ther.*, **215**, 77–81.
64. Nies, A.S., Gal, J., Fadul, S. and Gerber, J.G. (1983) Indomethacin–furosemide interaction: the importance of renal blood flow. *J. Pharmacol. Exp. Ther.*, **226**, 27–32.
65. Taylor, S.H. (1985) Diuretics in cardiovascular therapy. Perusing the past, practising in the present, preparing for the future. *Z. Kardiol.*, **74** (suppl. 2), 2–12.
66. Hamer, J. (1982) Complications of diuretic therapy. In *The Modern Management of Congestive Cardiac Failure*, Lloyd-Luke, London, pp.22–37.
67. Perez-Stable, E. and Caralis, P.V. (1983) Thiazide-induced disturbances in carbohydrate, lipid and potassium metabolism. *Am. Heart J.*, **106**, 245–51.
68. Pruszczynski, W., Vahanian, A., Ardaillou, R. and Acar, J. (1984) Role of antidiuretic hormone in impaired water excretion of patients with congestive heart failure. *J. Clin. Endrocrinol. Metab.*, **58**, 599–605.
69. Orinius, E. (1984) Hyponatremia in congestive heart failure treated with diuretics. *Acta Pharmacol. Toxol.*, **54**, (Suppl. 1), 115–17.
70. Dzau, V.J. and Hollenberg, N.K. (1984) Renal response to captopril in severe heart failure: role of furosemide in natriuresis and reversal of hyponatremia. *Ann. Intern. Med.*, **100**, 777–82.
71. Packer, M., Medina, N. and Yushak, M. (1984) Correction of dilutional hyponatremia in severe chronic heart failure by converting-enzyme inhibition. *Ann. Intern. Med.*, **100**, 782–9.
72. Nardone, D.A., McDonald, W.J. and Girard, D.E. (1978) Mechanisms in hypokalemia: clinical correlation. *Medicine*, **57**, 435–46.
73. Whang, R. and Aikawa, J.K. (1977) Magnesium deficiency and refractoriness to potassium repletion. *J. Chronic Dis.*, **30**, 65–8.
74. Wasnigh, R.D., Benfante, R.J., Yano, K., Heilburn, L. and Vogel, J.M. (1983) Thiazide effect on the mineral content of bone. *N. Engl. J. Med.*, **309**, 344–7.
75. Yendt, E.R. and Cohanim, M. (1978) Prevention of calcium stones with thiazides. *Kidney Int.*, **13**, 379–409.
76. McNabb, W.R., Noormohamed, F.H. and Lant, A.F. (1984) Acute and chronic effects of piretanide in congestive cardiac failure. In *Diuretics, Chemistry, Pharmacology and Clinical Applications* (eds J.B. Puschett, & A. Greenberg) Elsevier, New York, pp.355–8.
77. Steele, T.H. and Oppenheimer, S. (1969) Factors affecting urate excretion following diuretic administration in man. *Am. J. Med.*, **47**, 564–74.
78. Brooks, B.A., Lant, A.F., McNabb, W.R. and Noormohamed, F.H. (1984) Renal actions of a uricosuric diuretic, racemic indacrinone, in man: comparison with ethacrynic acid and hydrochlorothiazide. *Br. J. Clin. Pharmacol.*, **17**, 497–512.
79. Berglund, G. and Andersson, O. (1981) Beta blockers or diuretics in hypertension? A six year follow-up of blood pressure and metabolic side effects. *Lancet*, i, 744–7.
80. Murphy, M.B., Lewis, P.J., Kohner, E., Schumer, B. and Dollery, C.T. (1982)

Glucose intolerance in hypertensive patients treated with diuretics; a fourteen year follow-up. *Lancet*, **ii**, 1293–5.

81. Tasker, P.R.W. and Mitchell-Heggs, P.F. (1976) Non-ketotic diabetic precoma associated with high dose frusemide therapy. *Br. Med. J.*, **1**, 626–7.

82. Lasser, N.L., Grandits, G., Cutler, J.A., Kuller, L.H. and Sherwin, R.W. (1984) Effects of antihypertensive therapy on serum lipids and lipoproteins in the Multiple Risk Factor Intervention Trial. *Am. J. Med.*, **76**(2A), 52–66.

8 Antihypertensive drugs

ANN ERRICHETTI and BRIAN F. JOHNSON

8.1 Introduction

Epidemiological studies have shown that that there is a linear rise in mortality with increasing levels of systolic and diastolic blood pressure (BP) [1]. Although there is no threshold at which mortality rates suddenly accelerate, several studies demonstrate increased morbidity and mortality associated with diastolic BP above 90 mmHg [2, 3]. Since the major goal in treating patients with hypertension is to prevent the morbidity and mortality attributable to high BP, this means the reduction of elevated BP to the extent that excess cardiovascular risk is minimized.

In most western societies, more than 25% of men and women aged 35–65 years have diastolic BP levels of 90 mmHg or more. Because 75% of all hypertensives have mild hypertension (defined as a diastolic BP between 90 and 104 mmHg), this group of patients contributes more to total cardiovascular morbidity and mortality than more severely hypertensive patients. Whether all patients with mild hypertension should be treated routinely with drugs poses an important health problem with important social and economic implications. However, the benefits of therapy may not outweigh the risk of placing all patients in pharmacological therapy; especially since the 5-year survival rate exceeds 97% in this group of patients even when untreated [3]. Certainly, financial expense and non-severe adverse effects would be justified if it could be shown that drug therapy is effective in preventing cardiovascular complications.

In fact, the results of three recent, large-scale clinical trials show that antihypertensive therapy is least effective in preventing atherosclerotic complications including coronary artery disease, which is the major complication in mild hypertension. The question arises as to whether drug-related factors may even predispose to or favour the development of coronary disease, thereby outweighing the beneficial effects of BP reduction [4]. These and similar problems need to be resolved before treatment goals can be more conclusively identified.

Nonetheless, these trials reconfirm the value of drug therapy for those with diastolic pressure greater than 100 mmHg. However, for the larger number of hypertensives with diastolic pressures in the 90–100 mmHg range, these studies suggest the need for a more cautious and individualized approach with repeated measurements over a 3–6 month period before initiating drug therapy. Certainly the decision to initiate therapy in any patient requires consideration of at least two factors; the severity of the BP elevation and the presence of target-organ effects or additional risk factors for coronary artery disease. Current recommendations suggest that if the BP falls below 100 mmHg on repeated determinations, no drug therapy is advised but close observation should be carried out. However, when the value exceeds 95 mmHg after several months of observation, treatment is warranted. If the diastolic pressure remains below 95 mmHg, measurement of BP and follow-up every 3–6 months is recommended. In patients with all levels of hypertension, careful attention should be paid to non-pharmacological therapy as an initial intervention and also as an adjunct to drug therapy. Weight reduction, salt restriction, exercise, low-fat diets and cessation of smoking are all valuable in some patients.

The available antihypertensive drugs differ greatly in their mechanism and duration of action, haemodynamic effects, frequency and type of adverse effects, cost and relative potency. This chapter will discuss the clinical pharmacology of these various agents, as well as their clinical effectiveness.

8.2 Diuretics

Diuretics may be classified as (1) thiazides and related drugs, (2) high-ceiling loop diuretics and (3) potassium-sparing diuretics.

8.2.1 THIAZIDES

The benzothiadiazines and related sulphonamide derivatives are so similar that they may be considered together. All act after excretion in the proximal tubules to inhibit sodium reabsorption in the thick cortical segment of the ascending limb of the loop of Henle. The varying degree of carbonic anhydrase inhibition is of historical interest as leading to the discovery of the drugs, but does not contribute to the diuretic mechanism. The increased excretion of Na^+, Cl^- and water leads to contraction of plasma volume and stimulation of the renin–angiotensin–aldosterone system which contributes to the increase in K^+ excretion [5].

Thiazides are rapidly absorbed from the gut with moderate bioavaila-

238

bility (60–90%), and are extensively protein bound with a high volume of distribution. A long duration of action is associated with greater protein binding and renal tubular reabsorption.

A short-term antihypertensive effect due to volume depletion is followed by an autoregulatory adjustment of cardiac output towards normal with a fall in BP and peripheral resistance [6, 7]. Reversal of the response on withdrawal of long-term treatment shows a sharp increase in plasma volume, followed by a gradual rise in BP [7].

All thiazides and related drugs are equally effective antihypertensives at equivalent diuretic doses, the chief differences being cost and duration of action. The flat dose–response curve is related to an increased incidence of side effects above the recommended maximum dose. A single morning dose produces a 24 hour antihypertensive action. Very small doses such as hydrochlorothiazide 12.5 mg daily may produce optimum fall in BP with minimal side effects [8], and may be useful in the elderly who are liable to side effects [9].

Moderate Na^+ restriction enhances the hypotensive effect of the thiazides and may minimize K^+ loss [10], whereas a high Na^+ intake produces less response and more K^+ loss. Severe Na^+ restriction produces K^+ wastage secondary to hyperaldosteronism [11].

Side effects include the expected electrolyte disturbances, metabolic effects and unusual skin [12] or haematological disturbances [13]. There seems little difference between the various drugs. In the recent MRC study, bendrofluazide treatment was associated with male impotence.

The fall in serum K^+ averages 0.6 mmol/l [14] and changes little over 2 years' treatment [15] and there is little change in total body potassium. Serum K^+ levels below 3.0 mmol/l are found in 2–4% of patients on diuretics [16], and may be associated with increased ventricular ectopic activity, abolished by correcting serum K^+ with spironolactone. Ectopic activity may be related to the presence of myocardial disease [17]. A moderate reduction in serum K^+ to between 3.5 and 3.0 mmol/l is usually well tolerated and requires no intervention, unless there is known myocardial disease or digoxin is being used and the effect can be potentiated. Dietary supplementation requires KCl as bicarbonate and citrate tend to increase metabolic alkalosis. Hyponatraemia may occur with excessive dosage in the elderly.

Urate excretion is reduced but produces gout only in the susceptible. Symptomless hyperuricaemia requires no treatment, but gout may be treated with allopurinol or uricosuric agent while continuing diuretic treatment. Hypercalcaemia may be accentuated in predisposing conditions such as primary hyperparathyroidism [18].

A mild reversible impairment of glucose tolerance is usual on thiazide treatment and frank diabetes may be precipitated in the predisposed.

Antihypertensive drugs

Control of established diabetes may be disturbed, perhaps by a diuretic-induced insulin resistance, but the relation to hypokalaemia has been disputed [19]. Increased plasma triglycerides and cholesterol [20, 21] may be related to the diabetic tendency and may have adverse cardiovascular effects offsetting the benefits obtained by lowering BP.

Thiazides inhibit the excretion of lithium and may potentiate its effects [22].

Metolazone is structurally related to the thiazides but shares in part the profound diuretic effect of the loop diuretics, remaining effective in larger doses in renal failure. An apparent advantage in terms of K^+ loss does not seem sustained on long-term treatment [23].

Indapamide is a thiazide analogue with high lipid solubility [24]. It reduces BP in the absence of diuretic effect [24] and it may act as a calcium antagonist.

Xipamide is a potent antihypertensive diuretic, but behaves similarly to the thiazides.

Some phenoxyacetic acid derivatives, such as *tienilic acid*, have uricosuric properties and could be useful in gouty hypertensives, as they resemble thiazides in other ways. Tienilic acid has been withdrawn because of a high frequency of liver and renal damage [25]. *Indacrinone* is similar as it is an effective diuretic but without these adverse effects [26]. Uricosuria carries the risk of crystal deposition and should be avoided by stopping other diuretics a few days before the start of treatment and by providing a high fluid intake.

8.2.2 HIGH POTENCY LOOP DIURETICS

High potency is associated with action on the ascending limb of the loop of Henle. These drugs are less effective than thiazides in hypertension [27] presumably because of the brief duration of action. They have a steep dose–response curve and are effective in advanced renal failure. Combination with thiazides may give an augmented response [28], presumably as they act on different sites in the renal tubule. Prostaglandins are involved in the action [29] and may account for a venous vasodilatory effect in heart failure. By blocking prostaglandin synthesis, non-steroidal anti-inflammatory drugs antagonize the effects of frusemide [30].

A local renin effect may be involved in an intrarenal redistribution of blood flow [31]. Electrolyte and metabolic effects are similar to the thiazides.

Frusemide, a sulphonamide analogue, may have cross-reactions with the thiazides, and produces similar hypersensitivity reactions. Ototoxicity and nephrotoxicity are reported in combination with aminoglycosides

[32] but are dose dependent and usually reversible; this effect is commonly related to intravenous use in renal failure.

Bumetamide is a related diuretic with greater potency and better bioavailability than frusemide (80% v 40%) [33], but adverse reactions seem similar. *Piretanide* is a similar new analogue [34].

Ethacrynic acid behaves similarly but is an aryloxyacetic acid. Adverse effects seem similar to frusemide with which there is no additive effect [35]. It rarely produces hypersensitivity reactions and may have less effect on glucose tolerance than the sulphonamide derivatives [32].

8.2.3 POTASSIUM-SPARING DIURETICS

(a) Spironolactone

Spironolactone, an aldosterone antagonist, is a moderate diuretic with a long duration of action which produces K^+ retention rather than loss by specific competitive inhibition of aldosterone action in the distal tubule and collecting duct. The effects are mainly due to the active metabolite, canrenone, which accumulates over three to four days on daily dosing with spironolactone. It has specific use in the treatment of the hypertension of primary hyperaldosteronism [36], pre-operatively or in patients not candidates for surgery. Effect is related to the circulating level of aldosterone [37], but spironolactone is effective when aldosterone is not in excess, so its use is not confined to hyperaldosteronism. Although only a mild diuretic as a single agent, it may be useful as a second drug to arrest thiazide-induced K^+ loss [38], but may be dramatically effective if the patient is refractory due to secondary hyperaldosteronism [39]. There is a steep dose–response curve over the usual range of dose from 25 to 100 mg daily [40]. It is usually given as a fixed dose combination of 25 mg spironolactone with 25 mg hydrochlorothiazide.

Side effects are relatively frequent [41]. Hyperkalaemia is a major hazard if there is renal insufficiency or K^+ supplements are given. Hyponatraemia and nausea or other gastrointestinal symptoms are frequent. An antiandrogen effect produces gynaecomastia, impotence or reduced libido in 1.2% of men during long-term use and menstrual changes or breast soreness have been reported in women; there is no definite association with breast cancer.

(b) Triamterene

Triamterene is chemically unrelated to aldosterone and has an independent direct effect on distal tubular Na^+ and K^+ exchange. It is generally used as a second drug to prevent K^+ loss and can produce hyperkalaemia in renal failure or on K^+ supplements [42]. The hormonal effects of spironolactone are not seen and side effects are uncommon. A weak action as a folic acid anatagonist can produce megaloblastic anaemia in predisposed patients such as cirrhotics.

(c) Amiloride

Amiloride is another different non-steroidal drug which antagonizes the Na^+ and K^+ exchange. It is more potent than triamterene [5]. It has only slight diuretic and antihypertensive effects as a single agent and is usually used to prevent K^+ loss on thiazides, with a small additive effect on BP. The dose–response curve is flat between 5 and 15 mg daily, and side effects are infrequent as with triamterene.

8.3 Peripheral adrenergic neurone blockade

Adrenergic neurone blocking agents are antihypertensive by interfering with the vasoconstrictor response to adrenergic stimulation by various mechanisms, such as depletion of stores of neurotransmitter (noradrenaline) in adrenergic terminals or preventing release. Many drugs of this class have been developed empirically and may act by more than one mechanism. Agents acting generally at autonomic ganglia are mainly of historical interest since the development of drugs which selectively block sympathetic function without the unwanted and often dangerous effects of parasympathetic blockade.

8.3.1 RESERPINE

Reserpine, the most used and best studied of the alkaloids of *Rauwolfia serpentina* acts both centrally and peripherally to prevent sympathetic discharge [43]. Brain catecholamines and serotonin are depleted, which may account for sedative and depressant effects, but a peripheral action may be of greater antihypertensive significance. Reserpine blocks the uptake of noradrenaline by the storage sites of the adrenergic nerve terminals, depleting catecholamine stores and interfering with transmission of the nerve impulse. The effect is maximal within 24 hours. Chronic administration depletes myocardial stores and may precipitate heart failure in susceptible patients. There is usually only slight bradycardia and cardiovascular reflexes are also only partially inhibited, so that orthostatic hypotension is uncommon. Renal blood flow and glomerular filtration are somewhat reduced. There may be hypersensitivity to exogenous catecholamines.

Gastrointestinal absorption is rapid but incomplete [44] and there is slow metabolic elimination [44]. About 10% of the dose is recovered in the urine.

Reserpine was the original second-line drug in the Veterans Administration study [45] and the more recent HDFP trial. In doses up to 0.5 mg daily reserpine has limited effect, reducing mean BP by only 5 mmHg. In combination with a diuretic, BP reduction was 12 mmHg [45], equal to thiazide plus either beta-blockers or methyldopa.

The effect is slowly cumulative over four to six weeks. Doses up to 2 mg daily have been used for severe hypertension, at the cost of a greater incidence of side effects, or intravenously in hypertensive emergencies. This use is not recommended because of the delayed onset of action and accompanying sedation which can make clinical evaluation difficult.

Untoward responses to reserpine at usual therapeutic doses are primarily in the central nervous system and the gastrointestinal tract. The more common include nasal congestion, drowsiness, reduced libido, impotence, unpleasant dreams, nausea and fluid retention. Hypotensive episodes are uncommon with doses below 1 mg daily but elderly patients with cardiovascular disease may be sensitive. Increased intestinal motility may cause abdominal cramps or diarrhoea. Gastric secretion is increased and reserpine is contraindicated in peptic ulcer. Even doses as small as 0.25 mg daily can produce nightmares and depression which may lead to suicide, and reserpine should not be used in patients with anxiety-depressive state. Extrapyramidal effects are seen with prolonged high dosage. A suggested relation to breast cancer has not been confirmed [46].

Hypertension may occur if reserpine is given to patients receiving monoamine oxidase inhibitors. The action of indirect sympathomimetic amines, e.g. ephedrine and amphetamine, may be diminished. New patients should not be started on reserpine, but patients on satisfactory treatment may be continued.

8.3.2 ADRENERGIC NEURONE BLOCKERS

(a) Guanethidine

Guanethidine may be regarded as the typical compound of this group. It is actively taken up by the noradrenaline re-uptake mechanism and so inhibits the release of noradrenaline from post-ganglionic adrenergic neurones [47]. The action is reduced by the tricyclic antidepressants which block the membrane amine pump [48]. Hypotension may follow withdrawal of tricyclics. Phenothiazines have similar, less marked, effects. Guanethidine does not prevent the release of catecholamines in phaeochromocytoma and may cause a severe hypertensive response analogous to the transient pressor effect which may follow acute administration. Indirect sympathetic amines (e.g. ephedrine and amphetamine) used as appetite suppressants or nasal decongestants may cause therapeutic failure.

The fall in BP is due in part to venodilation and decreased venous return. BP is therefore more effectively lowered in the upright position or after exertion. A direct depressant effect on myocardial performance through noradrenaline depletion reduces cardiac output and heart rate [49], though the cardiac output tends to recover with chronic treatment, probably as a result of fluid retention. Renal blood flow and glomerular filtration follow these cardiac output changes [49]. As guanethidine does not readily cross the blood–brain barrier, brain catecholamines and serotonin are not depleted and the central effects of reserpine are not seen.

Guanethidine is slowly absorbed from the gastrointestinal tract and undergoes extensive first-pass liver metabolism. Blood levels are very variable [50]. Forty per cent is metabolized and eliminated by the liver and 60% excreted in the urine. In renal failure guanethidine will accumulate and produce an exaggerated hypotensive response.

Guanethidine has been used for moderate and severe hypertension [51]. With the advent of better-tolerated drugs, it is presently used only when combinations of other drugs have failed. Management is made difficult by the steep dose–response curve and increments should not exceed 10 mg each week, with postural hypotension as the therapeutic end-point, except in carefully supervised in-patients. Differences in absorption account for part of the wide variability in dose [52]. Fluid retention is common and may result in resistance to the antihypertensive effect. Added diuretics may restore sensitivity and reduce dosage requirements [53]. Tolerance on prolonged administration may be due to postsynaptic supersenstivity. Diarrhoea is a common side effect from increased intestinal motility. Failure of ejaculation is frequent and impotence not uncommon. Other side effects include dizziness, stuffy nose, syncope and a subjective weakness which usually relates to BP reduction.

(b) Guanadrel sulphate

Guanadrel sulphate acts similarly to guanethidine, but is well obsorbed orally with fairly rapid urinary excretion so that side effects are reversed rapidly. It is effective at all levels of hypertension [54] with the expected side effects at higher doses.

(c) Bethanidine

Bethanidine acts similarly to guanethidine but is rapidly and extensively absorbed and excreted [55]. It produces less diarrhoea than guanethidine but is otherwise similar in effect.

244

(d) Debrisoquine

Debrisoquine is similar to bethanidine in side effects and efficacy [56]. It is well absorbed from the gut and metabolized in the liver. Hydroxylation to 4-hydroxydebrisoquine is polymorphic with slow metabolism inherited as an autosomal recessive [57]. There is much variability in dosage requirement, but the plasma level of unchanged drug correlates with the hypotensive response [58]. Many patients require increases in dose on maintenance therapy due to enhanced metabolic degradation.

(e) Trimethaphan

Trimethaphan is a rapidly acting ganglion blocker useful intravenously in hypotensive anaesthesia, and in hypertensive emergencies such as aortic dissection. It also has direct vasodilatory properties. Intravenous infusion of 2 g/l at 1 mg/min may be increased up to 15 mg/min. Head up tilt may add a postural fall in BP. Careful monitoring is needed to avoid a precipitous fall in BP and the infusion should be tapered gradually. Patients may become refractory after several days.

8.4 Alpha-adrenergic blockers

Alpha- and beta-receptors [59] are defined by their response pattern to stimulation by various catecholamines. Alpha-adrenergic receptors, which mediate smooth muscle contraction in arterioles and veins, respond maximally to adrenaline (epinephrine) and noradrenaline (norepinephrine) and much less so to isoprenaline. Conversely, beta-adrenergic receptors respond maximally to isoprenaline. Beta-adrenergic receptors are subdivided into $beta_1$-receptors which mediate increased heart rate and contractility, and $beta_2$-receptors which mediate vascular and bronchial smooth muscle relaxation. In recent years, two subtypes of alpha-receptors have also been identified. In general, alpha-receptors located postsynaptically on the vascular smooth muscle cell are the $alpha_1$-subtype, whereas receptors which are located presynaptically on the sympathetic nerve ending are of the $alpha_2$-subtype. Blockade of the postsynaptic $alpha_1$-receptor results in relaxation of vascular smooth muscle with a resultant fall in BP. Noradrenaline release from adrenergic nerve terminals is controlled by the rate of firing of the neurone. Subsequent stimulation of the presynaptic $alpha_2$-receptor by noradrenaline in the synaptic cleft reduces further noradrenaline release from the nerve ending [60]. When high concentrations of noradrenaline are present, subsequent nerve impulses release less noradrenaline. Thus, the presynaptic $alpha_2$-receptor forms part of an autoregulatory feedback loop which maintains the local level of sympathetic activity and thereby vascular tone.

The morphologic definition of alpha-receptors as pre- or postsynaptic may be of less significance than their relative affinities for various agonists and antagonists [61]. It is now recognized that both pre- and postsynaptic alpha-receptors may be of either the alpha$_1$- or alpha$_2$-subtype, or a mixture of both [61]. Since increased vascular sensitivity to vasoconstrictor stimuli has been implicated in the pathogenesis of hypertension, alpha-adrenergic receptor blockers were specifically developed for clinical use. These include the non-selective alpha-blockers, phentolamine and phenoxybenzamine, and selective alpha$_1$-blockers such as prazosin, trimazosin and indoramin.

8.4.1 PHENOXYBENZAMINE AND PHENTOLAMINE

(a) Mode of action

Administration of phenoxybenzamine and phentolamine results in non-selective blockade of alpha-adrenergic receptors. Although these drugs exert their main effect on alpha$_1$-receptors, they also enhance norepinephrine release in response to sympathetic stimulation via an alpha$_2$-blocking effect. Phenoxybenzamine alkylates alpha-adrenergic receptors irreversibly [62], whereas phentolamine is a short-acting competitive antagonist, and also has a direct vasodilator effect on arteriolar smooth muscle [63]. Antagonism to serotonin, histamine and acetylcholine occurs in some tissues, but does not contribute to their effect at commonly employed doses. Neither drug has a significant central nervous system action.

The haemodynamic effects of non-selective alpha-blockade are vasodilatation, tachycardia, increased cardiac output and variable fall in BP [64]. Plasma renin and catecholamine levels are raised. Beta-adrenergic effects predominate as alpha-receptors are effectively blocked.

Phenoxybenzamine is poorly absorbed (20–30%) after oral administration. It is highly lipid soluble and is only slowly released from fat deposits giving a duration of effect of 24 hours [65] with a cumulative effect over a week on daily administration.

Phentolamine is usually given intravenously with a peak action at 5 minutes and a duration of effect of 30–60 minutes. Orally phentolamine is well absorbed, but extensive and rapid first-pass metabolism in intestinal wall or liver reduces availability to less than 20% and it is virtually undetectable in plasma after 3 hours.

Non-selective alpha-adrenergic blockers are disappointing in the treatment of hypertension as the fall in BP is unreliable and associated with severe side effects. Their main place is in the pre-operative management of patients with phaeochromocytoma. Intravenous phentolamine is also useful in the severe rebound hypertension induced by clonidine withdrawal or in the reaction to tyramine-containing foods in a patient receiving a monoamine oxidase inhibitor. An intravenous bolus of 1–5 mg is followed by 20 mg in 500 ml of 5% dextrose at 2–50 mg/hour.

Phenoxybenzamine 1 mg/kg diluted in 250–500 ml and infused over at least one hour is effective in the pre-operative management of phaeochromocytoma. It may be given 36 and 12 hours before surgery [65]. Oral phenoxybenzamine is useful for chronic treatment because it produces irreversible alpha-blockade. Treatment begins with 16–30 mg daily as a single dose and increments of 10 mg are made at 1–4 day intervals. Most patients require 40–80 mg daily. Because of the marked orthostatic effect, standing BP should be used as the end-point for dose titration.

Addition of propranolol blunts the reflex tachycardia, but a beta-blocker must not be added until alpha-blockade is effective, as unopposed alpha-adrenergic vasoconstriction will produce a hypertensive crisis. Combination therapy is useful in patients unsuitable for surgical treatment or with unresectable metastatic lesions.

The main side effect of unselective alpha-blockade is postural hypotension, as vasoconstriction is attenuated in both arteries and veins. Reflex tachycardia may progress to arrhythmias. Phentolamine has prominent gastrointestinal side effects due to a muscarinic action which can be blocked by atropine. Other side effects include small pupils, nasal congestion and failure of ejaculation. Sedation, fatigue and lethargy occur with therapeutic doses of phenoxybenzamine. Hyperventilation, motor excitability and even seizures have been associated with rapid injection of large intravenous doses.

8.4.2 SELECTIVE ALPHA$_1$-BLOCKERS

(a) Prazosin

Prazosin may be regarded as the typical drug of this group as it has few complicating actions. The antihypertensive effect was originally attributed to a direct smooth muscle relaxant vasodilator effect, analogous to the chemically similar papaverine [66], or to other effects found only at prazosin concentrations several orders higher (e.g. 10^{-3}–10^{-4}M) than the concentration in vascular smooth muscle at the usual therapeutic doses (M10^{-6}–10^{-7}M) [67].

Antihypertensive drugs

The current hypothesis is that prazosin selectively blocks postsynaptic alpha$_1$-receptors [68]. The pressor response to angiotensin remains and presynaptic alpha$_2$-receptors are functional. This prevents a disproportionate increase in noradrenaline release, avoiding the increase in heart rate, cardiac output and renin release seen with less selective antagonists [66] and with the direct acting vasodilators. A combined venous and arterial dilator effect may prevent an increase in venous return seen with pure arterial vasodilators [69]. After intravenous prazosin there is a fall in BP and peripheral resistance with only slight tachycardia and little change in cardiac output, and this situation is maintained in chronic oral therapy. Reflex responses are unaffected [70] and renal blood flow is well maintained [71]. Tolerance may develop from fluid retention and reflex sympathetic activity [68] suggesting use as part of the stepped-care programme, after diuretics and beta-blockers.

Prazosin is well absorbed orally with an average bioavailability of about 60% [72] in spite of first-pass metabolism [67]. There are high concentrations in vascular smooth muscle [67]. The plasma half-life is between 2 and 6 hours [67, 72] and blood levels after intravenous use are related to the change in BP [72]. High drug levels and prolonged elimination are disputed in renal failure but are established in congestive heart failure perhaps due to dysfunction of the principal hepatic route of elimination [67].

Prazosin is effective in all degrees of hypertension [73], producing a significant and sustained reduction in BP, and is useful as a single agent in patients who cannot tolerate a diuretic or a beta-blocker. It has been most used with a diuretic or as a third-line drug where it has an additive effect, although the tendency to fluid retention is less than with hydralazine and other vasodilators. It has potentially beneficial effects on serum lipids [4], as opposed to thiazides which increase LDL-cholesterol and triglycerides, and beta-blockers which raise triglycerides and lower HDL-cholesterol [4].

The starting dose is 1 mg two or three times daily with an initial 0.5 to 1 mg dose at bed time to minimize the 'first-dose effect'. The dose is then gradually increased up to 20 mg daily. The usual dose is 6–15 mg daily but some patients have responded to larger doses. The optimum effect may not appear for several weeks and dose adjustments should be at 4–6 week intervals. A single large oral dose may achieve rapid control of severe hypertension.

The major side effect is the 'first dose effect' of acute postural hypotension [74] which may be accentuated be previous volume depletion with a diuretic or by a beta-blocker limiting tachycardia. Postural hypotension declines markedly during chronic therapy, perhaps from retention of presynaptic modifying alpha-activity. Other side effects are mild and infrequent, with headache, nausea, drowsiness, urinary frequency and sexual dysfunction the most apparent.

(b) Trimazosin

Trimazosin is an analogue of prazosin which may act as a direct arteriolar dilator rather than by postsynaptic alpha$_1$ blockade [75]. It seems effective in all grades of hypertension [76] at a dose of 50 mg twice daily increasing to 900 mg daily in three divided doses. It is not associated with a 'first-dose effect'. *Doxazasin* is another prazosin analogue under investigation, with the advantage of a long half-life allowing once daily dosing, and less tendency to a first-dose effect [77].

(c) Indoramin

Indoramin is a postsynaptic alpha$_1$-antagonist that also blocks histamine and serotonin (5H-T) receptors. Local anaesthetic effects are not associated with any cardiac depression at therapeutic doses [78]. The main effect is on standing BP and there is a bradycardia of unknown mechanism [78]. Postural hypotension is not commonly symptomatic and a first-dose effect is less likely than with prazosin.

Indoramin is well absorbed and metabolized by the liver with extensive first-pass effect [79]. It is effective in mild to moderate hypertension [80], and may be added to a diuretic or a beta-blocker, if either is inadequate alone [81]. The initial dose of 25 mg two or three times a day may be increased up to 200 mg daily unless limited by sedation, which may be combated by taking a larger dose in the evening than in the morning.

(d) Ketanserin

Ketanserin was developed as a pure antagonist of selected serotonin (5H-T$_2$) receptors in rat brain, but was also shown to have lesser alpha$_1$-blocking effects leading to speculation on the relation of the two classes of receptor in the peripheral arteriolar wall. It produces a useful fall in blood pressure without change in heart rate [82]. Intravenous and early oral treatment is associated with alpha-blockade, but in chronic treatment the hypotensive effect seems more than can be accounted for by this action alone. The fall in BP is related to plasma levels, and the kinetics allow once or twice daily treatment in steady-state conditions. There are few side effects on a dose of 40 mg twice daily as there is little central serotonin antagonism, but larger doses cause sedation. The part played by serotonin in maintaining peripheral vascular tone in hypertension remains a matter of speculation but action through modulation of alpha-adrenergic tone is suspected [83].

Antihypertensive drugs

8.5 Beta-adrenergic blocking drugs

The fall in BP noted by Prichard [84] while treating angina patients with an early beta-blocker, pronethalol, led to the use of these drugs in hypertension. A hypotensive effect is a common property of all beta-blockers, in spite of their differing ancillary properties (Chapter 2).

8.5.1 MODE OF ACTION

The first suggestion was that the hypotensive effect is related to the haemodynamic action of beta-blockade of slowing of the heart rate and reduced cardiac output with an adaptive reduction in peripheral resistance by autoregulation in the long-term [85], although the response is not related to the pretreatment cardiac output.

Block of renin secretion [86], a beta$_1$ effect in man, plays a part in the response [87], but low-renin hypertension does respond to higher doses [88] and renin suppression is not a necessary factor for the response. In a stepped-care programme renin suppression may be more important in patients receiving renin-stimulating drugs such as diuretics or vasodilators [89].

A third proposal is that beta-blockers interfere with central sympathetic outflow. This is demonstrated by intravertebral injection in animal work, but wide variation in central nervous system penetration of beta-blockers in relation to lipid solubility is not related to their effect in lowering BP (Chapter 2).

A fourth possibility is that beta-blockers prevent presynaptic beta$_2$ stimulation of noradrenaline release [60]. However, beta-blockers are strikingly free of the postural hypotension characteristic of adrenergic neurone blockade [90] and plasma noradrenaline levels tend to rise. The early suggestion that beta-blockers reset the baroreceptors [91] has had little experimental support, although it neatly describes the therapeutic situation of a lower BP with retained postural responses.

The cardioprotective actions of beta-blockers may play a part in the improved prognosis of cardiac infarction survivors on beta-blockade (Chapter 2), and there is a sanguine suggestion that a similar benefit may be found in susceptible patients with hypertension [92].

8.5.2 CLINICAL USE

Numerous well-controlled trials have demonstrated a modest effect alone or in combination with other drugs in all grades of hypertension. Comparative studies [93] have shown similar effect with all beta-blockers, but one or other drug may be preferred to minimize side effects. A reduction of 10–25 mmHg in mean arterial pressure of hypotensive patients is usual. More than 80% of patients respond if an adequate dose is given [88]. An effect is generally noted in a few days but may take several weeks to develop fully [85]. There is a wide margin between therapeutic and toxic doses and excessive hypotension and drug tolerance are rare.

There is growing support for the use of beta-blockers as initial therapy in mild to moderate hypertension. Some investigators have suggested that patients should be scheduled prospectively for one or other therapeutic approach by renin-profiling [86], but long-term trials have failed to support the value of renin-profiling to identify responders to beta-blockers [87]. Beta-blockers seem ideal for younger patients with increased sympathetic drive. They are less effective than diuretics in the elderly [94] and in blacks [95].

In moderate hypertension, combination with another drug is usually required. The effect is markedly potentiated by a thiazide diuretic, and they are nearly always included in a regimen with a vasodilator drug to minimize reflex tachycardia. Concurrent use with clonidine increases the risk of hypertensive crisis if either drug is suddenly discontinued [96]. Compliance is encouraged by the once daily use of slowly excreted drugs such as nadolol or atenolol, or by the use of long-acting slow-release formulations of other beta-blockers. Complete 24-hour beta-blockade does not seem necessary for the hypotensive effect (Chapter 2).

Labetalol is the first of a new group of drugs with alpha- and beta-adrenergic blocking properties. At low doses beta-blockade predominates and the effect resembles propranolol. The alpha$_1$-blocking effects cause more fall in BP at higher doses [97]. Afterload reduction may minimize the adverse cardiac effects of beta-blockade. It is well tolerated in all degrees of hypertension in blacks and whites [98], and can quickly control hypertensive crises.

Labetalol is generally well tolerated at starting doses below 400 mg daily, but postural hypotension is frequent at larger doses [98], as are other effects of alpha-blockade such as impotence and failure of ejaculation. As antinuclear antibodies may appear [99], there might be a risk of drug-induced lupus.

8.6 Central andrenergic inhibitors

The immediate control of normal BP relies to a large extent on the baroreceptor reflex, which reduces peripheral vascular tone in response to a rise in pressure in the carotid sinus and related baroreceptors. The reflex is integrated by a vasomotor centre in scattered areas of the brain-stem and hypothalamus, largely mediated by alpha-receptors [100]. The reflex control remains intact but at a higher level of pressure in hypertension.

251

Antihypertensive drugs

Centrally acting antihypertensive drugs, such as methyldopa and clonidine, stimulate brain alpha-receptors to inhibit sympathetic outflow.

8.6.1 METHYLDOPA

Methyldopa was introduced as a synthetic analogue of DOPA (dihydroxy
phenylalanine, a precursor of dopamine and noradrenaline) to inhibit
dopa decarboxylase in adrenergic nerve terminals. It was later postulated
that alpha-methyldopa formed alpha-methylnoradrenaline which was
taken up by adrenergic terminals and acted as a false transmitter, blocking
the normal nerve impulses [101]. The main site of action seems to be the
central nervous system. Methyldopa rapidly penetrates and forms alpha-
methylnoradrenaline which blocks central alpha transmission.

The haemodynamic effects of methyldopa in hypertension are close to
ideal with a fall in peripheral resistance without change in cardiac output
or renal blood flow [102]. The reduced sympathetic tone leads to a fall in
heart rate and in plasma renin. Postural and exercise hypotension are
much less than with peripheral adrenergic blockers such as guanethidine.

Absorption of methyldopa is highly variable due to extensive (30–70%)
first-pass metabolism in the gut wall to an inactive metabolite [103]. Renal
excretion of the drug and metabolites is rapid, 80–90% being eliminated
in 48 hours with normal renal function. The hypotensive effect is not
related to plasma levels [103], suggesting that these do not reflect the
central action of the drug.

For many years methyldopa was the most widely used non-diuretic
antihypertensive agent, but it has been supplanted because of the high
incidence of side effects. It has been used in all degrees of hypertension,
often in combination with diuretics or other drugs. The good haemodynamic effect with little change in rate or cardiac output make it useful in
coronary or cerebrovascular disease and in pregnancy hypertension. The
starting dose of 250 mg two or three times a day is increased up to 3 g a
day, beyond which there is little further benefit and a high incidence of
side effects. Increased sensitivity in renal failure is not entirely due to
drug accumulation [104].

Adverse reactions are frequent, including weight gain due to fluid
retention (which may produce tolerance relieved by adding a diuretic),
drowsiness, nasal congestion and dizziness. Most effects are dose related
and may show tolerance with continued treatment, though lassitude
and drowsiness tend to persist [104]. An additive effect with laevodopa
may potentiate the antihypertensive effect and the improvement of
Parkinsonism.

Various autoimmune phenomena are described. A low-grade hepatitis
may progress to cirrhosis [105] and the drug should be avoided in liver

disease. A positive Coombs test is reported in 10–20% of patients on at least 1 g daily for more than 6 months, but only 0.2% develop haemolytic anaemia [106], and treatment can usually be continued. The action may be antagonized by sympathomimetic amines [107], tricyclics, some phenothiazines and monoamine oxidase inhibitors [108] by uptake blockade or direct competition at central alpha-adrenergic receptors. Rebound hypertension if methyldopa is suddenly withdrawn is less severe than with clonidine [109].

8.6.2 CLONIDINE

Clonidine stimulates several varieties of alpha-receptor. Myocardial alpha$_1$-receptors may contribute to the bradycardia produced, but stimulation of alpha$_2$-receptors in the medulla is the main cause of BP reduction [110] and bradycardia. Stimulation of postsynaptic alpha-receptors in vascular smooth muscle causes a transient pressor reponse after intravenous injection.

Supine cardiac output is depressed with little change in peripheral resistance. The latter falls on standing with a greater decline in BP. Sympathetic reflexes are preserved and postural hypotension is infrequent [111] and this situation is maintained with treatment for at least one year. Renal blood flow is maintained and decreased sympathetic activity may reduce renin release as a lesser factor in the response, though the fall in BP is not related to the renin changes.

Clonidine is well absorbed and reaches maximum effect after 2–4 hours, lasting up to 18 hours [112]. More than half is metabolized and the remainder excreted unchanged in the urine, with prolongation of the half-life in renal failure. High lipid solubility gives it a large volume of distribution and it easily penetrates the blood-brain barrier [112].

Clonidine is effective in all degrees of hypertension and is usually well-tolerated in spite of a fall in cardiac output. Fluid retention on long-term use may be combated by adding a diuretic with synergistic effect. The effect is similar to other sympatholytic drugs and their effects may not be additive [112]. A beta-blocker with clonidine may even worsen BP control.

Treatment is usually begun at 0.1 mg twice daily and increased at 1–2 week intervals to a maximum of 1.2 mg daily, minimizing side effects by giving a larger dose at bed time. The incidence of side effects is similar to methyldopa. The most frequent are dry mouth and sedation.

Rebound hypertension may occur when clonidine is abruptly discontinued [109]. Accompanying anxiety and tachycardia may simulate phaeochromocytoma, and suggest rapid and excessive return of catecholamine secretion which had been suppressed during treatment. The

Antihypertensive drugs

incidence is low in uncomplicated hypertension, but is accentuated by beta-blocker therapy. Many incidents are in poorly controlled, severe hypertension. It is best treated by reinstituting clonidine therapy or by a combination of alpha and beta-blockade such as phentolamine and propranolol. Gradual withdrawal of clonidine over 2–3 weeks generally avoids the syndrome.

Clonidine resistance may be produced by stimulation of peripheral alpha-receptors giving a pressor response to larger doses. Tricyclic anti-depressants can antagonize the effect of clonidine and should not be prescribed in combination.

8.6.3 OTHER CENTRAL ALPHA-AGONISTS

Guanabenz is a central alpha$_2$-agonist with similar effects to clonidine [113] and with similar side effects. A 10–20% decrease in serum cholesterol is reported on long-term use.

Guanfacine is a new type of antihypertensive compound with similar central alpha$_2$-receptor stimulation, but slower entry into the brain. Greater stimulation of presynaptic inhibitory alpha$_2$-receptors may contribute to its action. The long half-life makes a withdrawal syndrome less likely than with clonidine and only daily dosage is required [114]. Sedation and postural hypotension are less likely than with clonidine but paradoxical hypertension is seen at higher doses.

Lofexidine is a clonidine analogue which may produce less side effects [115].

Tiamidine is a similar analogue which suffers from the rebound phenomenon on withdrawal [116].

8.7 Renin–angiotensin blockers

The renin–angiotensin–aldosterone system plays an important part in the control of BP, mainly through the action of angiotensin II at receptor sites in vascular smooth muscle, the central nervous system, the adrenal cortex and within the kidney.

Renin is a proteolytic enzyme secreted by the juxtaglomerular apparatus of the kidney in response to hypovolaemia, hypotension, or sodium depletion. It reacts with a plasma glycoprotein to produce the relatively inactive decapeptide, angiotensin I, which is converted by antiotensin converting enzyme, found in vascular endothelial cells, (especially in the lungs) into the highly active octopeptide angiotensin II. This potent arterial vasoconstrictor raises BP by a direct action on arterioles and the central nervous system, and also stimulates aldosterone secretion to produce sodium retention. A direct action within the kidney may also inhibit sodium excretion. The resultant fluid retention and rise in BP have a negative feedback effect which prevents further renin release.

The system has been interfered with by direct angiotension II antagonists, such as saralasin, which are limited by partial agonist effects and are mainly used in diagnostic tests for renovascular hypertension [117]. A more useful approach has been inhibition of the converting enzyme, such as by teprotide, captopril and enalapril. Arising from analysis of the venom of the Brazilian pit viper (*Buthrops varacara*), a purified peptide, called teprotide, was effective in severe high BP but had to be given parenterally. The work of Ondetti *et al.* [118] has given rise to a series of orally absorbed di- and tripeptides which are active converting enzyme inhibitors.

8.7.1 CAPTOPRIL

The sulphide derivative, captopril remains the typical drug of this group, producing a reduction in plasma angiotensin II and aldosterone concentrations while plasma renin and angiotensin I levels increase considerably as negative feedback is removed. Although the acute effects of captopril are related to baseline plasma renin, the long-term response to captopril is unrelated [119] and renin profiling is not needed as a guide to captopril treatment.

There is evidence of a functional interaction between the renin–angiotensin system and sympathetic tone [120]. Further, angiotensin converting enzyme is synonymous with kininase II which inactivates the vasodilating peptide bradykinin [121]. Tissue bradykinin accumulation could potentiate the vasodilator effects, although direct measurement has been difficult. The hypotensive effect may also be due in part to the production of general intravascular and intrarenal vasodilator prostaglandins, which is attenuated by indomethacin [122]. A local formation of angiotensin II in the brain stem which produces sympathetic activation may also be blocked by captopril [123].

The antihypertensive action of captopril is associated with a reduction in peripheral vascular resistance. Venous capacitance increases, reducing cardiac preload [123] with little acute change in cardiac output or heart rate, suggesting a blunting of baroreceptor function. The relative lack of volume expansion may be explained by suppression of aldosterone secretion and increased renal blood flow which prevents the sodium retention usually produced by a fall in blood pressure [124]. Activation of the renin–angiotensin system by sodium depletion or a diuretic may enhance the antihypertensive effect of captopril [125].

Absorption is rapid after oral administration [126] with rapid onset of effect. Availability is 75% in fasting subjects, and plasma protein binding reaches 30%. It is 50% metabolized to inactive mixed disulphides [126] with rapid renal excretion of unchanged drug and disulphides in relation to renal function.

Captopril is effective and well tolerated in varying degrees of renovascular and essential hypertension [127]. Between 30 and 50% of patients require an additional diuretic for effective BP control, and the secondary hyperaldosteronism and hypokalaemia of diuretic treatment are inhibited.

Captopril has usually been used in patients with severe hypertension resistant to conventional triple therapy, but combination with other drugs seems to give little added benefit [128]. A large BP response to captopril has been used as a screening test for renal artery stenosis [129]. It is effective in the high renin hypertension of renal disease. The effect is well maintained on long-term treatment perhaps because there is no fluid retention, and the dose can sometimes be reduced, minimizing side effects [130]

The high renin patient, for instance with renal artery stenosis or after diuretic therapy, may be very sensitive and it is wise to begin with 6.25 mg three times a day under close observation. A dose of 25 mg three times daily 1 or 2 hours before meals may be adequate in mild hypertension but the more usual daily dose in severe hypertension is 75–150 mg, beyond which there is little further response. Twice daily treatment may give adequate long-term control [130]. Small infrequent doses are effective in severe renal dysfunction as excretion is impaired. Disasters have been reported in bilateral renal artery stenosis or a functional equivalent, as a dramatic fall in BP or loss of an intrarenal compensatory action of angiotensin II may provoke acute renal failure.

Subjective side effects are generally few on captopril and there are no problems in asthma, diabetes or liver disease. However, in severe hypertension with renal insufficiency there was a high incidence of adverse reactions [131], related to higher doses and cumulation in renal insufficiency. Significant proteinuria may rarely lead on to the nephrotic syndrome. As many patients had renal disease or were on other drugs the interpretation of these findings is difficult.

Neutropenia was seen in 0.3% of patients, but they usually recovered after treatment was discontinued and it is probably not an unduly high risk. Skin rash in 14% of patients on large doses [131] may be accompanied by fever in the first 2 weeks or after a dose increase. Taste disturbance or loss has been related to zinc binding and may be dose dependent. Precautionary screening procedures for neutropenia or nephrotic syndrome can be reserved for patients at high risk.

8.7.2 ENALAPRIL

As the major side effects of captopril resemble penicillamine and may be related to the sulphydryl group, newer derivatives without this component have been investigated. Enalapril is an example which produces extensive and long-lasting converting enzyme inhibition [132].

Enalapril may be regarded as a pro-drug, as its own effect is relatively weak. It is, however, well absorbed and converted by hepatic esterases into its diacid potent derivative (enalaprilat), the active form of the drug which is itself poorly absorbed [132]. Peak levels occur 3–4 hours after oral enalapril. The general effect seems similar to captopril [133] but the more sustained effect allows two daily doses. A starting dose of 2.5 or 5 mg is advisable in case of hypersensitivity in high-renin situations. Beyond 20 mg, larger doses have a greater duration of action but no more hypotensive effect [134]. There have been few side effects [133, 134].

8.8 Direct vasodilators

The major haemodynamic disturbance in essential hypertension is an abnormally high peripheral resistance. Many antihypertensive agents lower peripheral resistance by reducing sympathetic nervous activity or antagonizing vascular alpha-receptors. Direct-acting vasodilators specifically produce vasodilatation by inducing relaxation of vascular smooth muscle.

Hydralazine, diazoxide and minoxidil are used in hypertension for their main action on arteriolar resistance vessels, whereas nitrates act primarily on the venous circulation and are used in angina and congestive heart failure to reduce preload.

8.8.1 HYDRALAZINE

Hydralazine exerts its antihypertensive effect through direct relaxation of arteriolar smooth muscle, where it is concentrated [135]. The main effect is in cerebral, coronary, splanchnic and renal circulations rather than in skin and muscle, and cardiac reflexes remain intact minimizing postural hypotension. Hydralazine is equally effective in the upright and supine positions [136]. Baroreceptor responses to the fall in BP produce reflex increases in heart rate, cardiac output and plasma renin which may antagonize the hypotensive effect if the drug is given alone, and an increase in myocardial oxygen consumption may accentuate angina.

Hydralazine is rapidly and completely absorbed from the gut [137] with extensive first-pass metabolism [138]. Eighty five per cent of plasma hydralazine is bound by albumin. There is a continued antihypertensive action after the plasma levels fall with a half-life of 2–6 hours [137], probably on the basis of persistence of the drug in arteriolar smooth muscle [135]. High plasma levels persist in patients with renal insufficiency [138] as 90% of the drug is excreted in the urine, though mostly as metabolites [139].

Acetylation in the liver is one major route of metabolism [138] dependent on genetically determined activity of the enzyme. Patients are bimodally distributed as fast or slow acetylators. Acetylation is mainly a feature of the first pass, and this metabolism may be saturable in slow acetylators giving higher plasma levels in the steady state and a greater reduction in BP [139]. They are also more likely to develop antinuclear antibodies and drug-induced lupus [140]. General hepatic metabolism involves hydroxylation and gluconuridation in addition to acetylation.

The effectiveness of hydralazine is relatively modest as a single agent [141], but the effect is improved and side effects reduced by combination with a sympatholytic agent such as a beta-blocker to reduce the reflex effects [142], and a diuretic to prevent sodium retention, and it is the original third step in triple therapy [141].

The oral dose begins with 10 to 25 mg three to four times a day. Twice daily treatment may be effective in some patients. The dose is increased weekly but should not exceed 200 mg a day, especially in slow acetylators [142] as the risk of lupus is then increased. Hydralazine is useful in renal insufficiency as renal blood flow is increased, but accumulation may occur [139] and sodium retention is likely.

Chronic administration of higher doses produces an acute rheumatoid state in 10% of patients and a smaller number develop systemic lupus [141]. The joint changes are generally minor and slowly reverse when hydralazine is withdrawn, and in contrast to idiopathic disseminated lupus erythematosus there is little renal involvement and no joint deformities. The majority of patients have antinuclear antibodies [141].

8.8.2 MINOXIDIL

This potent vasodilator is usually reserved for severe hypertension. It has been shown to block calcium uptake into smooth muscle cell membranes [143] producing relaxation. As a potent vasodilator it provokes a sharp sympathetic response via baroreceptor reflexes which tend to antagonize the hypotensive effect. Renal blood blow may decrease causing an extensive fall in blood pressure [144] with retention of sodium and fluid.

Minoxidil is well-absorbed after oral administration and is mostly metabolized in the liver to a glucuronide which is excreted in the urine [145]. There is little plasma binding but it seems to bind to vascular smooth muscle. Plasma half-life is about 4 hours but the effect of a single dose may last 1 to 4 days [145]. There is no accumulation in renal insufficiency and no dose adjustment is required [145].

Minoxidil seems more potent than hydralazine [145] and a hypotensive response is found in 80% of patients when minoxidil is added [146]. It has been used effectively for up to 5 years [144] without drug tolerance or postural hypertension. The response seems independent of the cause of the hypertension [146]. The initial oral dose is 5 mg daily increasing weekly to 10–40 mg daily, usually in divided doses.

Many of the untoward effects of minoxidil relate to reflex sympathetic activation, and may occur at subtherapeutic doses [146]. Fluid retention is a major limiting feature not correlated with the dose of minoxidil, and often requires large doses of a loop diuretic, such as frusemide 400 mg daily. Hypertrichiosis is a frequent side effect which is not dose related and is easily reversed. This side effect is often unacceptable to women.

Extensive myocardial necrosis in animals has not been noted in man [147], but pericardial effusion is frequent and may need reduction in minoxidil dose and an increase in frusemide [148]. The frequent T wave flattening which tends to regress with continued therapy [149] may be a related phenomenon.

8.8.3 DIAZOXIDE

This non-diuretic thiazide analogue is a potent arteriolar vasodilator usually used intravenously for an acute effect on severe hypertension. It has complex effects on calcium ions in vascular smooth muscle [150]. The vasodilatation provokes sympathetic reflex effects and marked fluid retention requiring simultaneous use of frusemide.

The suggestion that rapid bolus injection of 300 mg was needed to overcome the high degree of protein binding [151] is now discredited, and the possible adverse effects of a sudden fall in BP suggest that it is better to titrate the fall in pressure with repeated smaller injections or slow infusion [152]. Care must be taken to avoid extravasation as the alkaline solution causes pain at the injection site.

Oral diazoxide is well absorbed with peak plasma levels at 2–5 hours. There is about 90% binding to plasma proteins and it may potentiate the effect of warfarin. About 60% of the drug is metabolized in the liver and excreted with the remaining unchanged drug in the urine, with a half-life of 20–30 hours if renal function is normal [151]. The oral dose is 200–1000 mg daily in 2 or 3 divided doses. It is usually restricted to severe hypertension because of the serious side effects which are not usually a problem in acute therapy.

Side effects recorded [153] include fluid retention, hyperglycaemia and hirsutism.

8.8.4 NITROPRUSSIDE

This powerful relaxant of vascular smooth muscle shares some nitrate properties in that it affects both arteries and veins, probably by interfering with intracellular release of calcium ions [154]. Its rapid onset and offset of effect make it useful as a flexible intravenous agent for hypertensive crises and for elective hypotensive anaesthesia. The chemical presence of a cyanide group in the molecule is usually dealt with by hepatic conversion into thiocyanate which is excreted in the urine over several days [155].

Because of the rapid action an infusion pump or microdrip regulator is needed, and the drip system must be protected from light as nitroprusside is photosensitive. A total of 50 mg is dissolved in 500 ml of 5% dextrose solution to give 100 µg/ml, and initial infusion at 1 µg/kg per min may be titrated up to 8 µg/kg per min for not more than 4 days to avoid central nervous system toxicity (such as confusion or fits) or hypothyroidism from a thiocyanate effect. The main side effects are due to excessive or too rapid fall in BP.

8.8.5 OTHER VASODILATORS

Guancydine resembles minoxidil, but also dilates capacitance vessels. It is limited by severe fluid retention and tachycardia [156].

Pinacidil, another guanidine, is 2 to 3 times more potent than hydralazine and produces similar side effects [157].

Prizidilol resembles hydralazine with a beta-blocker side-chain and suffers from being acetylated in the same way as hydralazine [158]. The heart rate changes after a single dose suggest an initial beta-blockade followed by later vasodilator action [158].

8.9 Calcium channel blockers

Abnormalities of calcium ion transport in vascular smooth muscle may be fundamental to the development and maintenance of hypertension [159]. Defects in red cell membrane cation transport have been described in hypertensives and in their normotensive relatives, and regulation of intracellular calcium by a sodium–calcium exchange mechanism suggests that an inherited defect of cell membrane Na^+ transport may underly the cell calcium changes producing the increased vascular tone of hypertension.

The calcium channel blockers, although originally described on the basis of negative inotropic effect on cardiac muscle (Chapter 3), also reduce peripheral vascular smooth muscle tone suggesting a specific effect on the postulated cause of hypertension. Experience in the treatment of hypertension with drugs of this group is practically confined to nifedipine, verapamil and more recently diltiazem, which are all structurally dissimilar. Although all acting as calcium channel blockers, they possess differing profiles of effects (Chapter 3). Unlike vasodilators the calcium channel blockers do not increase aldosterone secretion [160]. Calcium channel blockers are especially useful in hypertensive patients with coexisting disease interacting with other commonly used drugs, such as chronic obstructive airways disease, Raynaud's phenomenon, coronary artery disease or diabetes. They may be most valuable in older, low renin patients [161]. The fall in pressure is usually related to the pre-treatment level of pressure [162].

Nifedipine 10 to 30 mg produces a brisk effect 30 min after an oral dose [162] with cardiac sympathetic stimulation increasing the reflex output. The effect is sustained on chronic administration. The tachycardia and renin response are attenuated by adding propranolol, and nifedipine may also be used with a diuretic as part of a triple drug regimen [163].

Verapamil characteristically produces a sharp fall in BP when given by intravenous injection for arrhythmia control. Oral treatment produces a maximal response at 90–120 min, lasting for up to 4 hours. Tachycardia is not seen with oral verapamil as the sinus node is depressed, and there is little change in plasma renin or aldosterone [164]. Doses of 120–160 mg three times daily produce a consistent hypotensive effect. It produces a useful added effect with other drugs [165].

Diltiazem has been little used in hypertension, but seems to have similar effects with little change in heart rate [166] in doses of 30–60 mg every 8 hours increasing up to 360 mg daily.

The main drawback to long-term use of calcium channel blockers in hypertension is the need for frequent dosing. This is overcome by the development of sustained release formulations, which for nifedipine have been shown effective by 24 hour monitoring on twice daily dosing [167]. Nitrendipine, a nifedipine analogue, produces a 24 hour reduction of blood pressure on 20 mg or 40 mg once daily [168].

Both nifedipine and verapamil have been used for the rapid control of hypertensive emergencies using sublingual nifedipine 10 mg (as for relief of angina) or intravenous verapamil, 5 to 10 mg (as for the control of paroxysmal tachycardia) but there must be concern about the depressant effect of verapamil on myocardial contractility.

8.10 The selection of a drug regimen

The aim of antihypertensive therapy is to lower BP to normal levels with minimal side effects and inconveniences. Whereas single drug therapy may be sufficient, combination therapy is more often necessary to control moderate or severe hypertension. By taking advantage of the additive or synergistic interaction of various agents, combination therapy often reduces risks of adverse effects by utilizing smaller doses of individual drugs. The availability of effective antihypertensive agents offers considerable benefit for large numbers of hypertensives, though several practical problems prevent realization of their full potential. These problems include failure to detect hypertension, the use of inappropriate drugs or inadequate doses, and non-compliance. In particular, side effects discourage compliance. Many untreated hypertensives are asymptomatic, and may develop symptoms for the first time while taking antihypertensive drugs. The physician should make every effort to find a drug regimen which is not only effective but also well tolerated. Also, simplifying the regimen with drugs that can be taken once or twice daily will usually improve compliance.

The use of a diuretic as the first choice in therapy has been advocated by many experts. Objections have been raised, however, to the consistent use of a diuretic as the first drug, mainly on the basis of the observed side effects and potential hazards of diuretics [169]. Laragh [86] and others have advocated the initial use of a beta-blocking drug, at least in patients with high plasma renin activity. Some investigators advocate the combination of a diuretic and a beta-blocking drug as ideal initial therapy [170], whereas others suggest a beta-blocker for borderline and mild hypertensives and the combination of a thiazide-type diuretic and an adrenergic inhibitor, such as reserpine or guanethidine, in established hypertension [171].

A stepped-care approach has been widely recommended as a guide for treating hypertensives when drug therapy is indicated [172]. This approach, which allows individualization and flexibility in management, has been used effectively in most of the reported large-scale clinical trials of drug therapy. The stepped-care approach involves initiating therapy with a small dose of an antihypertensive drug, increasing the dose of that drug, and then adding or substituting one drug after another in gradually increasing doses until goal BP is achieved, side effects become intolerable, or the maximum dose of each drug has been reached. Initial drug therapy should be with either a thiazide or a beta-blocker, unless contraindications to both exist. A beta-blocker is often more effective than a diuretic in young whites, whereas diuretics are usually preferable in elderly blacks. If single agent therapy is not completely effective at doses that begin to produce side effects, a second drug should be added. If therapy was begun with a diuretic, it is recommended that a small dose of an adrenergic inhibiting agent be added; either a beta-blocker, a centrally acting inhibitor (e.g. clonidine, methyldopa), or an alpha$_1$-adrenergic blocker (e.g. prazosin). The choice of the second drug is arbitrary, since all antihypertensive agents have risks of side effects that are variably tolerated by different patients. However, on the basis of their established record of fewer side effects and better patient acceptance with equal efficacy, beta-blockers are most commonly preferred. Alternatively, if a beta-blocker has been used initially, a thiazide or related diuretic should be added. If BP control is still not achieved, in step 3 a drug which reduces peripheral resistance (e.g. hydralazine or prazosin) can be added. Alternatively, captopril or a calcium channel blocker may be substituted for the adrenergic inhibiting agent. If all three steps are ineffective, drugs which are powerful but usually associated with serious adverse effects may be necessary. Minoxidil is usually acceptable to men, while guanethidine is often preferable in women. Either drug should be given in the smallest dose possible, by using combinations with other agents. Before proceeding to each successive treatment step, possible causes of lack of response should be ruled out, including poor compliance, inadequate doses of drugs, excess dietary sodium intake, fluid retention, drug interactions, and unrecognized secondary causes of hypertension. If goal BP cannot be reached because of intolerable side effects in patients with moderate or severe hypertension, partial reduction to 90–100 mmHg diastolic pressure has been shown to decrease cardiovascular mortality and may have to be accepted [173,174].

There are currently no large-scale definitive data to document a substantial advantage for any drug in relation to efficacy or patient acceptance. Although diuretics are effective and well tolerated, their side effects may be of more serious consequence than was originally believed. In the major clinical trials which employed a diuretic, the lack of a clear improvement in cardiovascular mortality suggests that diuretics may possess a detrimental effect which counterbalances the beneficial effects of BP reduction on cardiovascular risks. One possibility is that asymptomatic hypokalaemia increases the risk of fatal arrhythmia.

The other possibility relates to evidence that diuretics cause long-term changes in plasma lipid concentrations that might accelerate the development of atherosclerosis. Beta-blockers, the principal alternative initial therapy, will reduce BP in about the same proportion of patients as achieved by diuretics. However, side effects or exclusion criteria preclude their use in approximately 25% of hypertensive patients [175]. As with diuretics, certain beta-blockers alter the plasma lipid profile in a potentially detrimental manner. One very important though unproven advantage of beta-blocking drugs is their cardioprotective effect. The use of these agents following a myocardial infarction reduces mortality during the next year. Whether they provide primary protection from first coronary events in hypertensives is unknown. The ongoing Medical Research Council Trial may provide more definitive evidence of any favourable effects of beta-blocking drugs versus diuretics.

Recently, the use of prazosin as initial therapy has been advocated, since it improves the blood lipid profile in a manner that might enhance its long-term effectiveness in reducing vascular disease. Thus, the long-term metabolic response may be one determinant of the overall effectiveness of treatment and a factor in the choice of an available antihypertensive agent.

Finally, the choice of the optimum treatment varies with age. Elderly patients may be more sensitive to volume depletion and sympathetic inhibition than younger patients because of impaired cardiovascular reflexes. For this reason, drug treatment should be initiated with smaller than usual doses, and smaller increments should be made at longer than usual intervals. Drugs that have a propensity to cause orthostatic hypotension (e.g. guanethidine, prazosin) should be avoided if possible.

Three recent studies in mild hypertension are reviewed in reference [176]. Large numbers are needed to show the relatively small benefit. A difference in effect between diuretics and beta-blockers must be considered in view of the metabolic effects of diuretics which may accentuate any cardiac mortality and the possible protective effect of beta-blockers seen after cardiac infarction which may spill over into hypertension.

The EWPHE study in the elderly, who may be a high risk group, showed a reduction in fatal cardiac infarction, widely acclaimed as a beneficial effect of preventing hypokalaemia with triamterene which may indicate a difference of behaviour in the elderly heart. There was a similar moderate reduction in strokes as in the MRC study and in the Australian study of more severe patients.

The MRC study looked at a younger age group, and were on the whole less severe, with fewer events. There was no difference in myocardial infarction rate which was not affected in the EWPHE study although mortality was less there. It needed 850 patient-years of treatment to prevent one stroke, so it is doubtful if treatment is cost-effective. The IPPPSH oxprenolol study showed no preference for beta-blockade where comparison was possible. No firm evidence arose of adverse effects of diuretics compared to beta-blockers which were contrasted in the MRC study. It still seems that control of the blood pressure may be more important than the drug used and consideration should be given to non-pharmacological approaches to the treatment of mild hypertension.

References

1. Kannel, W.B., Gordon, T. and Schwartz, M.S. (1971) Systolic versus diasto-

lic blood pressure and risk of coronary heart disease. The Framingham Study. *Am. J. Cardiol.*, **27**, 335.

2. Stamler, J. (1975) Epidemiology of hypertension: Achievements and challenges. In *Hypertension: A Practical Approach* (ed. M. Moser), Little, Brown, Boston.

3. Bulpitt, C.J. (1982) Prognosis of treated hypertension 1951–1981. *Br. J. Clin. Pharmacol.*, **13**, 73.

4. Lowenstein, J. and Neusy, A.J. (1982) The biochemical effects of antihypertensive agents and the impact on atherosclerosis. *J. Cardiovasc. Pharmacol.*, **3** (Suppl. 3), S256.

5. Francisco, L.F. and Ferris, T.F. (1982) The use and abuse of diuretics. *Arch. Intern. Med.*, **142**, 28.

6. Shah, S., Khatri, I. and Freis, E.D. (1978) Mechanism of antihypertensive effect of thiazide diuretics. *Am. Heart J.*, **85**, 611.

7. Tarazi, R.C., Dustan, H.P. & Frohlich, E.D. (1970) Long-term thiazide therapy in essential hypertension. *Circulation*, **41**, 709.

8. Berglund, G. and Andersson, O. (1981) Beta-blockade or diuretics in hypertension: A six year follow-up of blood pressure and metabolic side-effects. *Lancet*, **i**, 744.

9. McKenney, J.M. (1974) Antihypertensive drug therapy. *J. Am. Pharm. Assoc. M.S.*, **14**, 204.

10. Ram, C.V.S., Garrett, B.N. and Kaplan, N.M. (1981) Moderate sodium restriction and various diuretics in the treatment of hypertension. *Arch. Intern. Med.*, **141**, 1015.

11. Landmann-Suter, R. and Struyvenberg, A. (1978) Initial potassium loss and hypokalemia during chlorthalidone administration in patients with essential hypertension: The influence of dietary sodium restriction. *Eur. J. Clin. Invest.*, **8**, 155.

12. Arndt, K.A. and Jick, H. (1976) Rate of cutaneous reactions to drugs. *J. Am. Med. Assoc.*, **235**, 918.

13. Magil, A.B., Balloon, H.J., Cameron, E.C. and Rae, A. (1980) Allergic interstitial nephritis associated with thiazide diuretics: Clinical and pathologic observations in three cases. *Am. J. Med.*, **69**, 939.

14. Morgan, D.B. and Davidson, C. (1980) Hypokalemia and diuretics: An analysis of publications. *Br. Med. J.*, **280**, 905.

15. Hesp, R. and Wilkinson, P.R. (1976) Potassium supplementation of thiazide therapy. *Lancet*, **ii**, 1144.

16. Ramsay, L.E., Boyle, P. and Ramsey, M.H. (1977) Factors influencing serum potassium in treated hypertension. *Q. J. Med.*, **36**, 401.

17. Harrington, J.T., Isner, J.M. and Kassirer, J.P. (1982) Our national obsession with potassium. *Am. J. Med.*, **73**, 155.

18. Christenson, T., Hellstrom, K. and Wengle, B. (1977) Hypercalcemia and primary hyperparathyroidism: Prevalence in patients receiving thiazides as detected in a health screen. *Arch. Intern. Med.*, **137**, 1138.

19. Amery, A., Bulpitt, C., Schaepdryver, A., Fagard, R., Hellmans, J., Mutsers, A., Berthaux, P., Deruyttere, M., Dollery, C., Forette, F., Lund-Johansen, P. and Tuomilehto, J. (1978) Glucose intolerance during diuretic therapy: Results of the trial by the European working party on hypertension in the elderly. *Lancet*, **i**, 681.

20. Johnson, B.F., Bye, C., Labrooy, I., Munro-Faure, D. and Slack, J. (1974) The relation of antihypertensive treatment to plasma lipids and other vascular risk factors in hypertension. *Clin. Sci. Mol. Med.*, **47**, 9.

21. Ames, R.P. and Hill, P. (1976) Elevation of serum lipids during diuretic therapy of hypertension. *Am. J. Med.*, **61**, 748.

22. Petersen, V., Hvidt, S., Thomsen, K. and Schou, M. (1974) Effect of prolonged thiazide treatment on renal lithium clearance. *Br. Med. J.*, **3**, 143.

23. Lanzoni, V., Smith, G. and Chobanian, A.V. (1976) Influence of metolazone, hydrocholorothiazide, and spironolactone on potassium balance in hypertensive patients. In *Systemic Effects of Antihypertensive Agents* (ed. M.P. Sambhie), Stratton Intercontinental Medical Book Corporation, New York.

24. Campbell, D.B. and Moore, R.A. (1981) The pharmacology and clinical pharmacology of indapamide. *Postgrad. Med. J.*, **57**, (Suppl. 2), 7.

25. McLain, D.A., Garriga, F.J. and Kantor, O.S. (1980) Adverse reactions associated with ticrynafen use. *J. Am. Med. Assoc.*, **243**, 763.

26. Brooks, B.A., Blair, E.M., Finch, R. and Lant, A.F. (1980) Studies on the mechanism and characteristics of action on a uricosuric diuretic, indacrinone (MK-96). *Br. J. Clin. Pharmacol.*, **10**, 249.

27. Anderson, J., Godfrey, B.E., Hill, D.M., Munro-Faure, M.D. and Sheldon, J. (1971) A comparison of the effectiveness of hydrochlorothiazide and of furosemide in the treatment of hypertensive patients. *Q. J. Med.*, **160**, 541.

28. Wollam, G.L., Tarazi, R.C., Bravo, E.L. and Dustan, H.P. (1982) Diuretic potency of combined hydrochlorothiazide and furosemide therapy in patients with azotemia. *Am. J. Med.*, **72**, 929.

29. Abe, K., Yasusima, M., Chiba, S., Irokawa, N., Ito, T. and Yoshinaga, K. (1977) Effects of furosemide on urinary excretion of prostaglandin E in normal volunteers and patients with essential hypertension. *Prostaglandins*, **14**, 513.

30. Brater, D.C., Beck, J.M., Adams, B.V. and Campbell, W. (1980) Effect of indomethacin on furosemide-stimulated urinary PGE_2 excretion in man. *Eur. J. Pharmacol.*, **65**, 213.

31. Scherer, B. and Weber, P.C. (1979) Time-dependent changes in prostaglandin excretion in response to frusemide in man. *Clin. Sci.*, **56**, 77.

32. Cooperman, L.B. and Rubin, I.L. (1973) Toxicity of ethacrynic acid and furosemide. *Am. Heart. J.*, **85**, 831.

33. Brater, D.C., Chennavasin, P., Day, B., Burdette, A. and Anderson, S. (1983) Bumetanide and furosemide. *Clin. Pharmacol. Ther.*, **34**, 207.

34. Henderson, C.S., Beattie, T.J., Kennedy, A.C. and Dombey, S.L. (1982) Oral piretanide in chronic renal failure. *Br. J. Clin. Pharmacol.*, **14**, 857.

35. Hook, J.B. and Williamson, H.E. (1967) Addition of the saluretic action of furosemide to the saluretic action of certain other agents. *J. Pharmacol. Exp. Ther.*, **148**, 88.

36. Brown, J.J., Davies, D.L., Ferriss, J.B., Fraser, R., Haywood, E., Lever, A.F. and Robertson, J.I.S. (1972) Comparison of surgery and prolonged spironolactone therapy in patients with hypertension, aldosterone excretion, and low plasma renin. *Br. Med. J.*, **2**, 729.

37. Erbler, H.C., Wernze, H. and Hilfenhaus, M. (1976) Effect of the aldosterone

antagonist canrenone on plasma aldosterone concentration and plasma renin activity, and on the excretion of aldosterone and electrolytes by man. *Eur. J. Clin. Pharmacol.*, **9**, 253.

38. Ogilvie, R.I. and Ruedy, J. (1969) Treatment of hypertension with hydrochlorothiazide and spironolactone. *Can. Med. Assoc. J.*, **101**, 591.

39. Kincaid-Smith, P., Fang, P. and Laver, M.C. (1973) A new look at the treatment of severe hypertension. *Clin. Sci. Mol. Med.*, **45**, 75S.

40. McInnes, G.T., Perkins, R.M., Shelton, J.R. and Harrison, I.R. (1982) Spironolactone dose–response relationship in healthy subjects. *Br. J. Clin. Pharmacol.*, **13**, 513.

41. Greenblatt, D.J. and Koch-Weser, J. (1973) Adverse reactions to spironolactone: A report from the Boston Collaborative Drug Survey Program. *J. Am. Med. Assoc.*, **225**, 40.

42. Hansen, K.B. and Bender, A.D. (1967) Changes in serum potassium levels in patients treated with triamterene and a triamterene-hydrochlorothiazide combination. *Clin. Pharm. Exp. Ther.*, **8**, 392.

43. Ingentio, A.J., Barrett, J.P. and Procita, L. (1969) A centrally mediated peripheral hypotensive effect of alpha-methyldopa. *J. Pharmacol. Exp. Ther.*, **175**, 593.

44. Maass, A.R., Jenkins, B., Shen, Y. and Tannenbaum, P. (1969) Studies on absorption, excretion and metabolism of ^{3}H-reserpine in man. *Clin. Pharmacol. Exp. Ther.*, **10**, 366.

45. Veterans Administration Cooperative Study Group on Antihypertensive Agents (1962) Double-blind controlled study of antihypertensive agents. II. Chlorothiazide alone and in combination with other agents. *Arch. Intern. Med.*, **110**, 230.

46. Labarthe, D.R. and O'Fallon, W.M. (1980) Reserpine and breast cancer. *J. Am. Med. Assoc.*, **243**, 2304.

47. Mitchell, J.R. and Oates, J.A. (1970) Guanethidine and related agents. I. Mechanism of the selective blockade of adrenergic neurones and its antagonism by drugs. *J. Pharmacol. Exp. Ther.*, **172**, 100.

48. Meyer, J.F., McAllister, C.K. and Goldberg, L.I. (1970) Insidious and prolonged antagonism of guanethidine by amitryptiline. *J. Am. Med. Assoc.*, **213**, 1487.

49. Richardson, D.W., Wyso, E.U. Magee, J.H. and Cavell, G.C. (1960) Circulatory effects of guanethidine: Clinical, renal, and cardiac response to treatment with a novel hypertensive drug. *Circulation*, **22**, 184.

50. McMartin, C. and Simpson, P. (1971) Absorption and metabolism of guanethidine in hypertensive patients requiring different doses of drugs. *Clin. Pharmacol. Ther.*, **12**, 73.

51. Dollery, C.T., Emslie-Smith, D. and Milne, M.D. (1960) Clinical and pharmacological studies with guanethidine in the treatment of hypertension. *Lancet*, **ii**, 381.

52. Rahn, K.L. and Goldberg, L.I. (1969) Comparison of antihypertensive efficacy, intestinal absorption, and excretion of guanethidine in hypertensive patients. *J. Pharmacol. Exp. Ther.*, **10**, 858.

53. Dustan, H.P., Tarazi R.C. and Bravo, E.L. (1972) Dependence of arterial pressure on intravascular volume in treated hypertensive patients. *N. Engl. J. Med.*, **286**, 861.

Antihypertensive drugs

54. Dunn, M.I. and Dunlap, J.L. (1981) Guanadrel: A new anti-hypertensive drug. *J. Am. Med. Assoc.*, **245**, 1639.
55. Doyle, A.E. and Morley, A. (1965) Studies in the absorption and excretion of ^{14}C-labelled bethanidine in man. *Br. J. Pharmacol.*, **24**, 701.
56. Flammer, J., Weidman, P., Gluck, Z., Ziegler, W.H. and Reubi, F.C. (1979) Cardiovascular and endocrine profiling of adrenergic neurone blockade in normal and hypertensive man. *Am. J. Med.*, **66**, 34.
57. Mahgoub, A., Dring, L.G., Idle, T.R., Lancaster, R. and Smith, R.L. (1977) Polymorphic hydroxylation of debrisoquine in man. *Lancet*, **ii**, 584.
58. Silas, J.H., Lennard, M.J., Tucker, G.T., Smith, A.J., Malcolm, S.L. and Marten, T.R. (1977) Why hypertensive patients vary in their response to debrisoquine. *Br. Med. J.*, **1**, 422.
59. Ahlquist, R.P. (1948) A study of the adrenotropic receptor. *Am. J. Physiol.*, **153**, 586.
60. Langer, S.Z. (1981) Presynaptic regulation of the release of catecholamines. *Pharmacol. Rev.*, **32**, 337.
61. Hoffman, B.B. and Lefkowitz, R.J. (1981) Alpha-adrenergic receptor subtypes. *N. Engl. J. Med.*, **30**, 1390.
62. Nickerson M. (1957) Nonequilibrium drug antagonists. *Pharmacol. Rev.*, **9**, 246.
63. Taylor, S.H., Sutherland, G.R., McKenzie, G.T., Staunton, H.P. and Donald, K.W. (1965) The circulatory effects of intravenous phentolamine in man. *Circulation*, **31**, 741.
64. Fowler, N.O., Holmes, J.C. and Gaffney, T.E. (1970) Hemodynamic effects of phenoxybenzamine in anesthetized dogs. *J. Clin. Invest.*, **49**, 2036.
65. Nickerson, M. and Collier, B. (1975) Drugs inhibiting adrenergic nerves and structures innervated by them. In *The Pharmacologic Basis of Therapeutics*, (eds L.J. Goodman & A. Gilman) MacMillan, New York, pp. 533–64.
66. Lowenstein, J. and Steele, J.M. (1978) Prazosin. *Am. Heart. J.*, **95**, 262.
67. Wood, A.S., Bolli, P. and Simpson, F.O. (1976) Prazosin in normal subjects: Plasma levels, blood pressure and heart rate. *Br. J. Clin. Pharmacol.*, **3**, 19.
68. Graham, R.M., Oates, H.F. and Stoker, L.M. (1977) Alpha-blocking action of the antihypertensive agent, prazosin. *J. Pharmacol. Exp. Ther.*, **201**, 747.
69. Graham, R.M. and Pettinger, W.A. (1979) Prazosin. *N. Engl. J. Med.*, **300**, 232.
70. Mancia, G., Ferrari, A., Gregorini, L., Ferrari, M.C., Bianchini, D., Terzoli, L., Leonetti, G. & Zanchetti, A. (1980) Effects of prazosin on autonomic control of circulation in essential hypertension. *Hypertension*, **2**, 700.
71. Koshy, M.C., Mickley, D., Bourgoignie, J. and Blaufox, M.D. (1977) Physiologic evaluation of a new antihypertensive agent: Prazosin hydrochloride. *Circulation*, **55**, 533.
72. Bateman, D.N., Hobbs, D.C., Twoomey, T.M., Stevens, E.A. and Rawlins, M.D. (1979) Prazosin, pharmacokinetics and concentration effect. *Eur. J. Clin. Pharmacol.*, **16**, 177.
73. Bolli, P. and Simpson, F.O. (1975) Experience with prazosin in the treatment of hypertension. Prazosin Clinical Symposium. *Postgrad. Med. Spec.*, no. 69.
74. Stokes, G.S., Graham, R.M., Gain, J.M. and Davies, P.R. (1977) Influence of dosage and dietary sodium on the first-dose effects of prazosin. *Br. Med. J.*, **1**, 1507.

75. Constantine, J.W. and Hess, H.J. (1974) The cardiovascular effects of trimazosin. *Eur. J. Pharmacol.*, **74**, 227.
76. Pool, P.E., Seagren, J.C. and Salel, A.F. (1983) Clinical hemodynamic profile of trimazosin in hypertension. *Am. Heart J.*, **106**, 1237.
77. Elliot, H.L., Meredith, P.A., Sumner, D.J., McLean, K. and Reid, J.L. (1982) A pharmacodynamic and kinetic assessment of a new alpha-adrenoreceptor antagonist, doxazosin (UK 33274) in normotensive subjects. *Br. J. Clin. Pharmacol.*, **13**, 699.
78. Alps, B.J., Hill, M., Johnson, E.S. and Wilson, A.B. (1970) Autonomic blocking properties of WY 21901. *Br. J. Pharmacol.*, **40**, 1531.
79. Royds, R.B., Coltart, D.J. and Lockhart, J.D.F. (1972) Pharmacologic studies of indoramin in man. *Clin. Pharmacol. Ther.*, **13**, 380.
80. Draffan, G.H., Lewis, P.J., Firmin, J.L., Jordan, T.W. and Dollery, C.T. (1976) Pharmacokinetics of indoramin in man. *Br. J. Clin. Pharmacol.*, **3**, 489.
81. Stokes, G.S., Frost, G.W., Graham, R.M. and MacCarthy, E.P. (1979) Indoramin and prazosin as adjuncts to beta-adrenoceptor blockade in hypertension. *Clin. Pharmacol. Ther.*, **25**, 783.
82. Hedner, T., Persson, B., and Berglund, G. (1983) Ketanserin, a novel beta-hydroxytryptamine antagonist: monotherapy in essential hypertension. *Br. J. Clin. Pharmacol.*, **16**, 121–5.
83. Zabludowski, J.R., Zoccali, C., Isles, C.G., Murrary, G.D., Robertson, J.T.S., Inglis, G.C., Fraser, R. and Ball, S.G. (1984) Effect of the 5-hydroxytryptamine type 2 receptor antagonist, ketanserin, on blood pressure, the renin-angiotensin system and sympatho-adrenal function in patients with essential hypertension. *Br. J. Clin. Pharmacol.*, **17**, 309–16.
84. Prichard, B.N.C. (1964) Hypotensive action of pronethalol. *Br. Med. J.*, **1**, 1227.
85. Tarazi, R.C. and Dustan, H.P. (1972) Beta-adrenergic blockade in hypertension: Practical and theoretical implications of long-term hemodynamic variations. *Am. J. Cardiol.*, **29**, 633.
86. Laragh, J.H. (1973) Vasoconstriction-volume analysis for understanding and treating hypertension: The use of renin and aldosterone profiling. *Am. J. Med.*, **55**, 261.
87. Stokes, G.S., Weber, M.S. and Thornell, I.R. (1974) Beta-blockers and plasma renin activity in hypertension. *Br. Med. J.*, **1**, 60.
88. Zacharias, R.J., Cowen, K.J., Prestt, J., Vickers, J. and Wall, B.G. (1972) Propranolol in hypertension: A study of long-term therapy. *Am. Heart J.*, **83**, 755.
89. Zanchetti, A., Leonetti, G., Terzoli, L. and Sala, C. (1983) Beta-blockers and renin. *Drugs*, **25**, (Suppl. 2), 58.
90. Doyle, A.E. (1974) Use of beta-adrenoceptor blocking drugs in hypertension. *Drugs*, **8**, 422.
91. Prichard, B.N.C. and Gillam, P.M.J. (1964) The use of propranolol in the treatment of hypertension. *Br. Med. J.*, **2**, 725.
92. Beevers, D.G., Johnston, J.H. Larkin, H. and Davies, P.C. (1983) Clinical evidence that beta-adrenoceptor blockers prevent more cardiovascular complications than other antihypertensive drugs. *Drugs*, **25**, (Suppl. 2), 326.
93. Wilcox, R.G. (1978) Randomised study of six beta-blockers and a thiazide diuretic in essential hypertension. *Br. Med. J.*, **2**, 383.

Antihypertensive drugs

94. Buhler, F.R., Burkart, F., Benno, L.E., Ling, M., Marbet, G. and Pfisterer, M. (1975) Antihypertensive beta-blocking action as related to renin and age. A pharmacological tool to identify pathogenetic mechanisms in essential hypertension. *Am. J. Cardiol.*, **36**, 653.
95. Humphreys, G.S. and Devlin, D.G. (1968) Ineffectiveness of propranolol in hypertensive Jamaicans. *Br. Med. J.*, **2**, 601.
96. Bailey, R.R. and Neale, T.J. (1976) Rapid clonidine withdrawal with blood pressure overshoot exaggerated by beta-blockade. *Br. Med. J.*, **1**, 942.
97. Frishman, W.H. and Halprin, S. (1979) Clinical pharmacology of the new beta-adrenergic blocking drugs. Part 7. New horizons in beta-adrenoceptor blockade therapy: Labetalol. *Am. Heart J.*, **98**, 660.
98. Brogden, R.N., Heel, R.C., Speight, T.M. and Avery, G.S. (1978) Labetalol: A review of its pharmacology and therapeutic use in hypertension. *Drugs*, **15**, 251.
99. Waal-Manning, H.J. and Simpson, F. (1982) Review of long-term treatment with labetalol. *Br. J. Clin. Pharmacol.*, **13**, (Suppl. 1), 66S.
100. Kobinger, W. (1978) Central alpha-adrenergic systems as targets for hypotensive drugs. *Rev. Physiol. Biochem. Pharmacol.*, **81**, 39.
101. Kopin, I.J. (1968) False adrenergic transmitters. *Ann. Rev. Pharmacol.*, **8**, 377.
102. Dollery, C.T., Harrington, M. and Hodge, J.V. (1963) Haemodynamic studies with methyldopa: Effect on cardiac output and response to pressor amines. *Br. Heart J.*, **25**, 670.
103. Saavedra, J.A., Reid, J.L., Jordan, W., Rawlins, M.D. and Dollery, C.T. (1975) Plasma concentrations of alpha-methyldopa and sulphate conjugates after oral administration of methyldopa hydrochloride ethyl ester. *Eur. J. Clin. Pharmacol.*, **8**, 381.
104. Lawson, D.H., Gloss, D. and Jick, H. (1978) Adverse reactions to methyldopa with particular reference to hypotension. *Am. Heart J.*, **96**, 572.
105. Rodman, J.S., Deutsch, D.J. and Gutman, I. (1976) Methyldopa hepatitis: A report of six cases and review of the literature. *Am. J. Med.*, **60**, 941.
106. Lobuglio, A.F. and Jandl, S.H. (1967) The nature of the alpha-methyldopa red-cell antibody. *N. Engl. J. Med.*, **276**, 658.
107. McLaren, E.H. (1976) Severe hypertension produced by interaction of phenylpropanolamine with methyldopa and oxprenolol. *Br. Med. J.*, **2**, 283.
108. Van Zweiten, P.A. (1976) Reduction of the hypotensive effect of clonidine and alpha-methyldopa by various psychotropic drugs. *Clin. Sci. Mol. Med.*, **51**, 4115.
109. Houston, M.C. (1981) Abrupt cessation of treatment in hypertension: Consideration of clinical features, mechanism, prevention and management of the discontinuation syndrome. *Am. Heart J.*, **102**, 415.
110. Schmitt, H. and Schmitt, H. (1970) Interactions between 2-2, 6-dichlorophenylamino-2-imidazoline hydrochloride (CST-155, Catapresan) and alpha-adrenergic blocking drugs. *Eur. J. Pharmacol.*, **9**, 7.
111. Lund-Johanssen, P. (1974) Hemodynamic changes at rest and during exercise in long-term clonidine therapy of essential hypertension. *Acta Med. Scand.*, **195**, 111.
112. Rehbinder, D. (1970) *Catapresan in Hypertension*. (ed. M.E. Connolly), Butterworths, London, p. 227.
113. Walker, B.R., Hare, L.E. and Deitch, M.W. (1982) Comparative anti-

hypertensive effects of guanabenz and clonidine. *Int. Med. Res.*, **10**, 6.

114. Jerie, P. (1980) Clinical experience with guanfacine in long-term treatment of hypertension. *Br. J. Clin. Pharmacol.*, **10**, 37S.

115. Lopez, L.M. and Mehta, J.L. (1984) Comparative efficacy and safety of lofexidine and clonidine in mild to moderately severe systemic hypertension. *Am. J. Cardiol.*, **53**, 787.

116. Hansson, R.G. and Kokfelt, B. (1981) Changes in blood pressure, plasma catecholamines and plasma renin activity during and after treatment with tiamenidine and clonidine. *Br. J. Clin. Pharmacol.*, **1**, 73.

117. Case, D.B., Wallace, J.M., Keim, H.J., Weber, M.A. and Laragh, J.H. (1977) Possible role of renin in hypertension as suggested by renin-sodium profiling and inhibition of converting enzyme. *N. Engl. J. Med.*, **296**, 641.

118. Ondetti, M.A., Rubin, B. and Cushman, D.W. (1977) Design of specific inhibitors of angiotensin converting enzyme: New class of orally active antihypertensive agents. *Science*, **196**, 441.

119. Gavras, H., Brunner, H.R., Turini, G.A., Kershaw , G.R. Tifft, C.P., Cuttelod, S., Gavras, I., Vukovich, R.A. and McKinstry, D.N. (1978) Antihypertensive effect of the oral angiotensin converting enzyme inhibitor SQ 14825 in man. *N. Engl. J. Med.*, **298**, 991.

120. Clough, D.P., Collis, M.G., Conway, J., Hatton, R. and Keddie, J.R. (1982) Interaction of angiotensin converting enzyme inhibitors with the function of the sympathetic nervous system. *Am. J. Cardiol.*, **49**, 1410.

121. Erdos, E.G. (1975) Angiotensin I converting enzyme. *Circ. Res.*, **36**, 247.

122. Swartz, S.L. and Williams, G.H. (1982) Angiotensin converting enzyme inhibition and prostaglandins. *Am. J. Cardiol.*, **49**, 1405.

123. Fagard, R.H., Lijnen, P.J. and Amery, A.K. (1982) Hemodynamic response to captopril at rest and during exercise in hypertensive patients. *Am. J. Cardiol.*, **49**, 1569.

124. Atlas, S.A., Case, D.B., Sealey, J.E., Laragh, J.H. and McKinstry, D.N. (1979) Interruption of the renin–angiotensin system in hypertensive patients by captopril induces sustained reduction in aldosterone secretion, potassium retention and natriuresis. *Hypertension*, **1**, 274.

125. Vlasses, P.H., Rotmensch, H.H. Swanson, B.N., Mojaverian, P. and Ferguson, R.K. (1982) Low-dose captopril: Its use in mild to moderate hypertension unresponsive to diuretic treatment. *Arch. Intern. Med.*, **142**, 1098.

126. Kripalani, K.J., McKinstry, D.N., Singhvi, S.M., Willard, D.A., Vukovich, R. A. and Migdalof, B.H. (1980) Disposition of captopril in normal subjects. *Clin. Pharmacol. Ther.*, **27**, 636.

127. Brunner, H.R., Gavras, H., Waeber, B., Textor, S.C., Turini, G.A. and Wauters, J.P. (1980) Clinical use of an orally acting converting enzyme inhibitor: Captopril. *Hypertension*, **2**, 558.

128. Ferguson, R.K., Vlasses, P.H., Koplin, J.R., Shirinian, A., Burke, J.F. & Alexander, J.C. (1980) Captopril in severe treatment-resistant hypertension. *Am. Heart J.*, **90**, 579.

129. Laragh, J.H., Case, D.B., Atlas, S.A. and Sealey, J.E. (1980) Captopril compared with other antirenin systemic agents in hypertensive patients. *Hypertension*, **2**, 586.

130. Mimran, A. and Jover, G. (1982) Maintenance of the antihypertensive

efficacy of captopril despite consistent reduction in daily dosage. *Br. J. Clin. Pharmacol.*, **14**, 815.

131. Waeber, B., Favras, I., Brunner, H.R. and Gavras, H. (1981) Safety and efficacy of chronic therapy with captopril in hypertensive patients: An update. *J. Clin. Pharmacol.*, **21**, 508.

132. Patchett, A.P., Harris, E., Tristram, E.W., Wyvratt, M.J., Wu, M.T., Taub, D., Peterson, E.R., Ideler, T.S., Tenbrocke, J., Payne, L.G., Ondeyka, D.L., Thorsett, E.D., Greenlee, W.S., Lohr, N.S., Hoffsommer, R.D., Joshua, H., Ruyle, W.V., Rothrock, J.W., Aster, S.A., Maycock, A.L., Robinson, F.M., Firschmann, R., Sweet, C.S., Ulm, E.H., Gross, D.M, Vassil, T.L. and Stone, C.A. (1980) A new class of angiotensin converting enzyme inhibitors. *Nature*, **288**, 280.

133. Dunn, F.G., Digman, W., Ventura, H.O., Messerli, F.H., Kobrin, I. and Frohlich, E.D. (1984) Enalapril improves systemic and renal hemodynamics and allows regression of left ventricular mass in essential hypertension. *Am. J. Cardiol.*, **53**, 105.

134. Chrysant, S.G., Brown, R.D., Kem, D.C. and Brown, J.L. (1983) Antihypertensive and metabolic effects of a new converting enzyme inhibitor, enalapril. *Clin. Pharmacol. Ther.*, **33**, 741.

135. Moore-Jones, D. and Perry, H.M. (1966) Radioautographic localization of hydralazine-1-C^{14} in arterial walls. *Proc. Soc. Exp. Biol. Med.*, **122**, 576.

136. Ablad, B. (1963) A study of the mechanism of the hemodynamic effects of hydralazine in man. *Acta Pharm. Tox.*, **20**, (Suppl. 1), 1.

137. Lesser, J.M., Israili, Z.H., Davis, D.C. and Dayton, P.G. (1974) Metabolism and disposition of hydralazine-^{14}C in man and dog. *Drug Metab. Dispos.*, **2**, 351.

138. Reidenberg, M.M., Drayer, D., Demarco, A.L. and Bello, C. (1973) Hydralazine elimination in man. *Clin. Pharmacol. Ther.*, **14**, 970.

139. Talseth, T. (1976) Studies on hydralazine. I. Serum concentration of hydralazine in man after a single dose and at steady state. *Eur. J. Clin. Pharmacol.*, **10**, 183.

140. Perry, H.M. (1973) Late toxicity to hydralazine resembling systemic lupus erythematosus or rheumatoid arthritis. *Am. J. Med.*, **54**, 58.

141. Koch-Weser, J. (1976) Hydralazine. *N. Engl. J. Med.*, **295**, 320.

142. Zacest, R., Gilmore, E. and Koch-Weser, J. (1972) Treatment of essential hypertension with combined vasodilatation and beta-adrenergic blockade. *N. Engl. J. Med.*, **286**, 617.

143. Bonaccorsi, A., Franco, R., Garattini, S. and Chidsey, C. (1973) Mechanism of vasodilatory activity of the antihypertensive minoxidil. *Circulation*, **48** (Suppl. 4), 174.

144. Andersson, O. and Silvertsson, R. (1980) Renal function and vascular resistance during long-term minoxidil treatment of severe hypertension. *J. Cardiovasc. Pharmacol.*, **2** (Suppl. 2), 123S.

145. Gottlieb, J.B., Thomas, R.C. and Chidsey, C.A. (1972) Pharmacokinetic studies of minoxidil. *Clin. Pharmacol. Ther.*, **13**, 436.

146. Linas, S.L. and Nies, A.J. (1981) Minoxidil. *Ann. Intern. Med.*, **94**, 61.

147. Sobota, J.T., Martin, W.B., Carlson, R.G. and Feenstra, E.S. (1980) Minoxidil: Right atrial cardiac pathology in animals and in man. *Circulation*, **62**, 376.

148. Mitchell, H.C. and Pettinger, W.A. (1978) Long-term treatment of refractory

References

hypertensive patients with minoxidil. *J. Am. Med. Assoc.*, **239**, 2131.

149. Hall, D., Charocopos, F., Fruer, K.L. and Rudolph, W. (1979) Electrocardiographic changes during long-term minoxidil therapy for severe hypertension. *Arch. Intern. Med.*, **139**, 790.

150. Wohl, A.S., Hausler, L.M. and Roth, F.E. (1968) Mechanism of the antihypertensive effect of diazoxide: *In vitro* vascular studies in the hypertensive rat. *J. Pharmacol. Exp. Ther.*, **162**, 109.

151. Sellers, E.M. and Koch-Weser, J. (1969) Protein binding and vascular activity of diazoxide. *N. Engl. J. Med.*, **281**, 1141.

152. Ram, C.V. and Kaplan, N.M. (1979) Individual titration of diazoxide dosage in the treatment of severe hypertension. *Am. J. Cardiol*, **43**, 627.

153. Fang, P. MacDonald, I., Laver, M., Hua, P. and Kincaid-Smith, P. (1976) Oral diazoxide in uncontrolled malignant hypertension. *Med. J. Aust.*, **2**, 621.

154. Kreye, V.A.W., Baron, G.D. and Luth, V.B. (1975) Mode of action of sodium nitroprusside on vascular smooth muscle. *Naunyn Schmiedebergs Arch. Pharmakol.*, **288**, 381.

155. Cohn, J.N. and Burke, L.P. (1979) Nitroprusside. *Ann. Intern. Med.*, **91**, 752.

156. Clark, B.W. and Goldberg, L.I. (1972) Guancydine: A new antihypertensive agent used with quinethazone and guanethidine or propranolol. *Ann. Intern. Med.*, **76**, 579.

157. Ramsay, L.E. and Firestone, S. (1983) Preliminary evaluation of pinacidil in hypertension. *Br. J. Clin. Pharmacol.*, **16**, 336.

158. Larsson, R., Karlberg, B.E., Norlander, B. and Wirsen, A. (1981) Prizidolol, an antihypertensive with precapillary vasodilating and beta-adrenoceptor blocking actions in primary hypertension. *Clin. Pharmacol. Ther.*, **29**, 588.

159. Blaustein, M.P. (1977) Sodium ions, calcium ions, blood pressure regulation, and hypertension: A reassessment and a hypothesis. *Am. J. Physiol*, **232**, C165.

160. Lederballe Pedersen, O. Middelsen, E., Christensen, N.S., Kornerup, H.J. & Pedersen, E.B. (1979) Effect of nifedipine on plasma renin, aldosterone and catecholamines in arterial hypertension. *Eur. J. Clin. Pharmacol.*, **15**, 235.

161. Buhler, F.R. and Hulthen, L. (1982) Calcium channel blockers: A pathophysiologically based antihypertensive therapeutic concept for the future. *Eur. J. Clin. Pharmacol.*, **12**, 1.

162. Olivari, M.T. Bartorelli, C., Polese, A., Fiorentini, C., Moruzzi, P. and Guazzi, M.D. (1979) Treatment of hypertension with nifedipine, a calcium antagonist agent. *Circulation*, **59**, 1056.

163. Murphy, M.B., Scriven, A.S.I. and Dollery, C.T. (1983) Efficacy of nifedipine as a step 3 antihypertensive agent. *Hypertension*, **5**, (Suppl. 2), II-118.

164. Muiesan, G., Agabiti-Rosei, E., Alicandri, C., Beschi, M., Castellano, M., Orea, L., Fariello, R., Romanelli, G., Pasini, C. and Platto, L. (1981) Influence of verapamil on catecholamines, renin and aldosterone in essential hypertension patients. In *Calcium Antagonism in Cardiovascular Therapy: Experience with Verapamil* (eds Zanchetti and Krikler), *International Symposium*, Florence, 2–4 October 1980, Excerpta Medica, Amsterdam, pp. 238–49.

165. Lewis, G.R.J. (1980) Verapamil in the management of chronic hypertension. *Clin. Invest. Med.*, **3**, 175.

166. Bourassa, M.G., Cote, P., Theroux, P., Tubau, J.F., Genain, C. and Waters,

Antihypertensive drugs

P.D. (1980) Hemodynamics and coronary flow following diltiazem administration in anesthetized dogs and in humans. *Chest,* **787** (Suppl. I), 224.

167. Hornung, R.S., Gould, B.A., Jones, R.I., Sonecha, T.N. and Raftery, E.B. (1983) Nifedipine tablets for systemic hypertension: A study using continuous ambulatory intra-arterial recording. *Am. J. Cardiol.,* **51**, 1323.
168. Hansson, L., Andren, L., Oro, L. and Ryman, T. (1983) Pharmacokinetic and dynamic parameters in patients treated with nifedipine. *Hypertension,* **5**, (Suppl. 2), II-25.
169. Dollery, C.T. (1981) Does it matter how blood pressure is reduced? *Clin. Sci.,* **61**, 413S.
170. Finnerty, F.A. (1979) Diuretics as initial treatment for essential hypertension. *Br. J. Clin. Pharmacol.,* **7** (Suppl. S), 185S.
171. Messerli, F.H. (1981) Individualization of antihypertensive therapy: An approach based on hemodynamics and age. *J. Clin. Pharmacol.,* **21**, 517.
172. Joint National Committee on detection, evaluation and treatment of high blood pressure. The 1984 report of the Joint National Committee on detection, evaluation, and treatment of high blood pressure. *Arch. Intern. Med.,* **144**, 1045.
173. Australian Therapeutic Trial in Mild Hypertension (1980) Report by the management committee. *Lancet,* **i**, 1261.
174. Hypertension Detection and Follow-Up Program Cooperative Group (1979) Five-year findings of the Hypertension Detection and Follow-Up Program. I. Reduction in mortality of persons with high blood pressure, including mild hypertension. *J. Am. Med. Assoc.,* **242**, 2562.
175. Kaplan, N.M. (1983) Therapy for mild hypertension: toward a balanced view. *J. Am. Med. Assoc.,* **249**, 365.
176. Treatment of hypertension: the 1985 results (1985) *Lancet,* **ii**, 645–57.

9 Vasodilator therapy in congestive heart failure

JOHN HAMER

Vasodilator therapy was introduced with the somewhat naive idea that if a sick heart works less it should get better [1]. The use of the term 'unloading' subsconsciously suggests that a beneficial effect will be obtained. Confirmation of benefit was obtained as a result of the widespread practice of haemodynamic monitoring in the intensive care of seriously ill patients, which has allowed detailed study of the response to intravenous vasodilators in acute heart failure [2].

This approach arose from the evidence that the peripheral vasculature affected the heart [2] and that the increase in peripheral resistance to maintain perfusion in the face of a falling cardiac output might increase the load on the left ventricle, together with the Guyton concept that the venous return to each ventricle was adjusted by the body to produce an identical output from the two sides of the heart in spite of differing ventricular function (Starling) curves [3, 4]. Convincing data from acute studies with intravenous nitroprusside [5] have shown that vasodilator treatment reduces ventricular work and may be thought of as increasing myocardial efficiency by reducing myocardial oxygen consumption as left ventricular volume is reduced while external cardiac work is maintained. With this treatment we are seeking to make optimum use of the limited power output of the diseased heart.

It seems likely that the best response is obtained in patients showing maximal vasoconstrictor responses [6], leading me to formulate the concept of a 'stepped care' approach to heart failure [7] in which vasoconstrictor effects are induced by optimum diuretic treatment, before the introduction of vasodilator therapy. The differential activation of specific vasoconstrictor mechanisms, such as alpha-adrenergic vasoconstriction and the renin–angiotensin–aldosterone system, is responsible for some of the apparent tolerance to vasodilators and for rebound deterioration on withdrawal of treatment [6].

Vasodilator therapy in congestive heart failure

9.1 Preload effects

It is usual to consider two aspects of unloading in relation to the differential effects of vasodilators on the venous (capacitance) and arterial (resistance) systems, producing reduction in preload and afterload respectively. The main action of venous dilators, such as the nitrates, is on the capacitance vessels of the systemic venous system reducing left ventricular filling pressure, by removal of blood from the tense pulmonary venous system, but direct pulmonary venous dilatation may play a part in the response.

The main drugs used to reduce preload are the nitrates, though large doses or direct infusion can also produce arterial effects [8]. The main benefit from reduced preload is probably the reduction in left ventricular work that results from a smaller diastolic volume, through the law of Laplace [6]. Symptomatically, residual breathlessness may improve if there is reduction in pulmonary venous congestion. In severe failure the Starling curve is flat and there is little fall in output from the reduction in filling pressure; an adverse effect may occur in less severely affected patients with a steep Starling curve producing a dramatic fall in cardiac output [7] (Fig. 9.1). A similar effect may occur from increased regurgitation in mitral incompetence as preload is reduced [9] and regurgitant flow may increase at the expense of forward flow.

The tendency for a reduction in output as preload is reduced may be countered by improved myocardial function, expressed as movement to a higher Starling curve, as subendocardial flow improves following removal of the compressing effect of a raised diastolic pressure on the subendocardial regions of the left ventricle [10, 11].

It seems unlikely that the venous system responds uniformly to vasodilators [1]. The postural reservoirs which allow venous pooling on standing are under alpha-adrenergic arteriolar control, as shown by the development of postural hypotension after alpha-adrenergic blocking drugs. The easily accessible forearm veins are unlikely to be representative of the behaviour of the venous capacitance system as a whole. Animal work is complicated by the reactive hepatic venous sphincter, prominent in the dog, which easily produces portal pooling, and is vestigial in man. The venous capacitance which is important in determining ventricular filling pressure, and is affected by nitrates, is a weighted mean of the pressure and volume of all parts of the venous system, analogous to the hypothetical mean systemic pressure of Guyton [3], the static pressure in the circulation without flow and therefore not measurable in life. Changes here are dominated by alterations in the relatively large venous compartment.

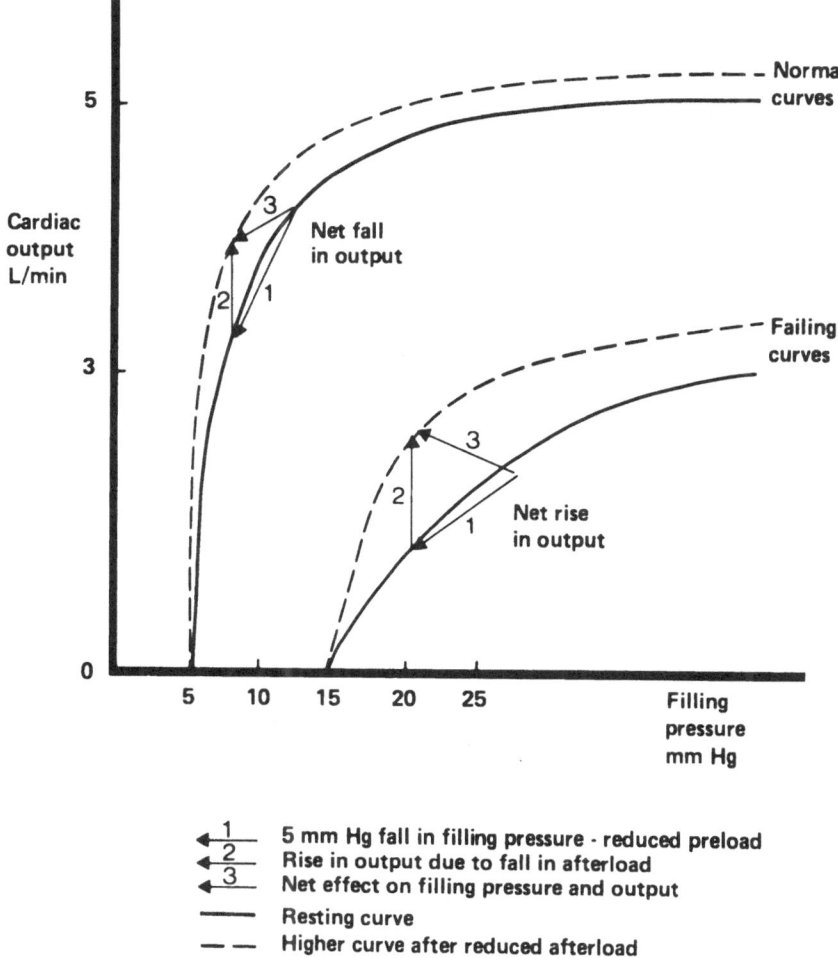

Fig. 9.1 Effect of vasodilators from the Starling curve. To show that a beneficial effect on output relates to the presence of a flat 'failing' curve and that vasodilatation with a steep 'normal' curve may produce deterioration with a fall in output. For an identical 5 mmHg fall in preload as filling pressure (arrow 1) the flat, failing curve produces less fall in output than the steep, normal curve. The beneficial effect of reduced afterload shifts the heart to a higher Starling curve (shown dotted) with a corresponding improvement in output (arrow 2). For the flat, failing curve the net effect (arrow 3) is a rise in output and a lower filling pressure, whereas in the steep normal curve the dramatic fall in output from reduced preload is not corrected and the net effect (arrow 3) is a fall in output with the lower filling pressure which may cause hypotension or reflex tachycardia. Reproduced with permission from [98].

Vasodilator therapy in congestive heart failure

9.2 Afterload effects

The work required for left ventricular ejection is rate-dependent and in theory the effect of vasodilators is best expressed in terms of an arterial impedance. However, the electrical analogy is not particularly useful here, and in terms of steady-flow impedance is dominated by the arteriolar resistance, the site of action of most vasodilator drugs. The vasoconstrictor response in heart failure, through the alpha-adrenergic sympathetic receptors or via angiotensin [6], operates at this level to raise peripheral resistance and maintain perfusion in the face of a falling cardiac output. This advantage is obtained at the expense of an impairment of left ventricular emptying and further increase in left ventricular work which may accentuate failure [2]. Arteriolar vasodilators reverse this process allowing more efficient emptying, so that the heart moves to a higher Starling curve [7] (Fig. 9.1) with a greater output for a given filling pressure. As a result of greater emptying, left ventricular diastolic volume is reduced, with further advantage in terms of reduced myocardial oxygen consumption [5].

As stroke volume increases there is usually no fall in blood pressure in spite of the arteriolar vasodilatation [12, 13] and coronary flow seems not to be impaired. Perhaps as a consequence of the absence of a fall in blood pressure and the general down-regulation of sympathetic receptors in failure [14] the reflex tachycardia which is a major feature of treatment with arterial vasodilators in hypertension is absent. The net result is increased cardiac output and improved tissue perfusion without an increase in left ventricular work.

Afterload reduction is often thought to be specific for low output effects such as fatigue or peripheral vasoconstriction [12], as opposed to preload reduction for persisting venous congestion producing dyspnoea. In many patients with a raised filling pressure, a combined effect on preload and afterload is needed [7], the improved output from reduced afterload with arteriolar vasodilatation helping to offset any reduction in output with reduced filling pressure from preload reduction by venous pooling (Fig. 9.1).

9.3 Vasodilator drugs

These may be classified as directly acting vasodilators which relax the smooth muscle of the vessels walls and those acting via specific block of the vasoconstrictor alpha sympathetic receptors or the action of angiotensin II [6]. Practically all the vasodilator drugs used in angina (Chapter 4) and hypertension (Chapter 8) have been tested for possible beneficial effect in congestive heart failure.

9.3.1 DIRECT VASODILATORS

This group of drugs includes both the nitrates, primarily used as preload-reducing venodilators, and hydralazine, an arteriolar dilator, widely used to reduce afterload. The division to venous and arteriolar dilators may be more apparent than real as both groups seem to operate by similar mechanisms in the smooth muscle cell, probably by increasing the level of cyclic guanosine monophosphate (cGMP) which inhibits contraction. Sodium nitroprusside, widely used intravenously in emergency work, acts similarly [6], and may have a dominant arteriolar effect because of its route of administration. The nitrates, though primarily thought of as venodilators can be shown to have arteriolar effects in higher concentrations or by parenteral injection [8].

Since the early studies by Mason and Braunwald [15] comparing nitroglycerine and amyl nitrite it has seemed likely that the vascular effect of all nitrates is similar, differences being due to variations in the rate of action and the briskness of the reflex sympathetic response. Similar considerations apply to the long-acting nitrates used in heart failure, in contrast to the short-acting drugs useful in acute prophylaxis of angina.

Early acute studies with intravenous nitroglycerine (=glycerol trinitrate) in pulmonary oedema were followed by the use of conventional sublingual nitroglycerine in other patients with acute ventricular failure [16]. The commonly used long-acting nitrate, isosorbide dinitrate, seems more easily prepared for intravenous use and may become the preferred nitrate for emergency work [17].

Attempts to prolong the nitrate action arose first for the long-term treatment of angina and have been applied to congestive heart failure. Isosorbide dinitrate is effective in doses of 5 mg chewed in the mouth or 30 mg orally to overwhelm hepatic metabolism with a large dose, compared to the standard 0.5 mg of sublingual glycerol trinitrate in angina. Controversy has been settled in favour of the main prolonged effect of isosorbide dinitrate being due to high plasma concentrations of the mononitrate metabolites [18]. Most work in heart failure has relied on chewable isosorbide dinitrate, though one study found a better output response with the larger oral doses [19], perhaps in relation to a better arteriolar action [8]. Efforts to prolong the nitrate effect by percutaneous absorption from ointment or controlled release skin pads [20] seem likely to be replaced by the discovery of good oral availability of the active metabolite 5-isosorbide mononitrate [21] which is probably largely responsible for the long effect of isosorbide dinitrate and is now available at an oral dose of 20–60 mg twice daily.

The possibility of tolerance to the effect of nitrates in congestive heart failure is raised by the rapid tolerance to the headache side effect seen in the treatment of angina, but the therapeutic action remains [22]. It is presumed that headache is due to arterial vasodilatation and the therapeutic effect to venous pooling. These observations have given rise to the suggestion that there is selective tolerance to the arterial effect; however, the relatively little published work suggests some attenuation of venous pooling [8]. Although persistence of the preload effect gives a continued clinical response, there is evidence of arterial tolerance after 3 months' treatment of heart failure [23]. A recent study of tolerance in angina finds a clear cut effect after 48 hours on oral isosorbide dinitrate, but the effect is difficult to localize as it is expressed in terms of blunting of the fall in blood pressure, and might represent arterial tolerance, though loss of anti-anginal effect suggests tolerance to venous pooling [24].

Good results are reported with oral isosorbide dinitrate in congestive heart failure [23] with long-term relief of symptoms of pulmonary congestion, such as breathlessness on exercise (8, 12). Submaximal exercise tolerance is improved [7]. A reduction in filling pressure is seen with sublingual chewable isosorbide dinitrate, but an arteriolar effect increasing output in acute studies seems to require the larger oral dose [19], though the evidence of tolerance to the arteriolar effect [23] gives support to the use of combination treatment with an arteriolar vasodilator such as hydralazine which gives an added output response [25].

The high mortality of congestive heart failure in patients still symptomatic after optimum diuretic treatment [26] makes assessment of improved survival difficult. Using hydralazine and isosorbide dinitrate there is evidence that clinical response is related to objective measurements of haemodynamic improvement [27]. Certainly there is no dramatic effect on survival as would be evident immediately with such a high mortality. Studies supporting [27] and refuting [28] improved survival have been reported. Unfortunately, both studies rely on comparison of 'responders' and non-responders, and there is a suspicion that the 'responders' may be a less severe group, being more stable and with less haemodynamic disturbance. Persistent treatment with an arterial dilator in non-responders may add a high output load to the left ventricle with adverse effects [6]. A reduction in myocardial cell size, indicating reduced hypertrophy, has been found in serial myocardial biopsies from patients treated with hydralazine alone or in combination with isosorbide dinitrate, but not on the nitrate alone [29], suggesting that benefit relates to afterload reduction.

9.3.2 SODIUM NITROPRUSSIDE

Nitroprusside has long been used intravenously as a mainly arterial vasodilator in hypotensive anaesthesia and in the flexible control of hypertensive crises [30]. Action on the vessel walls is probably similar to that of nitrate [6, 31], via cyclic GMP. The predominant arterial effect may be related to the need for intravenous administration. It has been widely used for left ventricular failure in myocardial infarction [32] where haemodynamic monitoring is available. If long-term treatment (more than 2–3 hours) is needed the risk of cyanide cumulation can be combated by adding sodium thiosulphate to the drip leading to the formation of harmless thiocyanate [33]. As there is some preload effect nitroprusside may be useful acutely in cases of congestive heart failure and it has been used at cardiac catheterization to predict the response to oral prazosin.

9.3.3 HYDRALAZINE

This widely used antihypertensive arteriolar vasodilator may have a basically similar action to the nitrates [6, 31]; the predominantly arterial action is attributed to reflex venoconstriction opposing any venous effect, so that the preload effect is small [31]. Local tissue oedema from disturbance of the Starling capillary equilibrium may produce resistance to vasodilation [6]. The dose needed is large in relation to that effective in hypertension and is often over 400 mg daily with added risk of drug-induced disseminated lupus. There is hope that the new analogue, endralazine, with different metabolism [34], may be similarly effective and free of this complication [35].

The presence of an additional positive inotropic effect from hydralazine [36] may contribute to the favourable haemodynamic changes, but departs from the pure concept of unloading and might tend to produce adverse effects in ischaemic heart disease. In non-ischaemic patients, hydralazine increased myocardial oxygen consumption by 33%, but coronary vasodilation easily compensated and the coronary arteriovenous oxygen difference decreased [37]. Apparent tolerance to hydralazine is usually due to fluid retention, but there may be a specific tachyphylaxis [38].

Many other potent vasodilators have been given a trial in congestive heart failure. Minoxidil, notorious for needing powerful associated loop diuretics in the treatment of hypertension, predictably had a similar effect in heart failure, producing severe fluid retention although the haemodynamic changes seem satisfactory [39]. A similar beneficial intravenous response to diazoxide is reported [40] and carries the possibility of oral use, although experience of side effects in hypertension is not encouraging. Even the relatively feeble vasodilator dipyridamole has been tried [41] and found to have a modest but brief effect. Trial of prostacyclin (epoprostenol) suspected of being the final common pathway of vasodilator action had the expected favourable effect [42], but seems impractical apart from emergency work as it requires intravenous infusion, though more stable analogues may be considered.

9.3.4 CALCIUM ANTAGONISTS

An alternative approach to vasodilatation in congestive heart failure is the calcium antagonists so useful in angina and hypertension [43], although they carry the potential adverse property of a negative inotropic effect, normally balanced by reflex sympathetic stimulation in patients with angina or hypertension. Nifedipine, perhaps the best vasodilator of the calcium antagonists showed dominantly arteriolar effects in patients with acute heart failure after myocardial infarction [44]. Although theoretically advantageous and giving [43] a satisfactory acute response, some unpredictable adverse effects with profound hypotension or pulmonary oedema [45], suggesting an adverse effect on the myocardium, indicate caution in its further use in heart failure. The lack of an effect on preload may account for some disappointment in the effects in an acute study [46].

Verapamil which may have even more negative inotropic effect has been tested on the basis that unloading will counteract any adverse effect on the myocardium [47], but this may be unduly optimistic and the prospect must be guarded. Ischaemia increases the sensitivity of the calcium channel to verapamil, but there was no evidence of the anticipated summation of ischaemia and verapamil on the inwards calcium current in this study [47]. New selective calcium antagonists without negative inotropic effect are under study (see felodipine, p. 95).

9.3.5 BETA-ADRENERGIC AGONISTS

The vasodilator effects of the beta$_2$-agonists, originally introduced for their bronchodilator action, has been applied to the treatment of heart failure. The relative failure of selectivity of some of these drugs may be associated at larger doses with some beta$_1$ myocardial stimulation producing an additional haemodynamic effect at the cost of a possible increase in myocardial work and adverse long-term effect, and some analogues, such as pirbuterol, have been developed as inotropic drugs with little effect on heart rate. The beta$_2$ vasodilator effect is mainly in skeletal muscle and may not improve flow in critically impaired regions such as the renal vascular bed. Intravenous salbutamol has been used in acute situations and may have inotropic effects by this route. There is disagreement as to whether oral treatment in heart failure produces benefit mainly by vasodilation [48] or inotropic action [49]; probably both play a part. There is suspicion that further down-regulation of beta receptors [14] will quickly lead to tolerance to these drugs.

9.3.6 COMPENSATORY VASOCONSTRICTOR MECHANISMS IN HEART FAILURE

There is evidence of activation of both the sympathetic and the renin systems in congestive heart failure [50], and either may be attacked selectively by vasodilator drugs. The sympathetic response may be a marker of serious haemodynamic disturbance, and contributes to increasing the resistance to left ventricular ejection [2]. Sympathetic stimulation may augment the renin release which seems largely independent [50]. The situation is complicated by down-regulation of sympathetic receptors [14] which makes them less responsive than usual to stimulation.

High renin levels are usual in acute exacerbations of failure or in patients with hyponatraemia [50], and we have found high plasma aldosterone, a marker of renin action, to increase with the intensity of diuretic treatment [51], giving the clue to the need for vasodilator treatment as the next step in management [7]. These vasoconstrictor responses lead to rebound deterioration when vasodilator treatment is suddenly discontinued [6].

These considerations have led to vasodilator treatment in heart failure with sympathetic blockers, such as prazosin, or angiotensin converting enzyme inhibitors, such as captopril. In the extreme situation of hyponatraemia, inappropriate antidiuretic hormone secretion may contribute to the pressor response [52].

Early work with *phentolamine* may be misleading as its alpha-blocking effects are seen only at high dose and its dominant action is as a direct arteriolar vasodilator [53].

9.3.7 PRAZOSIN

This post-synaptic alpha-blocker is comparable to intravenous nitroprusside, and seems to give the desirable balance of venous and arteriolar dilatation needed in the treatment of heart failure. There is wide experience of its use in hypertension. The first dose postural hypotensive effect seen in hypertension is rare in heart failure [54], presumably as it just adds a further component of preload reduction. However, impaired metabolism of prazosin in heart failure still suggests caution with initial doses [55].

The development of tolerance to prazosin has attracted much attention [56], and a placebo-controlled study could detect no benefit over 6 months [57] using clinical and relatively insensitive non-invasive tests. With haemodynamic measurement, the preload and afterload effects are attenuated [56], but the exercise response remains in keeping with

283

continued clinical benefit. Some of the tolerance may be related to compensatory renin-mediated fluid retention and can be combated by an increase in diuretic treatment, especially with an aldosterone antagonist [56]. However, Mason and colleagues [58] have identified a transient receptor tachyphylaxis to phenylephrine stimulation, lost after a few days, which explains the situation neatly. The analogue, trimazosin, introduced to avoid prazosin tolerance, seems to have similar action and showed no loss of effect over 3 months [59].

9.3.8   SELECTIVE RENAL VASODILATION

The renal vasodilator effect of dopamine acting on specific dopaminergic receptors is evident at low doses, i.e., below 5 mg/kg/min, before the effect is swamped by alpha-adrenergic vasoconstriction and beta-adrenergic tachycardia [60], suggesting that low-dose dopamine infusion may be useful to start a diuresis in refractory patients [61]. Propylbutyldopamine seems to be a useful selective analogue which stimulates the dopamine receptors without adrenergic vasoconstriction. At doses below 40/mg/kg min, there was no emetic effect and renal blood flow increased with some tachycardia, but no fall in blood pressure, suggesting that a similar analogue may be useful in heart failure [60].

9.3.9   ANGIOTENSIN BLOCKADE

The identification of activation of the renin system as a cause of apparent tolerance to sympathetic blocking and direct vasodilators leads naturally to consideration of block of this system as a further vasodilator effect [62], particularly when a high renin state is generated by intensive diuretic therapy. Angiotensin converting enzyme (ACE) inhibition prevents the conversion of angiotensin I into the active vasoconstrictor angiotensin II which mediates the effects of renin on vascular tone and aldosterone secretion. The early ACE inhibitor, teprotide (SQ 20,881) was used to evaluate this approach [62] and was shown to have similar haemodynamic effects to sodium nitroprusside [63]. The presence of a modest venodilator effect from ACE inhibition has caused surprise as angiotensin II was thought to act mainly as an arteriolar constrictor; it has been suggested that the venous effect may be mediated by other mechanisms [31]. Most work with ACE inhibitors in congestive heart failure has been carried out with the orally active analogue, captopril (SQ 14,225) which allows ambulant treatment [64]. Improvement was maintained at 6 months without fluid retention or late tolerance [64], presumably as compensatory hyperaldosteronism is blocked at the level of angiotension II by ACE inhibition, and captopril seems promising for use as a vasodila-

284

tor in heart failure in spite of troublesome side effects [65]. The absence of deterioration on withdrawal [66] suggests that the rebound seen with other vasodilators was largely mediated by the activation of the renin mechanism.

The haemodynamic response to ACE inhibitors involves a fall in general peripheral vascular resistance with an increase in cardiac output [67]. Perhaps as a secondary effect of the increase in output, there is a fall in plasma noradrenaline [68]. Hepatic blood flow fell, but renal blood flow increased considerably (60%) without change in glomerular filtration rate and there was a sharp increase in sodium excretion [67], suggesting reversal of a renin-mediated renal vasoconstriction with a possible intrarenal redistribution of blood flow. A possible adverse effect is suggested by the great sensitivity to ACE inhibition in high renin patients, leading to excessive vasodilatation and a fall in blood pressure which may reduce renal blood flow with an anti-diuretic effect [69], and care is needed in the initiation of treatment. A postural hypotensive response requiring saline infusion is reported in patients on intensive diuretic therapy [69], suggesting that a preliminary reduction in diuretic dose might be advisable. A hyperkinetic circulatory state preventing a satisfactory response to captopril [70] may be a non-specific side effect of the drug or merely a manifestation of the more general phenomenon of the effect of a high output stress from arteriolar vasodilatation in a non-responsive heart [6].

Good data show an inverse relation between plasma renin and serum sodium, and hyponatraemia is widely recognized as a marker of a high renin state [71] and probable responsiveness to captopril, with a warning of possible hypersensitivity. It may represent interference with a specific renin dependent control of free water excretion, perhaps through the countercurrent mechanism, or direct stimulation of antidiuretic hormone release through a renin mechanism as suggested by some animal work. Antidiuretic hormone may provide an additional vasoconstrictor process, blocked indirectly by ACE inhibition.

The serious toxic effects of captopril [65] have stimulated search for alternative ACE inhibitors with different chemical structure. Enalapril seems a good prospect with the expected effects on renin and angiotensin [72], and a slightly more prolonged effect than captopril; there was a good haemodynamic response over a few weeks.

Attempts have recently begun to explore the logical approach of combined vasodilator therapy with a conventional vasodilator and an ACE inhibitor. Adding nitroprusside to patients on captopril produced an additional response [73], but I would prefer to see the more logical sequential approach of adding captopril to conventional vasodilator therapy, when apparent tolerance due to activation of the renin mechanism begins to interfere with the response.

9.3.10 THE PULMONARY CIRCULATION

Because of the importance of pulmonary arteriolar vasoconstriction in the production of pulmonary hypertension there has been much interest in the possible use of arteriolar vasodilators to unload the right ventricle.

The common cause of right ventricular failure is cor pulmonale from chronic obstructive airways disease and here correction of the underlying hypoxia by controlled oxygen therapy will relieve the pulmonary vasoconstriction and pulmonary hypertension, providing an almost physiological form of afterload reduction for the right ventricle.

The basis of the pulmonary vasoconstriction is a disturbed homeostatic mechanism which teleologically seems designed to maintain appropriate ventilation-perfusion relations. In the presence of local impairment of ventilation, as in partial segmental collapse, alveolar hypoxia produces arteriolar constriction so that flow to the underventilated alveoli is reduced and ventilation-perfusion mismatch avoided. As flow in the remaining normal lung is normal or increased there is no fall in arterial oxygen tension. When the same process is invoked globally, in the whole lung, by diffuse obstructive airways disease, the generalized pulmonary arteriolar constriction produces pulmonary hypertension and right ventricular failure. A corollary of this process is that pulmonary vasodilatation may increase perfusion of underventilated alveoli, leading to a fall in arterial oxygen tension [74]. A similar minor effect has been noted in the congested lungs of heart failure after nitroprusside [1].

The other group of patients obviously candidates for pulmonary vasodilator treatment are those with the rare disease of primary pulmonary hypertension or the more complex situation of pulmonary hypertension producing cyanosis in patients with a cardiac septal defect or persistent ductus arteriosus (Eisenmenger's syndrome). Assessment of pulmonary vasodilator drugs is difficult because if pulmonary vascular resistance falls and cardiac output rises, the pulmonary artery pressure and right ventricular work may not change [74]. As many vasodilators also dilate the systemic arterioles, a fall in systemic arterial pressure may limit treatment [74]. If cardiac output rises as a result of systemic vasodilation, resistance will fall, and resistance measurements cannot be equated with a pulmonary vascular response.

In obstructive airways disease, intravenous nitroprusside reduced resistance and did not change output [75]. Pirbuterol, a beta agonist with little vasodilator effect [31], had a greater effect on resistance, and output rose with no fall in arterial oxygen tension over 6 weeks [75]. Other studies, however, show a fall in arterial oxygen saturation, compensated by an increase in cardiac output which maintained oxygen delivery [76]. The similarity of the response to oxygen and to nifedipine [77] suggests that the hypoxic vasoconstriction may be mediated by calcium ions and the calcium antagonists could selectively reverse this process. Partial correction of ventilation-perfusion mismatch leads to only a slight improvement in arterial oxygen tension and is clearly less satisfactory than relief of vasoconstriction with supplemental oxygen therapy. However, use of calcium antagonists, such as nifedipine, may offer a more convenient form of pulmonary vasodilatation than continuous oxygen therapy and have a useful part as an adjuvant treatment [77].

It seems unlikely that pirbuterol directly dilates the pulmonary vascular bed through its beta$_2$-agonist effect in these patients as implied [75, 76]. Beta$_2$-mediated bronchodilatation may produce such an effect secondary to relief of alveolar hypoxia. The fall in pulmonary vascular resistance is mainly due to an increase in cardiac output [75, 76] thought to be secondary to a vasodilator effect on raised systemic vascular resistance, or to the inotropic effect of pirbuterol [31]. Although the additional effect of pirbuterol may be useful in these patients [76], the primary attack must continue to be to reduce afterload by relief of alveolar hypoxia with bronchodilator treatment and controlled oxygen therapy.

Primary pulmonary hypertension, although rare, has been frequently studied as a relatively simple model of pulmonary vasoconstriction, urgently needing treatment because of the known bad prognosis. Hydralazine seemed to produce favourable response in some patients but not in others [78]. The responders had only moderate pulmonary hypertension and may be more easily reversible by vasodilatation. The non-responders seem to have more fixed pulmonary hypertension and tended to have a fall in systemic arterial pressure and a tachycardia. In another acute study [79] the systemic effect was seen and output increased but there was no change in pulmonary vascular resistance or pulmonary artery pressure in a variety of different types of pulmonary hypertension including 11 primary cases. Captopril has also been tried and showed a major effect on systemic resistance with little rise in output [80]. The hope with these mainly arteriolar vasodilators is that a better response will be seen in long-term treatment, though with hydralazine [79] no benefit was seen over 6 to 36 months. The prospects seem poor unless some more selective mechanism is discovered.

9.4 Problems of vasodilator therapy

9.4.1 PATIENT SELECTION

We have made little further progress in solving the challenging questions posed by Zelis and colleagues in 1979 [1]. The question of which patients respond to a vasodilator has been partly clarified in relation to reduction in preload and afterload. Mitral incompetence presents a problem as reduced preload from a nitrate effect may increase regurgitation with a sharp decrease in forward output [9]. However, afterload reduction with hydralazine was useful in patients with mitral regurgitation [81]. The fall in peripheral resistance was associated with an increase in cardiac output and fall in left ventricular filling pressure; similar effects persisted on exertion and the effect was maintained for several months in those with a satisfactory response. A similar beneficial effect is reported in severe aortic incompetence [82] with afterload reduction by nifedipine, although there was no change in the regurgitant fraction assessed angiocardiographically. In primary myocardial disease the reduction in left ventricular volume with vasodilation may reduce functional mitral incompetence [6].

A good response to preload reduction may rely on a flat Starling curve, so that there is little fall in output as filling pressure is reduced. Disaster may follow inappropriate reduction in preload with a more normal, steep, Starling curve [7] and such an adverse effect (Fig. 9.1) is usually signalled by the unusual occurrence of a tachycardia. Excessive treatment may produce postural hypotension [69].

Not surprisingly a good response to afterload reduction in an acute study with nitroprusside has been linked to a high peripheral resistance [83]. A high peripheral resistance must not necessarily be ascribed to increased arteriolar tone; it may represent primarily the effect of a low cardiac output. A similar study from France [84] relates the response to severity of left ventricular disease expressed as the ventricular pressure–volume curve, which may be looking at another aspect of poor left ventricular performance, more important from the point of view of preload reduction, and again related to a low cardiac output. Measurement of plasma hormone levels [50] may allow prediction of the most appropriate vasodilator for afterload reduction to act either on the sympathetic or the renin response or by a general vasodilator, but in practice treatment is likely to proceed on a sequential trial and error basis as described here.

9.4.2 DRUG TOLERANCE

An apparent tolerance is likely with vasodilation on the basis of the homeostatic response [85] as secondary mechanisms to maintain vasoconstriction come in to play when others are blocked [86]. Fluid retention is one such mechanism and may be renin-mediated, responding specifically to an aldosterone antagonist [55]. The introduction of captopril [64] might be thought a logical next step. In some patients the presence of oedema seems to impair the response to vasodilation [86], and could be relieved by additional diuretic therapy. Receptor down-regulation could lead to tolerance to the beta agonist vasodilators.

Nitrate tolerance has long been a matter for concern in the treatment of angina, but does not seem to interfere with effectiveness there [1]. The situation is less clear with isosorbide dinitrate, which seems to be subject to tolerance in angina [24]. The preload effect is retained in spite of the tolerance to arteriolar dilatation [22, 23], which does not seem important in the treatment of heart failure [1, 22], giving rise to the idea of adding an arteriolar dilator, such as hydralazine, if the nitrate effect becomes inadequate [25].

Hydralazine shows little evidence of tolerance in long-term treatment of heart failure (1), although a tachyphylactic effect independent of fluid retention has been suggested [38] and would be confirmed by a persisting arterial response to other drugs [85].

The major concern has been with prazosin where haemodynamic tolerance has been reported with a sustained clinical benefit, a situation explained by the finding of transient tachyphylaxis at receptor level [58]. The analogue trimazosin may be free of tolerance [59]. Tolerance to captopril does not seem to be frequent [86], unless the hyperkinetic circulatory state [70] can be regarded as such an effect, producing useless vasodilatation without improving ventricular function. Doubtless some other vasoconstrictor mechanism will be brought into play to counteract the effect of captopril in the presence of inadequate cardiac output, encouraging the search for a final common vasodilator pathway which can be blocked, or, as a final step in the stepped-care approach [7], the use of inotropic drugs to take advantage of the residual energy stores untapped even in the failing myocardium of the end-stage recipient hearts removed for transplantation [87]. Many of the best-known inotropic drugs [7] also have vasodilator effects, contributing to the apparently favourable acute haemodynamic response, although inotropic stimulation may have adverse long-term effects on the myocardium [7].

9.4.3 DISTRIBUTION OF BLOOD FLOW

The suspicion that the arteriolar vasodilator effects of drugs reducing afterload will increase cardiac output only to produce useless flow by feeding functional arteriovenous shunts rather than increasing perfusion of vital organs is refuted by objective studies [1, 6]. Hydralazine and captopril improve renal blood flow [31] which may make diuretic therapy more effective [1]. Captopril may have a specific intrarenal effect or block a local action of renin perhaps producing a change in the regional distribution of blood flow within the kidney [67].

Effects on the coronary circulation are of especial importance in pateints with coronary artery disease. Ischaemic effects are reported as frequent with hydralazine as opposed to nitroprusside [88]. They were not related to hypotension or reflex tachycardia, but it is suggested that preload may be increased, or that the known inotropic effect of hydralazine is playing a part. A study of hydralazine in non-ischaemic heart failure, presumably with normal coronary arteries, showed a greater fall in coronary vascular resistance than in general systemic resistance, so that coronary arteriovenous oxygen difference fell, although myocardial oxygen consumption increased [37] a loss of the usual autoregulation with possible ischaemic consequences through coronary steal in the presence of coronary artery disease.

Comparison of captopril, hydralazine and prazosin to similar haemodynamic effect on output and filling pressure in ischaemic heart failure, showed that only captopril reduced myocardial oxygen consumption [89]. A few patients had lactate production in each group, showing that local ischaemia can deteriorate [88], presumably if there are regions of critically impaired flow. A difference in haemodynamic effects of isosorbide and prazosin or hydralazine suggested that preload reduction reduced myocardial oxygen consumption and so coronary blood flow, whereas no change was seen with prazosin or hydralazine acting on afterload [89] suggesting a possible differential effect on survival [90].

Resting skeletal muscle blood flow, although unrelated to the exercise response [6], may be important in preventing the hypoxic stimulation of receptors that plays a part in the general sympathetic systemic arteriolar constriction [1].

9.4.4 IMPROVEMENT IN EXERCISE PERFORMANCE

Some disappointment was expressed [1] that maximal exercise tolerance was not increased in spite of improved resting haemodynamics after hydralazine and isosorbide [91]. However, there was an improvement on submaximal exercise which may be more relevant to an increase in normal daily activities and an improved quality of life. The normal sympathetic response to exercise seems to be preserved and there is no tendency to exercise syncope [1]. Presumably the increase in sympathetic tone in failure is so great that vasodilator treatment does not overwhelm the exercise response. In a short-term study with hydralazine alone, there was no increase in nutritional flow to muscle, so that oxygen uptake and lactate production were unaffected [92], leading to the implication that the increase in cardiac output is shunted away from nutritional vessels [1]. A study of isosorbide dinitrate alone, with a dominant effect on preload, suggests that relief of dyspnoea is due to a lower pulmonary venous pressure on exercise [93] as ejection fraction increases [91]. The exercise response to captopril seems similar to the other vasodilators without metabolic benefit to ischaemic skeletal muscle [94], and, as anticipated from block or the renin effect, fluid retention and late tolerance were not a feature in six-month studies [95].

9.4.5 PROGNOSIS

The assessment of minor improvement in prognosis in patients with such a high mortality [26] is difficult and much benefit is probably unlikely [1]. Recent studies with hydralazine plus isosorbide dinitrate [27, 28] give equivocal answers and make it clear that there is no dramatic effect [96]. Our main aim is improvement in quality of life, that is to allow the patient to be more active. There is some evidence [29] that afterload reduction may have a more favourable effect in reversing hypertrophy in cardiomyopathy than reduction of preload, refuting the expectation [90] of a better effect due to greater reduction in myocardial oxygen consumption from reduced preload in ischaemic heart disease. Perhaps different vasodilators are preferable in different situations. In keeping with the general response [96] is the lack of effect of hydralazine alone (reducing afterload) over 20 weeks in a placebo-controlled study [97]. Both groups improved their exercise tolerance, suggesting that greater attention and training may be helpful in these patients, whether or not they have vasodilator therapy.

The beneficial effect of reduced afterload with hydralazine in mitral regurgitation [81] may be useful in less severe patients or as a preliminary to valve replacement. A similar situation is found in aortic regurgitation [82].

Speculation [1] that vasodilators might become primary therapy for heart failure seem inappropriate as less-affected patients more often show adverse effects [7, 96], but in the context of the stepped-care approach for more severe patients, designed to increase the vasoconstrictor response as a preliminary to vasodilatation, vasodilators may well come before digitalis or inotropic drugs as the next step after adequate diuretic treatment [7].

References

1. Zelis, R., Flaim, S.F., Moskowitz, R.M. and Nellis, S.H. (1979) How much can we expect from vasodilator therapy in congestive heart failure? *Circulation*, **59**, 1092–7.
2. Cohn, J.N. (1981) Marriage of the heart and the peripheral circulation. *Progr. Cardiovasc. Dis.*, **24**, 189–90.

3. Guyton, A.C. (1963) *Circulatory Physiology: Cardiac Output and its Regulation.* W.B. Saunders, Philadelphia.

4. Shepherd, J.T. and Vanhoutte, P.M. (1978) Role of the venous system in circulatory control. *Mayo Clin. Proc.*, **53**, 247–55.

5. Thompson, D.S., Juul, S.M., Wilmshurst, P., Naqvi, N., Coltart, D.J., Jenkins, B.S. and Webb-Peploe, M.M. (1981) The effects of sodium nitroprusside on cardiac work, efficiency and substrate extraction in severe left ventricular failure. *Br. Heart J.*, **46**, 394–400.

6. Packer, M. and Le Jemtel, Th.H. (1982) Physiologic and pharmacologic determinants of vasodilator response: a conceptual framework for rational drug therapy for chronic heart failure. *Progr. Cardiovasc. Dis.*, **24**, 275–92.

7. Hamer, J. (1984) The modern management of congestive heart failure. In *Recent Advances in Cardiology* – 9 (ed. D.J. Rowlands), Churchill-Livingstone, Edinburgh, pp. 275–288.

8. Packer, M. (1983) New perspectives on therapeutic application of nitrates as vasodilators agents for severe chronic heart failure. *Am. J. Med.*, **74** (6B), 61–72.

9. Petrovich, L.J., Selvan, A., Welton, D., Nahormek, P.A., Adyanthaya, A. and Alexander, J.K. (1978) Pre-load reduction in mitral regurgitation: detrimental hemodynamic effects. *Am. J. Cardiol.*, **41**, 382.

10. Moir, T.W. and DeBra, D.W. (1967) Effect of left ventricular hypertension, ischemia and vasoactive drugs on the myocardial distribution of coronary flow. *Circ. Res.*, **21**, 65–74.

11. Hoffman, J.I.E. and Buckberg, G.D. (1978) The myocardial supply: demand ratio – a critical review. *Am. J. Cardiol.*, **41**, 327–32.

12. Mason, D.T. (1978) Afterload reduction and cardiac performance. Physiologic basis of systemic vasodilators as a new approach in treatment of congestive heart failure. *Am. J. Med.*, **65**, 106–25.

13. Chatterjee, K. and Parmley, W.W. (1977) Vasodilator treatment for acute and chronic heart failure. *Br. Heart J.*, **39**, 706–20.

14. Kent, R.S. and Shand, D.G. (1981) Adrenergic receptor regulation. In *Recent Advances in Cardiology* – 8 (ed. J. Hamer and D.J. Rowlands), Churchill Livingstone, Edinburgh, London, Melbourne, New York.

15. Mason, D.T. and Braunwald, E. (1965) The effect of nitroglycerin and amyl nitrite on arteriolar and venous tone in the human forearm. *Circulation*, **32**, 755–66.

16. Cottrell, J.E. and Turndorf, H. (1978) Intravenous nitroglycerin. *Am. Heart J.*, **96**, 550–3.

17. Gwilt, D.J., Petri, M. and Reid, D.S. (1983) Intravenous isosorbide dinitrate in acute left ventricular failure – a dose response study. *Eur. Heart J.*, **4**, 712–17.

18. Chasseaud, L.F., Down, W.H. and Grundy, R.K. (1975) Concentrations of the vasodilator isosorbide dinitrate and its metabolites in the blood of human subjects. *Eur. J. Clin. Pharmacol.*, **8**, 157–60.

19. Figueras, J., Taylor, W.R., Ogawa, T., Forrester, J.S., Singh, B.N. and Swan, H.J.C. (1979) Comparative haemodynamic and peripheral vasodilator effects of oral and chewable isosorbide dinitrate in patients with refractory congestive heart failure. *Br. Heart J.*, **41**, 317–24.

20. Shaw, J.E. and Urquhart, J. (1981) Transdermal drug administration – a nuisance becomes an opportunity. *Br. Med. J.*, **283**, 875–6.

References

21. Bodigheimer, K., Nowak, F.G. and Delius, W. (1981) Comparative invasive study of the actions of isosorbide 5-mononitrate in chronic heart failure. *Med. Welt.*, **32**, 543–7.
22. Abrams, J. (1980) Nitrate tolerance and dependence. *Am. Heart J.*, **99**, 113–23.
23. Leier, C.V., Huss, P., Magorien, R.D. and Unverferth, D.V. (1983) Improved exercise capacity and differing arterial and venous tolerance during chronic isosorbide dinitrate therapy for congestive heart failure. *Circulation*, **67**, 817–22.
24. Parker, J.O., Fung, H.-L., Ruggirello, B.S. and Store, J.A. (1983) Tolerance to isosorbide dinitrate: rate of development and reversal. *Circulation*. **68**, 1074–80.
25. Chatterjee, K., Massie, B., Rubin, S., Gelberg, H., Brundage, B.H. and Ports, T.A. (1978) Long-term outpatient vasodilator therapy of congestive heart failure. Consideration of agents at rest and during exercise. *Am. J.Med.*, **65**, 134–45.
26. Franciosa, J.A., Wilen, M., Ziesche, S. and Cohn, J.N. (1983) Survival in men with severe chronic left ventricular failure due to either coronary heart disease or idiopathic dilated cardiomyopathy. *Am. J. Cardiol.*, **51**, 831–6.
27. Massie, B., Ports, T., Chatterjee, K., Parmley, W., Ostland, J., O'Young, J. and Haughom, F. (1981) Long-term vasodilator therapy for heart failure: clinical response and its relationship to haemodynamic measurements. *Circulation*, **63**, 269–78.
28. Walsh, W.F. and Greenberg, B.H. (1981) Results of long-term vasodilator therapy in patients with refractory congestive heart failure. *Circulation*, **64**, 499–505.
29. Unverferth, D.V., Mehegan, J.P., Magorien, R.D., Unverferth, B.J. and Leier, C.V. (1983) Regression of myocardial cellular hypertrophy with vasodilator therapy in chronic congestive heart failure associated with idiopathic dilated cardiomyopathy. *Am. J. Cardiol.*, **51**, 1392–8.
30. Palmer, R.F. and Lasseter, A.Z. (1975) Drug therapy; sodium nitroprusside. *N. Engl. J. Med.*, **292**, 294–7.
31. Miller, R.R., Fennell, W.H., Young, J.B., Palomo, A.R. and Quinones,M.A. (1982) Differential systemic arterial and venous actions and consequent cardiac effects of vasodilator drugs. *Prog. Cardiovasc. Dis.*, **24**, 353–74.
32. Pohl, J.E.F. (1980) The clinical use of sodium nitroprusside infusion. In *Topics in Therapeutics* 6 (ed. H.F. Woods), Pitman Medical, Tunbridge Wells, Kent, UK, pp.165–73.
33. Pasch, T., Schulz, V. and Hoppelshauser, G. (1982) Nitroprusside-induced formation of cyanide and its detoxication with thiosulfate during deliberate hypotension. *J. Cardiovasc. Pharmacol.*, **5**, 77–85.
34. Holmes, D.G., Bogers, W.A.J.L., Wideroe, T.-E., Huunan-Seppala, A. and Wideroe, B. (1983) Endralazine, a new peripheral vasodilator: absence of effect of acetylator status on antihypertensive effect. *Lancet*, **i**, 670–1.
35. Quyyumi, A.A., Wagstaff, D. and Evans, T.R. (1981) Acute hemodynamic effects of endralazine: a new vasodilator for chronic refractory congestive heart failure. *Am. J. Cardiol.*, **51**, 1353–7.
36. Leier, C.V., Desch, C.E., Magorien, R.D., Triffon, D.W., Unverferth, D.V., Boudoulas, H. and Lewis, R.P. (1980) Positive inotropic effects of hydralazine in human subjects: comparison with prazosin in the setting of congestive

heart failure. *Am. J. Cardiol.*, **46**, 1039–44.

37. Magorien, R.D., Brown, G.P., Unverferth, D.V., Nelson, S., Boudoulas, H., Bombach, D. and Leier, C.V. (1982) Effects of hydralazine on coronary blood flow and myocardial energetics in congestive heart failure. *Circulation*, **65**, 528–33.

38. Packer, M., Meller, J., Medina, N., Yushak, M. and Gorlin, R. (1982) Hemodynamic characterization of tolerance to long-term hydralazine therapy in severe chronic heart failure. *N. Engl. J. Med.*, **306**, 57–62.

39. Nathan, M., Rubin S.A., Siemienczuk, D. and Swan, H.J. (1982) Effects of acute and chronic minoxidil administration on rest and exercise haemodynamics and clinical status in patients with severe, chronic heart failure. *Am. J. Cardiol.*, **50**, 960–6.

40. Massie, B.M., Stern, R., Hanlon, J.T. and Haughom, F. (1982) Beneficial hemodynamic effects of intravenous diazoxide in refractory congestive heart failure. *Am. Heart J.*, **104**, 581–6.

41. Packer, M., Gorlin, R., Meller, J. and Medina, N. (1982) Central hemodynamic effects of dipyridamole in severe heart failure: comparison with hydralazine. *Clin. Pharm. Ther.*, **32**, 54–61.

42. Yui, Y., Nakajima, H., Kawai, C. and Murakami, T. (1982) Prostacyclin therapy in patients with congestive heart failure. *Am. J. Cardiol.*, **50**, 320–4.

43. Prida, X.E., Kubo, S.H., Laragh, J.H. and Cody, R.J. (1983) Evaluation of calcium-mediated vasoconstriction in chronic congestive heart failure. *Am. J. Med.*, **75**, 795–800.

44. Cantelli, F., Pavesi, P.C., Nacarella, F. and Bracchetti, P. (1981) Comparison of acute haemodynamic effects of nifedipine and isosorbide dinitrate in patients with heart failure following acute myocardial infarction. *Int. J. Cardiol.*, **1**, 151–63.

45. Brooks, N., Cattell, M., Pidgeon, J. and Balcon, R. (1980) Unpredictable response to nifedipine in severe cardiac failure. *Br. Med. J.*, **281**, 1324.

46. Elkayam, U., Weber, L., Torkan, B., Berman, D. and Rahimtoola, S.H. (1983) Acute hemodynamic effect of oral nifedipine in severe chronic congestive heart failure. *Amer. J. Cardiol.*, **52**, 1041–5.

47. Ferlinz, J. and Citron, P.D. (1983) Hemodynamic and myocardial performance characteristics after verapamil use in congestive heart failure. *Am. J. Cardiol.*, **51**, 1339–45.

48. Poole-Wilson, P.A., Bourdillon, P.D.V., Foale, R.A., Timms, A.D. and Sutton, G.C. (1979) Salbutamol in treatment of heart failure. *Br. Heart J.*, **41**, 380.

49. Sharma, B. and Goodwin, J.F. (1978) Beneficial effect of salbutamol on cardiac function in severe congestive cardiomyopathy. Effect on systolic and diastolic function of the left ventricle. *Circulation*, **58**, 449–60.

50. Levine, T.B., Francis, G.S., Goldsmith, S.R., Simon, A.B. and Cohn, J.N. (1982) Activity of the sympathetic nervous system and renin–angiotensin system assessed by plasma hormone levels and their relation to hemodynamic abnormalities in congestive heart failure. *Am. J. Cardiol.*, **49**, 1659–66.

51. Knight, R.K., Miall, P.A., Hawkins, L.A., Dacombe, J., Edwards, C.R.W. and Hamer, J. (1979) Relation of plasma aldosterone concentration to diuretic treatment in patients with severe heart disease. *Br. Heart J.*, **42**, 316–25.

52. Szatalowicz, V.L., Arnold, P.E., Chaimovitz, C., Bichet, D., Berl, T. and Schrier, R.W. (1981) Radioimmunoassay of plasma arginine–vasopressin in hyponatremic patients with congestive heart failure. *N. Engl. J. Med.*, **305**, 263–6.

53. Richards, D.A., Woodings, E.P. and Prichard, B.N.C. (1978) Circulatory and alpha-adrenoceptor blocking effects of phentolamine. *Br. J. Clin. Pharamcol.*, **5**, 507–13.

54. Rouleau, J.-L., Warnica, J.W. and Burgess, J.H. (1981) Prazosin and congestive heart failure: short and long-term therapy. *Am. J. Med.*, **71**, 147–52.

55. Jaillon, P., Rubin, P.,Yee, Y.-G., Ball, R., Kates, R., Harrison, D. and Blaschke, T. (1979) Influence of congestive heart failure on prazosin kinetics. *Clin. Pharmac. Ther.*, **25**, 790–4.

56. Desch, C.E., Magorien, R.D., Triffon, D.W., Blanford, M.F., Unverferth, D.V. and Leier, C.V. (1979) Development of pharmacodynamic tolerance to prazosin in congestive heart failure. *Am. J. Cardiol.*, **44**, 1178–82.

57. Markham, R.V., Corbett, J.R. Gilmore, A., Pettinger, W.A. and Firth, B.G. (1983) Efficacy of prazosin in the management of chronic congestive heart failure: a 6-month randomized, double-blind, placebo-controlled study. *Am. J. Cardiol.*, **51**, 1346–52.

58. Mason, D.T., Awan, N.A., Needham, K.E., Evenson, M. and Amsterdam, E.A. (1981) Mechanism of transient prazosin hemodynamic 'tachyphylaxis' in heart failure: acute, subacute and late serial evaluation of alpha receptor responses with phenylephrine by cardiac catheterization during prolonged oral prazosin therapy. *Am. J. Cardiol,* **47**, 389 (abstr.).

59. Ports, T.A., Chatterjee, K., Wilkinson, P., Avakian, D. and Parmley, W.W. (1983) Trimazosin in chronic congestive heart failure: improved left ventricular function at rest and during exercise. *Am. Heart J.*, **106**, 1036–42.

60. Fennell, W.H., Taylor, A.A., Young, J.B., Brandon, T.A., Ginos, J.Z., Goldberg, L.I. and Mitchell, J.R. (1983) Propybutyldopamine: hemodynamic effects in conscious dogs, normal human volunteers and patients with heart failure. *Circulation*, **67**, 829–36.

61. Beregovich, J., Bianchi, C., Rubler, S., Lomnitz, E., Cagin, N., and Levitt, B. (1974) Dose-related hemodynamic and renal effects of dopamine in congestive heart failure. *Am. Heart J.*, **87**, 550–7.

62. Turini, G.A., Brunner, H.R., Ferguson, R.K., Rivier, J.L. and Gavras, H. (1978) Congestive heart failure in normotensive man. Haemodynamics, renin and angiotensin II blockade. *Br. Heart J.*, **40**, 1134–42.

63. Vrobel, T.R. and Cohn, J.N. (1980) Comparative hemodynamic effects of converting enzyme inhibitor and sodium nitroprusside in severe heart failure. *Am. J. Cardiol.*, **45**, 331–6.

64. Awan, N.A., Amsterdam, E.A., Hermanovich, J., Bommer, W.J., Needham, K.E. and Mason, D.T. (1982) Long-term hemodynamic and clinical efficacy of captopril therapy in ambulatory management of severe chronic congestive heart failure. *Am. Heart J.*, **103**, 474–9.

65. Atkinson, A.B. and Robertson, J.I.S. (1979) Captopril in the treatment of clinical hypertension and cardiac failure. *Lancet*, **ii**, 836–9.

66. Ikram, H., Nicholls, M.G., Espiner, E.A. and Maslowski, A.H. (1981) Absence of rebound deterioriation in cardiac function upon withdrawal of captopril for heart failure. *Lancet*, **i**, 844.

Vasodilator therapy in congestive heart failure

67. Creager, M.A., Halperin, J.L., Bernard, D.B., Faxon, D.P., Melidossian, C. D., Gavras, H. and Ryan, T.J. (1981) Acute regional circulatory and renal hemodynamic effects of converting-enzyme inhibition in patients with congestive heart failure. *Circulation*, **64**, 483–9.
68. Cody, R.J., Franklin, K.W., Kluger, J. and Laragh, J.H. (1982) Sympathetic responsiveness and plasma norepinephrine during therapy of chronic congestive heart failure with captopril. *Am. J. Med.*, **72**, 791–7.
69. Cody, R.J., Franklin, K.W. and Laragh, J.H. (1982) Postural hypotension during tilt with chronic captopril and diuretic therapy of severe congestive heart failure. *Am. Heart J.*, **103**, 480–4.
70. Fouad, F.M., Salcedo, E.E., Saragoca, M., Bravo, E.L. and Tarazi, R.C. (1981) Hyperkinetic circulation associated with captopril therapy for congestive heart failure. *N. Engl. J. Med.*, **305**, 405–6.
71. Levine, T.B., Franciosa, J.A, Vrobel, T. and Cohn, J.N. (1982) Hyponatraemia as a marker for high renin heart failure. *Br. Heart J.*, **47**, 161–6.
72. Fitzpatrick, D., Nicholls, M.G., Ikram, H. and Espiner, E.A. (1983) Haemodynamic, hormonal and electrolyte effects of enalapril in heart failure. *Br. Heart J.*, **50**, 163–9.
73. Cody, R.J., Franklin, K.W. and Laragh, J.H. (1983) Combined vasodilator therapy for chronic congestive heart failure. *Am. Heart J.*, **105**, 575–80.
74. Rich, S., Martinez, J., Lam, W., Levy, P.S. and Rosen, K.M. (1983) Reassessment of the effects of vasodilator drugs in primary pulmonary hypertension: Guidelines for determining a pulmonary vasodilator response. *Am. Heart J.*, **105**, 119–27.
75. MacNee, W., Wathen, C.G., Hannan, W.J., Flenley, D.C. and Muir, A.L. (1983) Effect of pirbuterol and sodium nitroprusside on pulmonary haemodynamics in hypoxic cor pulmonale. *Br. Med. J.*, **287**, 1169–72.
76. Peacock, A., Busst, C., Dawkins, K. and Denison, D.M. (1983) response of pulmonary circulation to oral purbuterol in chronic airflow obstruction. *Br. Med. J.*, **287**, 1178–80.
77. Kennedy, T.P., Michael, J.R., Huang, C.-K., Kallman, C.H., Zahka, K., Schlott, W. and Summer, W. (1984) Nifedipine inhibits hypoxic pulmonary vasoconstriction during rest and exercise in patients with chronic obstructive pulmonary disease. *Am. Rev. Resp. Dis.*, **129**, 544–51.
78. Kadowitz, P.J. and Hyman, A.L. (1982) Hydralazine and the treatment of primary pulmonary hypertension. *N. Engl. J. Med.*, **306**, 1357–9.
79. McGoon, M.D., Seward, J.B., Vlietstra, R.E., Choo, M.H., Moyer, T.P. and Reeder, G.S. (1983) Haemodynamic response to intravenous hydralazine in patients with pulmonary hypertension. *Br. Heart J.*, **50**, 579–85.
80. Leier, C.V., Bambach, D., Nelson, S., Hermiller, J.B., Huss, P., Magorien, R., D. and Unverferth, D.V. (1983) Captopril in primary pulmonary hypertension. *Circulation*, **67**, 155–61.
81. Greenberg, B.H., DeMots, H., Murphy, E. and Rahimtoola, S.H. (1982) Arterial dilators in mitral regurgitation: effects at rest and exercise hemodynamics and long-term clinical follow-up. *Circulation*, **65**, 181–7.
82. Fioretti, P., Benussi, B., Klugman, S. and Camerini, F. (1983) Acute hemodynamic effects of nifedipine at rest and during stress in severe aortic incompetence. *Eur. Heart J.*, **4**, 110–6.
83. Lukes, S.A., Romero, C.A. and Resnekov, L. (1979) Haemodynamic effects of

sodium nitroprusside in 21 subjects with congestive heart failure. *Br. Heart J.*, **41**, 187–91.

84. Merillon, J.P., Motte, G., Aumont, M.C., Prasquier, R. and Gourgon, R. (1979) Study of left ventricular pressure–volume relations during nitroprusside infusion in human subjects without coronary artery disease. *Br. Heart J.*, **41**, 325–30.

85. Meggs, L.G. and Hollenberg, N.K. (1980) When is loss of responsiveness to a vasodilator agent in the patient with congestive heart failure due to tachyphylaxis? *Am. Heart J.*, **100**, 753–4.

86. Colucci, W.S., Williams, G.H., Alexander, R.W. and Braunwald, E. (1981) Mechanisms and implications of vasodilator tolerance in the treatment of congestive heart failure. *Am. J. Med.*, **71**, 89–99.

87. Bristow, M.R., Ginsberg, R., Minobe, W., Cubicciotti, R.S., Sageman, W.S., Lurie, K., Billingham, M.E., Harrison, D.C. and Stinson, E.B. (1982) Decreased cathecholamine sensitivity and beta-adrenergic-receptor density in failing human hearts. *N. Engl. J. Med.*, **307**, 205–11.

88. Packer, M., Meller, J., Medina, N., Yushak, M. and Gorlin, R. (1981) Provocation of myocardial ischemic events during initiation of vasodilator therapy for severe chronic heart failure. *Am. J. Cardiol.*, **48**, 939–46.

89. Rouleau, J.-L., Chatterjee, K., Benge, W., Parmley, W.W. and Hiramatsu, B. (1982) Alterations in left ventricular function and coronary hemodynamics with captopril, hydralazine and prazosin in chronic ischaemic heart failure. A comparative study. *Circulation*, **65**, 671–8.

90. Parmley, W.W., Rouleau, J.-L. and Chatterjee, K. (1982) Vasodilators in heart failure secondary to coronary artery disease. *Am. Heart J.*, **103**, 625–32.

91. Franciosa, J.A. and Cohn, J.N. (1975) Hemodynamic responsiveness to short and long-acting vasodilators in left ventricular failure. *Am. J. Med.*, **65**, 126–33.

92. Rubin, S.A., Chatterjee, K., Ports, T.A., Gelberg, H.J., Brundage, B.H. and Parmley, W.W. (1979) Influence of short-term oral hydralazine therapy on exercise hemodynamics in patients with severe chronic heart failure. *Am. J. Cardiol.*, **44**, 1183–9.

93. Hecht, H.S., Karahalios, S.E., Schnugg, S.J., Ormiston, J.A., Hopkins, J.M., Rose, J.G. and Singh, B.N. (1982) Improvement in supine bicycle exercise performance in refractory congestive heart failure after isosorbide dinitrate: radionuclide and hemodynamic evaluation of acute effects. *Am. J. Cardiol.*, **49**, 133–40.

94. Kugler, J., Maskin, C., Frishman, W.H., Sonnenblick, E.H. and LeJemtel, T.H. (1982) Regional and systemic metabolic effects of angiotensin-converting enzyme inhibition during exercise in patients with severe heart failure. *Circulation*, **66**, 1256–61.

95. Awan, N.A., Amsterdam, E.A., Hermanovich, J., Bommer, W.J., Needham, K.E. and Mason, D.T. (1982) Long-term hemodynamic and clinical efficacy of captopril therapy in ambulatory management of severe chronic congestive heart failure. *Am. Heart J.*, **103**, 474–9.

96. Braunwald, E. and Colucci, W.S. (1984) Vasodilator therapy of heart failure: Has the promisory note been paid? *N. Engl. J. Med.*, **310**, 459–61.

97. Franciosa, J.A., Weber, K.T., Levine, T.B., Kinasewitz, G.T., Janicki, J.S., West, J., Henis, M.M.J. and Cohn, J.N. (1982) Hydralazine in the long-term

treatment of chronic heart failure: lack of difference from placebo. *Am. Heart J.*, **104**, 587–94.
98. Hamer, J. (1981) Vasodilatation in the treatment of congestive heart failure. *Br. J. Clin. Pharmacol.*, **12**, 23S–26S.

10 Prostaglandins and cardiovascular medicine

J. O'GRADY and S.G. MOODY

10.1 Introduction

It is more than 50 years since activity attributable to prostaglandins was reported in the literature and almost precisely 50 years since von Euler gave the name 'prostaglandin' to an extract of sheep seminal vesicles which stimulated smooth muscles and caused hypotension in experimental animals. The biology of the 1930s was in advance of the chemistry and it was not until the post-war years that Bergstrom and his colleagues isolated two distinct compounds, prostaglandin E_1 and prostaglandin $F_{1\alpha}$, from the extract, and even that depended not only on technical achievement but the ability to collect sheep vesicular glands from half Scandinavia! By the 1960s six prostaglandins had been identified and it was becoming clear that they were much more widely biologically distributed than previously thought. Research into their biology and possible therapeutic role was inhibited by the inability to synthesize them on a large scale, and although for a time much of the world's supply was derived from coral polyps of the *Gorgonia* genus, it was not until the early 1970s that fully synthetic methods were availiable for the manufacture of prostaglandins [1].

In man, the major source of prostaglandins is arachidonic acid (Fig. 10.1) which is itself derived from the essential dietary fatty acid, linoleic acid. Arachidonic acid is an important component of the phospholipids of cell membranes. Prostaglandins are not stored but released on demand through cleavage of arachidonic acid from the cell membrane by phospholipase A_2. The conversion of arachidonic acid into the known prostaglandins is illustrated in Fig. 10.2.

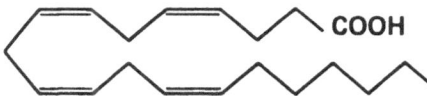

Fig. 10.1 Arachidonic acid.

299

Prostaglandins and cardiovascular medicine

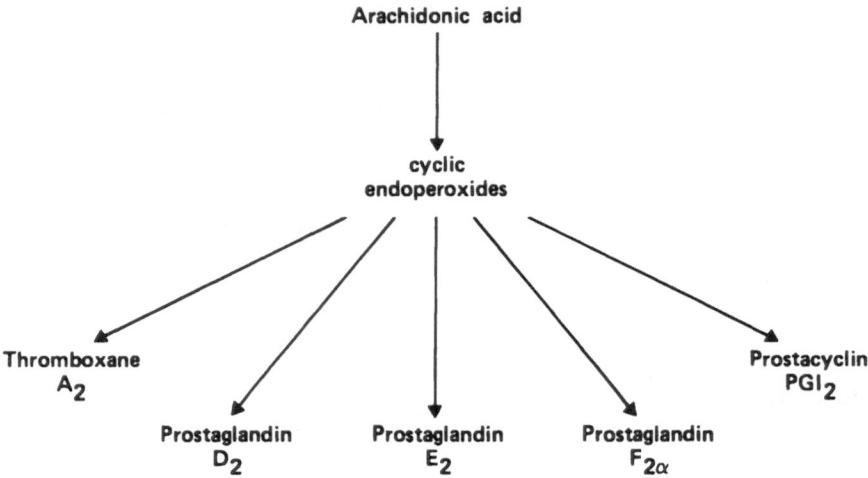

Fig. 10.2   Prostaglandins derived from arachidonic acid.

The nomenclature of the prostaglandins may appear daunting to the unwary and less than logical when it is considered that the first ones isolated were called E and F, but this nomenclature was due to the solubility of these compounds in buffers containing ethanol and phosphate (spelt in Swedish with an 'f') respectively.

All the prostaglandins have 20 carbon atoms and these are numbered from the carboxyl terminal (see Fig. 10.3). The prostaglandins derived from arachidonic acid have two double bonds at position 5–6 and 13–14 and are hence sometimes called '2' series prostaglandins. The alphabetic descriptor is derived from the substitutions on the cyclopentane ring at positions 9 and 11. The E prostaglandins have a keto group at position 9 and a hydroxy at position 11, whereas the F prostaglandins have a hydroxy at both these positions. The α in prostaglandin $F_{1\alpha}$ refers to the stereochemistry of the hydroxy group at position 9. The β form is not known to occur naturally [2].

Besides the production of the classical prostaglandins shown in Fig 10.2 arachidonic acid is the source of a considerable number of other highly active compounds. In the platelet, the main product of arachidonic acid is a substance called thromboxane A_2 a short lived but highly potent stimulator of platelet aggregation and a vasoconstrictor (Fig. 10.4). It was whilst investigating the ability of tissues to synthesize thromboxane A_2 that Vane and his colleagues discovered another arachidonic acid product, not manufactured in the platelet but in the blood vessel wall and having properties directly opposed to those of thromboxane A_2. PGI_2, or prostacyclin as this substance was popularly called, was the most potent

300

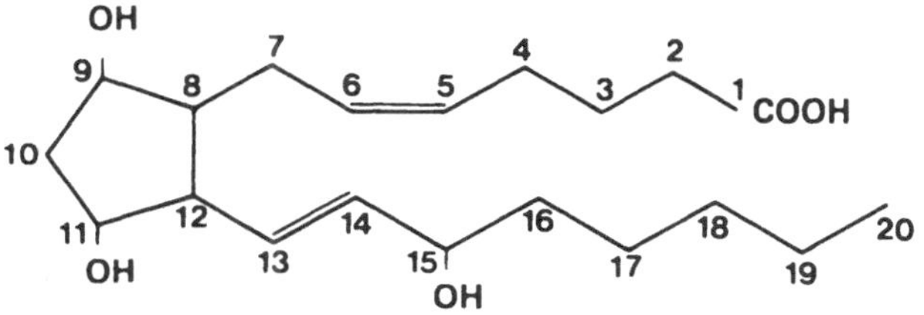

Fig. 10.3 PGF$_{2\alpha}$

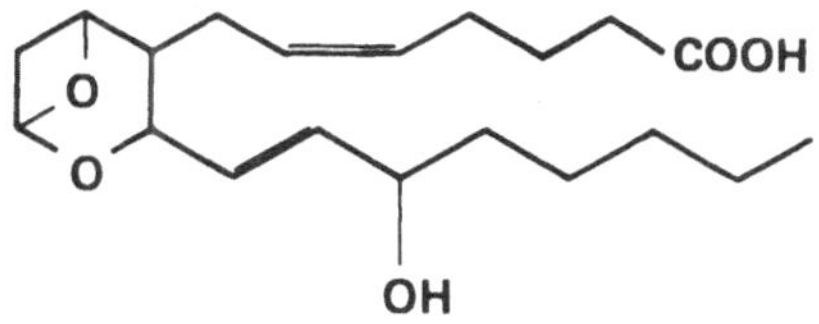

Fig. 10.4 Thromboxane A$_2$

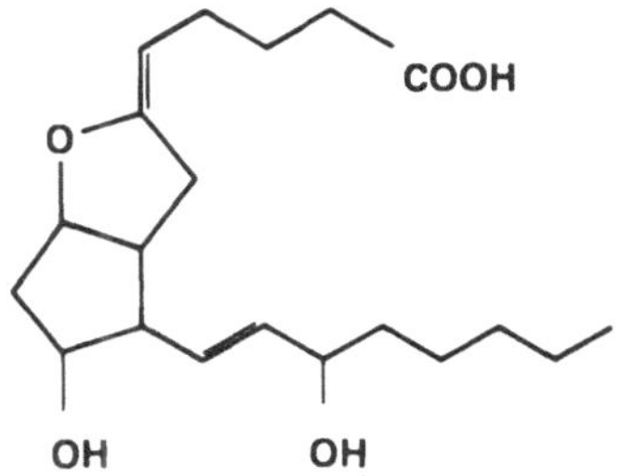

Fig. 10.5 Prostacyclin

inhibitor of platelet aggregation known (Fig. 10.5). It seemed likely that these two substances formed a biological compliment since release of PGI$_2$ from the vessel wall could prevent platelet deposition on the endothelium except when injury to the vessel revealed more thrombogenic tissue below and a platelet plug was permitted to form. Original theories of a Yin/Yang balance between thromboxane A$_2$ and PGI$_2$ and the possibility that PGI$_2$ might be a circulating antithrombotic hormone have proved a fruitful stimulus to investigation of thrombosis and haemostasis [3].

The other major products of arachidonic acid are the leukotrienes, so called because of their chemical structure and their derivation from leukocytes (Fig. 10.6). Understanding of their biology is slowly emerging. They appear to be mediators of the symptoms of asthma, they can constrict bronchioles and stimulate mucous production and are also involved in the pathophysiology of immediate hypersensitivity reactions. They are also chemoattractants for leukocytes during inflammation. It

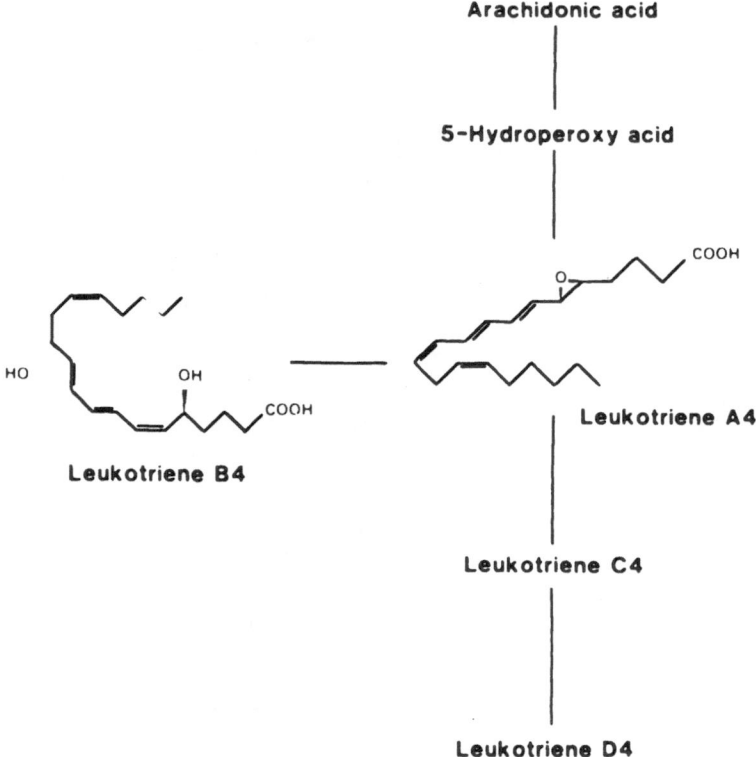

Fig. 10.6 Leukotrienes

remains to be seen whether inhibition of their production will have important medicinal consequences [4].

There is almost no tissue that does not release prostaglandins under the appropriate stimulus and it is clear they have a multitude of biological functions. Not least of these is their role as mediators of inflammation. Although aspirin has been used as an anti-inflammatory and anti-pyretic since before the turn of the century, its mode of action was unknown. However, in the early 1970s, it was shown that aspirin potently inhibits the enzyme cyclo-oxygenase, which is responsible for the generation of prostaglandins and thromboxane A_2 from arachidonic acid, a property shared with the other aspirin-like, non-steroidal, anti-inflammatory drugs. The anti-thrombotic properties of aspirin were also attributed to its ability to block thromboxane A_2 synthesis although PGI_2 synthesis is blocked at the same time [3].

Although the ability to block prostaglandin synthesis has become medically important, the prostaglandins themselves have disappointingly few therapeutic niches. Prostaglandins E_2 and $F_{2\alpha}$ are predominantly employed in obstetrics for ripening the cervix and stimulating the uterus; of the remainder, PGE_1 and PGI_2 are the only ones having any impact on cardiovascular medicine.

PGE_1 (also alprostadil) is derived from bishomo-γ-linolenic acid, the precursor of the type 1 prostaglandins, and was one of the earliest prostaglandins isolated whilst PGI_2 (also prostacyclin or epoprostenol) was not discovered until 1976. These two represent opposite ends of an exciting era in the discovery of naturally occurring prostaglandins.

10.2 Clinical pharmacology

10.2.1 PLATELET AGGREGATION

PGI_2 is the most potent known inhibitor of platelet aggregation induced by ADP, collagen and thrombin *in vitro* whilst PGE_1 is about thirty times less potent [5]. In *ex vivo* tests of platelet aggregation, where platelets are removed from subjects who have received infusions of prostaglandins and exposed to known doses of aggregant, it has proved more difficult to demonstrate the platelet inhibitory activity of PGE_1. Intravenous PGE_1 100 ng/kg/min was well tolerated by healthy male volunteers but no evidence of *ex vivo* platelet aggregation inhibition was demonstrated [6]. However, in anaesthetized patients undergoing cardiopulmonary bypass, PGE_1 50 ng/kg/min was not only associated with *ex vitro* inhibition of platelet aggregation but, in addition, substantial falls in blood pressure [7]. It is possible, however, that differences in potency existed between material extracted from animal sources used in the early experiments and later material manufactured chemically.

Intravenous administration of PGI_2 to man inhibits platelet aggregation with a threshold dose of about 4 ng/kg/min [8]. Higher doses have been reported to disaggregate circulating platelet clumps but at doses not normally tolerated by conscious volunteers.

Both PGE_1 and PGI_2 inhibit platelet aggregation by stimulating platelet adenylate cyclase leading to an increase in cyclic AMP levels in platelets. PGI_2 is more potent than PGE_1 in this respect and also produces a more persistent elevation of the cyclic AMP. Both prostaglandins interact with the same receptor on the platelet membrane [9,10].

10.2.2 CARDIOVASCULAR EFFECTS

The predominant effects in man of an infusion of PGE_1 10–100 ng/kg/min or PGI_2 2–8 ng/kg/min are an increase in heart rate and a fall in diastolic blood pressure [8,11]. These cardiovascular changes are almost inevitably accompanied by facial flushing and headache (see below). Usually the increase in heart rate is accompanied by an increase in cardiac output and a fall in systemic vascular resistance. The increase in cardiac output is probably due to an increase in stroke volume as well as the increase in heart rate, but minor direct chronotropic or inotropic activity of either agent cannot be excluded [11–13]. Neither cardioselective β-blockade nor atropine modify the PGI_2-induced tachycardia suggesting that it is not due to increased sympathetic drive in response to hypotension or withdrawal of vagal tone [14].

10.2.3 SIDE EFFECTS

PGE_1 and PGI_2 have a very similar profile of side effects in volunteers and patients. Both drugs have been reported to cause facial flushing, tachycardia, hypotension and headache, probably as a result of their vasoactive properties. Other effects include erythema over the infused vein and gastrointestinal effects, including abdominal cramps and nausea [2, 8, 15, 16]. It has been suggested that PGE_1 causes fewer side effects than PGI_2 but at doses causing similar pharmacological effects there is probably little difference between them. PGE_1 causes swelling of the extremities in some patients, a symptom hitherto unreported for PGI_2, and has also been reported to raise body temperature [17]. PGI_2 may induce sudden bradycardia with pallor and sweating, possibly a Bezold-Jarisch-type vagal reflex [16]. PGI_2 has been reported to increase blood glucose levels, particularly after acute glucose loading [18,19], but without an effect on insulin release [20], in contrast to PGE_1 which appears to inhibit insulin release and slow glucose uptake [21]. Most side effects reverse rapidly on cessation of the infusion.

10.3 Metabolism

Both PGE_1 and PGI_2 are subject to metabolic degradation along the conventional pathways for prostaglandins, although PGI_2 is normally hydrolysed to the inactive 6-keto $PGF_{1\alpha}$ before enzymic degradation occurs. Initial metabolism of PGE_1 occurs through dehydrogenation at the 15–OH position (refer to Fig. 10.3), giving rise to a 15-keto derivative. The 13–14 double bond is then reduced to give the corresponding dihydro compound. Both side chains may be subjected to attack, successive β-oxidation of the carboxyl results in 2-3 dinor 13–14 dihydro 15-keto PGE_1, whilst ω-oxidation of the methyl side chain gives the corresponding dicarboxylic acid. There is potential for direct conversion of PGI_2 via

9-OH dehydrogenase to 6-keto PGE_1 which also inhibits platelet activity, but this does not seem to be an important pathway in man. The non-enzymic product of PGI_2, 6-keto-$PGF_{1\alpha}$ is subject to the same metabolic processes as those described above for PGE_1 [22, 23].

Using tritiated PGE_1 and thin-layer chromatography, it can be shown that about 80% of an intravenously administered dose is removed on single passage through the lungs, the predominant metabolite being 15-keto PGE_1. In contrast, PGI_2 does not appear to be a good substrate for the pulmonary membrane transport system and is little affected by passage through the lungs. When 11β-[^{3}H] PGI_2 was given intravenously to volunteers the major route of excretion was the urine with only minor amounts of radioactivity being detected in the faeces. At least 16 urinary products of PGI_2 have been identified by gas chromatography – mass spectrometry (GC-MS), but compounds with the 6-keto PGE_1 structure were notable by their absence [23]. In the plasma the major metabolite is believed to be 6-keto $PGF_{1\alpha}$ but significant amounts of dinor 6,15-diketo 13,14-dihydro 20-carboxyl $PGF_{1\alpha}$ and dinor 6,15-diketo 13,14-dihydro $PGF_{1\alpha}$ were detected by GC-MS following administration of [^{3}H] PGI_2 to normal subjects. Urinary excretion of 2,3 dinor 6-keto $PGF_{1\alpha}$ has been used as an index of the endogenous production rate of PGI_2.

PGE_1 and PGI_2 are rapidly converted into inactive forms after intravenous administration. Although PGI_2 is not metabolized by the lungs, this advantage may be offset by the rapid spontaneous hydrolysis to 6-keto $PGF_{1\alpha}$. The kinetics of disappearance of PGI_2 in the blood are poorly investigated, non-enzymatic conversion to 6-keto $PGF_{1\alpha}$ proceeds with a half-life of only a few minutes, but PGI_2 binding to albumin may prolong its circulating life.

The primary site of metabolism of PGE_1 is the lungs with subsidiary metabolism occurring in the liver and kidneys, most breakdown products appearing in the urine [22]. PGI_2 is probably metabolized in the major vascular beds, although 6-keto $PGF_{1\alpha}$ is also subject to hepatic and renal degradation.

10.4 Therapeutic role

10.4.1 EXTRACORPOREAL CIRCULATIONS

Cardiopulmonary bypass and other forms of extracorporeal circulation expose the blood to non-endothelialized surfaces which cause platelet activation, thrombocytopenia and release of platelet vasoactive secretory proteins. Platelet aggregates released during cardiopulmonary bypass have been implicated in the aetiology of the cerebral dysfunction associated with this procedure.

Prostaglandins and cardiovascular medicine

PGE_1 has been investigated in animals and in man for its ability to prevent platelet activation during cardiopulmonary bypass. When rhesus monkeys were subjected to cardiopulmonary bypass in the presence and absence of PGE_1 it was claimed that PGE_1 preserved platelet numbers and prevented platelet secretion. The bleeding time was normalized at the end of bypass after heparin neutralization [24]. This is in contrast to the experience with patients where platelet-active doses proved difficult to administer in the face of severe hypotension and cardiovascular instability and PGE_1 is not indicated for use in extracorporeal circulations [7].

PGI_2 has been used successfully in cardiopulmonary bypass to preserve platelet numbers and function [25]. A priming dose of 10 ng/kg/min is given prior to the start of bypass and 20 ng/kg/min is given during the remainder of the procedure. Using this regimen, one investigator was able to show a reduced blood loss in the twenty-four hour period following bypass [26]. Higher doses than those quoted give problems with hypotension similar to those seen with PGE_1 [27]. PGI_2 has also been used successfully in other extracorporeal circuits to control platelet activation [28].

10.4.2 PGE₁ AND THE DUCTUS ARTERIOSUS

In 1973 Coceani and Olley showed that PGE_1 (and PGE_2) relaxed isolated strips of lamb ductus arteriosus under anaerobic conditions and speculated that PGE_1 and PGE_2 may have a role in maintaining ductus patency *in utero* [29]. The ductus is much less sensitive to PGI_2 than PGE_1 although like all vascular tissue the ductus is able to manufacture large quantities of PGE_2. It is possible the natural regulator of ductus tone is PGE_2, of which the placenta may be an important source.

In the fetus the ductus arteriosus shunts blood from the pulmonary artery to the descending aorta and bypasses the high resistance pulmonary circulation. After birth the vascular resistance of the lungs falls and the ductus closes by mechanisms not fully defined. There are two main groups of congenital heart defects where maintenance of a patent ductus is the only way of providing at least a partially effective circulation. In some cyanotic defects pulmonary blood flow is restricted and incomplete oxygenation of the blood occurs. Such conditions include pulmonary atresia or stenosis, tetralogy of Fallot (with pulmonary stenosis) and tricuspid atresia. In the relevant acyanotic conditions the pulmonary circulation is unimpaired but systemic blood flow is restricted by interruption of the aortic arch or coarctation of the aorta. In the cyanotic conditions the maintenance of the patent ductus reverses the fetal right to left shunt to allow blood to flow through the ductus to the pulmonary artery improving oxygenation, whereas in the acyanotic conditions maintenance of the right to left shunt is the only means of providing flow in the descending aorta, albeit from the pulmonary artery. In addition in the special case of transposition of the great arteries a patent ductus may be able to contribute to arterio-venous mixing by virtue of creating a bi-directional shunt between the aorta and the pulmonary artery and thus help prevent hypoxia and acidaemia.

The use of PGE_1 to maintain the patency of the ductus in these conditions has been reviewed [30]. A total of 492 cases are included, of which 385 were infants with cyanotic disease, the remainder had aortic arch anomalies. The majority of the children treated were less than 4 days old; after this age the effect of PGE_1 is much reduced, probably because closure of the ductus is almost complete and the tissue is no longer pharmacologically active. PGE_1 was infused either through an intra-arterial catheter or an intravenous catheter, usually placed at cardiac catheterization, initial dosage was 0.1 µg/kg/min. PGE_1 infusion was associated with a significant increase in PaO_2 for all diagnoses, in the patients younger than 96 hours the increase in PaO_2 was inversely proportional to the initial PaO_2. Route of administration had no bearing on the clinical outcome, but a birth weight of greater than 4 kg was significantly associated with a lack of response to PGE_1.

In uncomplicated pulmonary atresia, pulmonary stenosis and tricuspid atresia, PGE_1 is indicated to improve arterial oxygen content. In transposition of the great arteries it has also been of benefit but it should not be administered prior to balloon atrial septostomy since it may contribute to closure of the foramen ovale and thus reduce atrial mixing of systemic and arterial blood. There is also a risk of precipitating congestive failure if there is no atrial mixing but increased pulmonary blood flow [31].

Although the number of acyanotic defects reviewed was fewer than the cyanotic cases improvements in lower body perfusion and femoral arterial pulse volume were noted. In aortic arch interruption, and juxta ductal coarctation of the aorta, these improvements in perfusion were associated with increased urine flow and correlation of metabolic acidaemia [30].

A review of the case reports of the 492 patients who received PGE_1 showed that just over 40% had an intercurrent medical event (IME) although only 50% of these were considered to be 'related' or 'probably related' to administration of PGE_1 [32]. Respiratory depression or apnoea was seen in 10–12% of cases, mostly in those infants having a birth weight of less than 2 kg. It is recommended that PGE_1 should only be administered when facilities are available for assisted ventilation. The majority of IMEs did not, however, require withdrawal of treatment. Cutaneous vasodilation often with local oedema was seen in 11% of cases receiving intra-arterial administration, compared with 3% of patients who received intravenous PGE_1. Since the clinical outcome is not affected by the route of administration, the intravenous route is preferred. As previously described [17], PGE_1 had a thermogenic effect in a small number of cases. Central nervous system incidents including seizure-like activity accounted for 16% of all incidents reported. The overall mortality of patients treated with PGE_1 was 34% which is about half that previously reported, but such an improvement may be partially due to improvements in surgical techniques and the management of the critically ill neonate. Nevertheless, prolonged survival of the critically ill neonate may allow a less hurried approach to surgery in a more stable patient.

Chronic infusion of PGE_1 for up to 100 days has been associated with cortical hyperostosis or laminar periosteal thickening of the long bones. However, after cessation of the infusion, the bony alterations were improved. The aetiology of these changes in unknown [33].

The structure of the ductus and pulmonary artery may also be altered by chronic infusion. After 12 days' PGE_1 for pulmonary atresia, reductions in pulmonary smooth muscle have been noted. Lacerations and weakness of the ductus have also been identified after PGE_1 infusion, but may represent natural pathology in an artificially dilated organ rather than specific responses to PGE_1 [34, 35].

10.4.3 ANGINA AND MYOCARDIAL INFARCTION

After coronary artery occlusion, survival of the acutely ischaemic myocardium depends on collateral blood supply, myocardial oxygen demands and other metabolic and cellular processes. After acute permanent occlusion of the mid left circumflex coronary artery in conscious dogs PGE_1 0.5 µg/kg/min or PGI_2 0.5 µg/kg/min into the left atrium from 5 minutes to 6 hours after occlusion was associated with a reduced infarct size and an increased collateral blood flow. The reduction in infarct size is believed to be due not only to the increased collateral flow but clearance of platelet aggregates from the ischaemic area. It is also possible that cytoprotective properties of prostaglandins may be important since PGI_2 has also been shown to reduce CPK loss from ischaemic areas as a result of maintaining cellular integrity and preventing lysosomal disruption [36].

In patients with acute myocardial infarction of less than 12 hours duration intravenous PGE_1 3–21 ng/kg/min for 90 minutes resulted in decreases in mean systemic arterial pressure and mean pulmonary pressure and relief of left ventricular function without significant tachycardia or other side effects [37]. PGI_2 in recent myocardial infarction (less than 14 hours from onset) was also well tolerated in the dose range 2–5 ng/kg/min [38]. Further clinical work is obviously necessary to evaluate this indication. In left ventricular failure more than three months after myocardial infarction, intravenous PGE_1 augmented left ventricular function, increasing cardiac index and stroke volume and decreasing total systemic vascular resistance [39]. Essentially similar results were found with PGI_2. In patients with congestive failure following myocardial infarction or proven coronary artery disease acute haemodynamics improved and peripheral perfusion increased [40].

Angina has a complex aetiology but it has been suggested that temporary coronary vasospasm due to increased vascular sensitivity to vasoconstrictor stimuli secondary to a reduction in local PGI_2 production in atherosclerotic vessels could be involved. It is possible that transient vasospasm may be precipitated by thromboxane A_2 locally released by aggregating platelets. In patients with variant angina, intravenous PGI_2 did not reduce the incidence of spontaneous ischaemic episodes [41]. In contrast, in stable angina PGI_2 increased pacing time to angina and improved lactate metabolism [42]. In unstable angina the clinical findings to date are less clear. In one study PGI_2 was reported to precipitate sichaemic episodes, decrease lactate extraction and increase negative ST segment changes [43], whilst in another study a sustained benefit from PGI_2 infusion was found for 3 months [44]. PGE_1 in unstable angina has properties similar to PGI_2 and was reported to reduce the incidence of ischaemic episodes in some patients [45].

PGI_2 has been safely infused alone into the coronary vessels of patients with coronary artery disease [46] and in combination with fibrinolytic agents [47,48] in an attempt to recanalize occluded vessels during early myocardial infarction. Published data to date are only preliminary but sustained recanalization was achieved with minimal effects on the heart and systemic circulation.

10.4.4 PULMONARY HYPERTENSION

Primary pulmonary hypertension presents a difficult therapeutic challenge. Oral vasodilators may be of benefit but are associated with troublesome side effects. PGI_2 has been shown preferentially to dilate the pulmonary vasculature of hypoxic neonatal lambs. In a human neonate with pulmonary vasoconstriction due to persistent fetal circulation PGI_2 infusion successfully dilated the hypoxic pulmonary circulation and returned pulmonary signs to normal [49]. Similarly in an 8-year-old girl with idiopathic pulmonary artery hypertension PGI_2 reduced pulmonary artery pressures and resistance without changing systemic vascular resistance and was more effective than conventional vasodilators or 100% oxygen [50]. In adult primary pulmonary hypertension the results have been more variable. In four patients with pulmonary vascular disease, no selective effects of PGI_2 on the pulmonary vasculature could be demonstrated [51], whilst in seven others, total pulmonary resistance was decreased by more than 20% in all cases with increases in cardiac output and stroke volume; heart rate was only moderately raised. In several patients these effects were sustained during 24–48 hour infusions [52]. Whether in the adult the pulmonary circulation is more sensitive to PGI_2 or whether the effects are due to loss of activity of the PGI_2 before it reaches the systemic circulation remains to be elucidated. A single case report of a patient with severe primary pulmonary hypertension being successfully managed on continuous ambulatory PGI_2 for more than 12 months raises the hope that PGI_2 might help to maintain such patients until heart–lung transplant surgery becomes available [53].

10.5   Other prostaglandins

PGE_2 has similar pharmacological effects to PGE_1 on the ductus arteriosus and indeed may be the endogenous controller of ductus tone. Oral PGE_2 has been used successfully to maintain a patent ductus in neonates with right-sided obstructions. Initial dosing at 20–25 ng/kg every hour was well tolerated although diarrhoea was more of a problem than with PGE_1. The changes in PaO_2 after oral dosing with PGE_2 were similar to those after PGE_1 and treatment was continued for several weeks without problems. The more mature babies are claimed to present a reduced operative risk [54].

PGE_2 has also been reported to have an antiarrhythmic effect after intravenous infusion [55] and after intravaginal administration for induction of labour [56]. Prostaglandin $F_{2\alpha}$ has also been reported to have antiarrhythmic activity. The mechanism of action of the antiarrhythmic effect is unclear but is unlikely to be of clinical significance [57].

Prostaglandin A_1 is a chemically derived product of prostaglandin E_2 lacking the hydroxyl at C-11 and having a double bond at C-10–C-11. It causes vasodilation, natriuresis and has inotropic activity in animals. It has been used as an acute treatment for hypertensive crisis [58] and generally lowers blood pressure in patients with essential hypertension through peripheral arteriolar dilation and sodium diuresis [59]. PGA_1 has also been used to control hypertension in labour [60]. High doses of PGA_1 may cause bradycardia [59].

10.6   Prostaglandin inhibition and the patent ductus arteriosus

As previous stated the modulators of ductus tone are thought to be endogenous prostaglandins, possibly prostaglandin E_2 of placental origin. Closure of the ductus is thought to occur through the withdrawal of the natural regulator at birth. Inhibition of prostaglandin production by indomethacin also results in closure of the ductus *in vitro* and *in vivo* further suggesting the importance of prostaglandins in the physiology of the ductus arteriosus [61].

In the premature infant the ductus arteriosus frequently remains patent and a left to right shunt occurs which increases pulmonary blood flow and pulmonary artery pressure, ultimately reducing lung compliance and exacerbating respiratory distress. Surgical ligation of the patent ductus is associated with significant mortality and morbidity. The clinical use of indomethacin to close the patent ductus in the premature infant with a risk or significant left to right shunt and evidence of respiratory distress has gained ground in recent years although the absolute criteria for its use remain to be defined. Since a significant proportion of cases of patent ductus will close spontaneously during conventional medical therapy it has been claimed indomethacin may be used effectively after failure of conventional therapy and before surgery is attempted even when shunting has occurred [61]. In this large study birth weight did not affect the outcome whereas others have reported that in infants of less than 1000g birth weight indomethacin is more [63] or less [64] effective at closing the ductus than other forms of therapy, although in these cases intervention was started before significant shunting had occurred. Complications of indomethacin include transitory reductions in renal function and bleeding problems. The long-term consequences of pharmacological closure of the ductus compared with surgical intervention have yet to be evaluated. Indomethacin appears to be at least as good as surgery and may reduce duration of oxygen therapy, decrease retrolental fibroplasia [62], and the time to regain birthweight [63].

10.7 Summary

Prostaglandins, although widely distributed biologically active compounds, have made relatively little impact on cardiovascular medicine. PGE_1 clearly has an established and important role in the maintenance of a patent ductus in certain kinds of congenital heart disease. PGI_2 has been used successfully as a platelet protective agent in extra corporeal circuits and there are hints that it may have a place in the management of severe primary pulmonary hypertension. Many major potential uses for the prostaglandins remain to be evaluated; peripheral vascular disease, stroke, myocardial infarction and angina all may yet prove to be indications for which the prostaglandins may have a use, but major clinical trials and large investment will be necessary to evaluate them fully.

Prostaglandins and cardiovascular medicine

Whilst the need for continuous intravascular administration persists, their widespread use may be limited, but this should be resolved by the development of orally active analogues.

References

1. Bergstrom, S. (1983) The prostaglandins: from the laboratory to the clinic (Nobel lecture). *Angew. Chem. Int. Ed. Engl.*, **22**, 858–66.
2. Bergstrom, S., Carlson, L.A. and Weeks, J.R. (1968) The prostaglandins: a family of biologically active lipids. *Pharamcol. Rev.*, **20**, 1–48.
3. Moncada, S. (1983) Biology and therapeutic potential of prostacyclin. *Stroke*, **14**, 157–68.
4. Bach, M.K. (1984) Prospects for the inhibition of leukotriene synthesis. *Biochem, Pharmacol.*, **33**, 515–21.
5. Moncada, S., Gryglewski, R., Bunting, S. and Vane, J.R. (1976) An enzyme isolated from arteries transforms prostaglandin endoperoxides to an unstable substance that inhibits platelet aggregation. *Nature*, **263**, 663–5.
6. Carlson, L.A., Irion, E., and Oro, L. (1968) Effect of infusion of prostaglandin E_1 on the aggregation of blood platelets in man. *Life Sci.*, **7**, 85–90.
7. van den Dungen, J.J.A.M., Velders, A.J., Karliczek, G.F., Homan van der, Heide, J.N. and Wildevuur, Ch.R.H. (1980) Platelet preservation during cardiopulmonary bypass (CPB) with prostaglandin E_1 (PGE_1) and prostacyclin (PGI_2). *Trans. Am. Artif. Intern. Organs*, **26**, 481–6.
8. Data, J.L., Molony, B.A., Meinzinger, M.M. and Gorman, R.R. (1981) Intravenous infusion of prostacyclin sodium in man: clinical effects and influence on platelet adenosine diphosphate sensitivity and adenosine 3':5'-cyclic monophosphate levels. *Circulation*, **64**, 4–12.
9. Moncada, S. (1982) Prostacyclin and arterial wall biology. *Arteriosclerosis*, **2**, 193–207.
10. Marquis, N.R., Vigdahl, R.L. and Tavormina, P.A. (1969) Platelet aggregation 1. Regulation by cyclic AMP and prostaglandin E_1. *Biochem. Biophys. Res. Commun.*, **36**, 965–72.
11. Eklund, B. and Carlson, L.A. (1980) Central and peripheral circulatory effects and metabolic effects of different prostaglandins given i.v. to man. *Prostaglandins*, **20**, 333–47.
12. Eklund,B., Joretag, T. and Jaijser, L. (1981) Dissimilar effects of prostacyclin on cardiac output and forearm blood flow in healthy men. *Clin. Physiol.*, **1**, 123–30.
13. Warrington, S.J., Smith, P.R. and O'Grady, J. (1980) Noninvasive assessment of the cardiovascular effects of prostacyclin (PGI_2) in man. *Eur. J. Cardiol.*, **12**, 73–80.
14. Hassan, S., Pickles, H., Fish, A., Burke, C., Warrington, S. and O'Grady, J. (1982) The cardiovascular and platelet effects of epoprostenol (prostacyclin, PGI_2) are unaffected by β-adrenoceptor blockade in man. *Br. J. Clin. Pharmacol.*, **14**, 369–77.
15. Carlson, L.A., Ekelund, L.G. and Oro, L. (1968) Clinical and metabolic effects of different doses of prostaglandin E_1 in man. *Acta Med. Scand.*, **183**, 423–30.

16. Pickles, H. and O'Grady, J. (1982) Side effects occurring during administration of epoprostenol (prostacyclin, PGI₂) in man. *Br. J. Clin. Pharmacol.*, **14**, 177–85.

17. Dieppe, P.A., Clifford, P.C., Martin, M.F.R., Wicher, J.T. and Baird, R.N. (1982) Intravenous infusions of prostaglandins E₁ and I₂ for the treatment of small artery ischaemia and peripheral vasospasm. In *Prostaglandins in Clinical Medicine* (eds K. Wn & E. Rossi), Year Book Medical Publishers, pp. 215–23.

18. Szczeklik, A., Pieton, R., Siederadzki, J. and Nizankowski, R. (1980) The effects of prostacyclin on glycemia and insulin release in man. *Prostaglandins*, **19**, 959–68.

19. Dembinska-Kiec, A., Kostka-Trabka, E., Grodzinska, L., *et al.* (1981) Prostacyclin and blood glucose levels in humans and rabbits. *Prostaglandins*, **21**, 113–21.

20. Patrono, C., Pugliese, F., Ciabattoni, G. *et al.* (1981) Prostacyclin does not affect insulin secretion in humans. *Prostaglandins*, **21**, 379–85.

21. Giugliano, D. and Torella, R. (1978) Prostaglandin E₁ inhibits glucose-induced insulin secretion in man. *Prostaglandins Med.*, **1**, 165–6.

22. Golub, M., Zia, P., Matsuno, M. and Horton, R. (1975) Metabolism of prostaglandins A₁ and E₁ in man. *J. Clin. Invest.*, **56**, 1404–10.

23. Brash, A.R., Jackson, E.K., Saggese, C.A. Lawson, J.A., Oates, J.A., and Fitzgerald, G.A. (1983) Metabolic disposition of prostacyclin in humans, *J. Pharmacol. Exp. Ther.* **226**, 78–87.

24. Addonizio, V.P., Strauss, J.F., Macarak, E.J., Colman, R.W. and Edmunds, L.H. (1978) Preservation of platelet number and function with prostaglandin E₁ during total cardiopulmonary bypass in rhesus monkeys. *Surgery*, **83**, 619–25.

25. Walker, I.D., Davidson, J.F., Faichney, A. *et al.* (1981) A double blind study of prostacyclin in cardiopulmonary bypass surgery. *Br. J. Haematol.*, **49**, 415–23.

26. Longmore, D.B., Hoyle, P.M. Gregory, A. *et al.* (1981) Prostacyclin administration during cardiopulmonary bypass in man. *Lancet*, **i**, 800–4.

27. Radegran, K., Aren, C., Teger-Nilsson, A.C., and Hall, D.P. (1982) Prostacyclin infusion during extracorporeal circulation for coronary bypass. *J. Thor. Cardiovasc. Surg.*, **83**, 205–11.

28. Turney, J.H., Fewell, M.R., Williams, L.C., *et al.* (1980) Platelet protection and heparin sparing with prostacyclin during regular dialysis therapy. *Lancet*, **ii**, 219–22.

29. Coceani, F. and Olley, P.M. (1973) The response of the ductus arteriosus to prostaglandins. *Can. J. Physiol. Pharmacol.*, **51**, 220–5.

30. Freed, M.D., Heyman, M.A., Lewis, A.B., Roehl, S.L. and Kensey, R.C. (1981) Prostaglandin E₁ in infants with ductus arteriosus – dependent congenital heart disease. *Circulation*, **64**, 899–905.

31. Driscoll, D.J., Jugler, J.D., Nihill, M.R. and McNamara, D.G. (1979) The use of prostaglandin E₁ in a critically ill infant with transposition of the great arteries. *J. Pediatr.*, **95**, 259–61.

32. Lewis, A.B., Freed, M.D., Heymann, M.A., Roehl, S.L. and Kensey, R.C. (1981) Side effects of therapy with prostaglandin E₁ in infants with critical congenital heart disease *Circulation*, **64**, 893–8.

33. Ueda, K., Saito, A., Nakano, H. *et al.* (1980) Cortical hyperostosis following

long-term administration of prostaglandin E_1 in infants with cyanotic congenital heart disease. *J. Pediatr.*, **97**, 834–6.

34. Haworth, S.G., Sauer, U. and Buhlmeyer, K. (1980) Effect of prostaglandin E_1 on pulmonary circulation in pulmonary atresia. *Br. Heart J.*, **43**, 306–14.

35. Silver, M.M., Freedom, R.M., Silver, M.D., and Olley, P.M. (1981) The morphology of the human new born ductus arteriosus. *Hum. Pathol.*, **12**, 1123–6.

36. Jugdutt, B.I., Hutchins, G.M., Bulkley, B.H., and Becker, L.C. (1981) Dissimilar effects of prostacyclin, prostaglandin E_1 and prostaglandin E_2 on myocardial infarct size after coronary occlusion in conscious dogs. *Circ. Res.*, **49**, 685–700.

37. Popat, K.D. and Pitt, B. (1982) Hemodynamic effects of prostaglandin E_1 infusion in patients with acute myocardial infarction and left ventricular failure. *Am. Heart J.*, **103**, 485–9.

38. Edhag, O., Henriksson, P. and Wennmalm, A. (1983) Prostacyclin infusion in patients with acute myocardial infarction (preliminary report). *N. Engl. J. Med.*, **308**, 1032–3.

39. Awan, N.A., Evenson, M.K. and Mason, D.T. (1981) Cardiocirculatory and myocardial energetic effects of prostaglandin E_1 in severe left ventricular failure due to chronic coronary heart disease. *Am. Heart J.*, **102**, 703–9.

40. Yui, Y., Nakajima, H., Kawai, C. and Murakami, T. (1982) Prostacyclin therapy in patients with congestive heart failure. *Am. J. Cardiol.*, **50**, 320–4.

41. Chierchia, S., Patrono, C., Crea, F. *et al.* (1982) Effects of intravenous prostacyclin in variant angina. *Circulation*, **65**, 470–7.

42. Bergman, G., Atkinson, L., Richardson, P.J. *et al.* (1981) Prostacylin: haemodynamic and metabolic effects in patients with coronary artery disease. *Lancet*, **i**, 569–72.

43. Bergman, G., Kiff, P.S., Atkinson, L. and Jewitt, D.E. (1983) Failure of intravenous prostacyclin to influence the initial progress of patients with unstable angina. *Circulation*, **68**, (Suppl. 3), 397.

44. Szczeklik, A., Szczeklik, J., Nizankowski, R., and Gluszko, P. (1980) Prostacyclin for acute coronary insufficiency. *Artery*, **8**, 7–11.

45. Nemerovski, M. and Shell, W.E. (1982) Prostaglandin E_1 therapy in unstable angina pectoris. In *Prostaglandins in Clinical Medicine* (eds K. Wu & E. Rossi), Year Book Medical Publishers, pp. 295–309

46. Hall, R.J.C. and Dewar, H.A. (1981) Safety of coronary arterial prostacyclin infusion. *Lancet*, **i**, 949.

47. Blasko, G., Berentey, E., Harsanyi, A. and Sas, G. (1983) Intracoronarily administered prostacyclin and streptokinase for treatment of myocardial infarction *Adv. Prostaglandin Thromboxane Res.*, **11**, 385–90.

48. Uchida, Y., Hanai, T., Hasegawa, K., Kawamura, K. and Oshima, T. (1983) Recanalization of obstructed coronary artery by intracoronary administration of prostacyclin in patients with acute myocardial infarction. *Adv. Prostaglandin Thromboxane Res.*, **11**, 377–83.

49. Lock, J.E. Olley, P.M., Coceani, F., Swyer, P.R. and Rowe, R.D. (1979) Use of prostacyclin in persistent foetal circulation. *Lancet*, **i**, 1343.

50. Watkins, W.D., Peterson, M.B., Crone, R.K., Shannon, D.C. and Levine, L. (1980) Prostacyclin and prostaglandin E_1 for severe idiopathic pulmonary artery hypertension. *Lancet*, **i**, 1083.

51. Guadagni, D.N., Ikram, H. and Maslowski, A.H. (1981) Haemodynamic effects of prostacyclin (PGI_2) in pulmonary hypertension. *Br. Heart J.*, **45**, 385–8.

52. Rubin, L.J., Groves, B.M., Reeves, J.T., Frosolono, M., Handel, F. and Cato, A.E. (1982) Prostacyclin-induced acute pulmonary vasodilation in primary pulmonary hypertension. *Circulation*, **66**, 334–8.

53. Higenbottam, T., Wells, F., Wheeldon, D. and Wallwork, J. (1984) Long-term treatment of primary pulmonary hypertension with continuous intravenous epoprostenol (prostacyclin). *Lancet*, **i**, 1046–7.

54. Silove, E.D., Coe, J.Y., Shiu, M.F. *et al.* (1981) Oral prostaglandin E_2 in ductus dependent pulmonary circulation. *Circulation*, **63**, 682–8.

55. Mest, H.J., and Rausch, J. (1983) The antiarrhythmic effect of PGE_2 on premature ventricular beats (PVBs) in man. *Prostaglandins Leukotrienes Med.*, **10**, 279–87.

56. Mohr, D.N., Davis, S. and Markis, J.E. (1981) Clinical evidence of prostaglandin E_2 antiarrhythmic properties. *Am. Heart J.*, **102**, 123–4.

57. Mann, D., Meyer, H.G. and Forster, W. (1973) Preliminary clinical experience with the antiarrhythmic effect of $PGF_{2\alpha}$. *Prostaglandins*, **3**, 905–12.

58. Slotkoff, L.M. (1974) Prostaglandin A_1 in hypertensive crisis. *Ann. Intern. Med.*, **81**, 345–7.

59. Westura, E.E., Kannegiesser, H., O'Toole, J.D. and Lee, J.B. (1970) Antihypertensive effects of prostaglandin A_1 in essential hypertension. *Circ. Res*, **26/27**, (Suppl 1), 131–40.

60. Toppozada, M.K., Shaala, S.A. and Moussa, H.A. (1983) Therapeutic use of PGA_1 infusions in severe pre-eclampsia – a major clinical potential. *Clin. Exp. Hypertens.* [B], **2**, 217–32.

61. Clyman, R.I. (1980) Ontogeny of the ductus arteriosus response to prostaglandins and inhibitors of their synthesis. *Semin. Perinatol.*, **4**, 115–24.

62. Gersony, W.M., Peckham, G.J., Ellison, R.C., Miettimen, O.S. and Nadas, A.S. (1983) Effects of indomethacin in premature infants with patent ductus arteriosus: Results of a national collaborative study. *J. Pediatr.*, **102**, 895–906.

63. Mahony, L., Heymann, M.A., Carnero, V., Brett, C. and Clyman, R.I. (1983) When to treat the patent ductus arteriosus with indomethacin in very-low-birth-weight infants. *Adv. Prostaglandin Thromboxane Leukotriene Res.*, **12**, 491–4.

64. Friedman, W.F., Kurlinski, J., Jacob, J., Disessa, T.G., Gluck, L., Merritt, T.A. and Feldman, B.H. (1980) The inhibition of prostaglandin and prostacyclin synthesis in the clinical management of patent ductus arteriosus. *Semin. Perinatol.*, **4**, 125–33.

315

11 *Antithrombotic agents*

J.R.A. MITCHELL

11.1 Introduction

When a blood vessel is breached, liquid blood rushes out until its flow is arrested by a complex three-stage process known as haemostasis [1]. The first two steps are almost instantaneous – a change in vessel tone which produces vasoconstriction; activation of blood platelets so that they can stick to the wound edges and to each other to form the initial haemostatic plug. This plug is then slowly reinforced, as concrete is strengthened by steel wires, by fibrin strands. These are deposited because activation of the clotting system generates thrombin which turns a soluble circulating plasma protein (fibrinogen) into the insoluble threads of fibrin which scaffold the plug. The clotting system is an amplifying cascade whereby substrates are converted into enzymes, which in turn catalyse the conversion of the next substrate. It can be triggered by external thromboplastic materials released from the injured tissues or by activation of clotting factors when they come into contact with injured or foreign surfaces. The first of these coagulation pathways (the extrinsic system, initiated by phospholipid tissue thromboplastins) is more rapid than the contact-activated intrinsic system which may take at least 10 minutes to generate fibrin. A powerful feed-back loop is provided in that the thrombin generated by these processes initiates further platelet and clotting activation to reinforce the plug.

Our lives thus depend on a deceptively simple sequence of events:

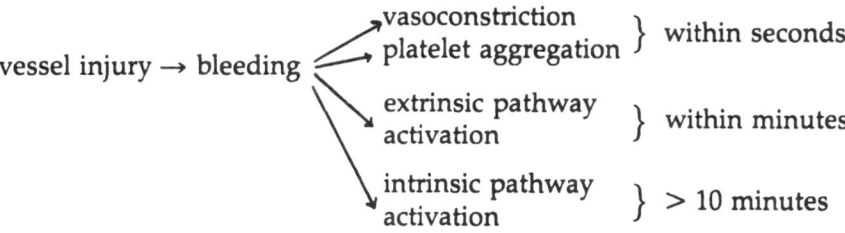

317

Antithrombotic agents

If blood does not solidify after injury we would bleed to death, so why should anyone wish to tamper with these protective pathways?

11.2 The theoretical basis for contemporary antithrombotic regimes

If liquid, flowing blood solidifies inside blood vessels, then blood flow is locally impaired or the growing mass can break off and block vessels in distant sites. This process of thrombosis and embolization [2] constitutes the most serious of all the threats to life and health in the developed world, in that more people are harmed by its consequences than by any other disease, including cancer. In England and Wales, some 160 000 people die each year from heart attacks caused by thrombi forming in their coronary arteries, blocking them and producing ischaemic necrosis of the myocardium (myocardial infarction). Occlusion of brain arteries by thrombi or emboli produces cerebral infarction and such strokes kill 80 000 annually, disabling at least twice this number. Blockage of a leg artery produces disability by causing ischaemic limb necrosis and such gangrenous limbs require amputation. Finally, the formation of thrombi in the big leg veins is almost universal after serious injuries or operations in the elderly and is all too common even after lesser insults in younger people. These leg-vein thrombi may whirl off centrally, pass through the heart and lodge in major pulmonary arteries. Pulmonary embolization kills some 20 000 people annually in England and Wales, so if one adds together the deaths from arterial and venous thrombo-embolism and ignores the even more tragic problem of residual disability, one perceives that they kill some 300 000 per year. In public health terms we need to contrast this with conditions such as road accidents and breast cancer, each of which kills only 10 000 annually, but for which major public education campaigns, backed by seat-belt legislation for road deaths and screening programmes for breast cancer, are being mounted. Why, then are we not mounting similar campaigns against thrombotic disease? The harsh answer is that we do not know how to prevent thrombosis, for although we know what the thrombi are made of, we are not privy to the assembly instructions. Analogies have therefore been drawn between the harmful blood solidification we call thrombosis and the life-saving solidification which we require for haemostasis [1, 3]. The use of manipulators of clotting and platelet behaviour in an attempt to prevent thrombosis derives from these beliefs.

11.2.1 IS THROMBOSIS CLOTTING IN THE WRONG PLACE?

Scrutiny of arterial and venous thrombi shows that fibrin strands provide

318

them with the same sort of reinforcement as in the haemostatic plug. In slow-flow systems such as the leg veins or fibrillating atria, the fibrin network is often fine and randomly arranged, whereas in fast-flow major arteries the fibrin is coarse and laminated, forming the 'Lines of Zahn'. The resemblance between haemostatic plugs and thrombi led to the belief that thrombosis was due to inappropriate clotting, triggered by the release of thromboplastins from damaged vessel walls, thereby activating the extrinsic pathway, or activation of the intrinsic pathway by contact between clotting proteins and vessel walls which had lost their protective endothelium and which were therefore providing the equivalent of an unnatural surface.

The truth of this theory was immaterial until 1916 when a Canadian medical student found that if he added extracts of liver to freshly drawn blood, it did not clot [4]. The possibility of using this direct anticoagulant, named heparin because of its original source, to modify 'harmful clotting', opened up the era of anticoagulant therapy, but the need to give heparin by injection limited its perceived applicability. The discovery in the 1930s that the reason why cows in North America were bleeding to death was that the badly stored sweet clover hay on which they were fed was generating an orally active anticoagulant, paved the way for much wider use of anticoagulants [5]. By 1939, this active natural material had been characterized as a coumarin and crystallized by Link's team in Wisconsin. They went on to synthesize hundreds of related compounds and in 1948, one compound was found to be particularly active and because it was water soluble, tasteless and odourless it rapidly became a most successful rodenticide. It was a coumarin whose discovery had been made by the Wisconsin Alumni Research Foundation so it was named warfarin and is now the most widely used oral anticoagulant in human clinical practice. Unlike heparin, the addition of coumarins to blood does not impede clotting so they are indirect anticoagulants and we shall describe later how their anticoagulant action is produced. We shall then test the hypothesis that thrombosis is clotting in the wrong place by asking whether the agents currently available to modify the clotting cascade (the direct anticoagulant, heparin, or the indirect coumarin anticoagulants) have any therapeutic value in vascular disease?

11.2.2 IS THROMBOSIS PLATELET ACTIVATION IN THE WRONG PLACE?

Fibrin is not the only thrombus-building material, for the fibrin network contains masses of aggregated platelets, surrounded by polymorphonuclear leukocytes [3]. Initially, the only known platelet activator was the thrombin which had been generated by the clotting cascade, so it was assumed that effective anticoagulation would also prevent platelet participation. In the 1960s it was realized that platelets could also be activated by materials which did not derive from the clotting system [6]; some of them were contained within the platelets themselves (adenosine diphosphate; serotonin; catecholamines) while others, such as collagen and other subendothelial structures, could be provided by damaged vessel walls. Stimulation of the platelets leads to the release of further supplies of aggregating agents thus providing a powerful amplifying feed-back loop for incorporating additional platelets into the mass. It was postulated that platelet abnormalities could be responsible for thrombosis, so the hunt was on for agents which would reduce adhesion, aggregation and the release reactions. We now need to assess whether any of the ready-made agents (dipyridamole; aspirin; sulphinpyrazone) have been shown to possess antithrombotic activity. We also need to take note of the subsequent discovery that an entirely novel system could profoundly modify platelet behaviour; as described in Chapter 10, platelets use their membrane lipids to synthesize a powerfully pro-aggregatory, vasoconstrictor material (thromboxane A_2; TXA_2) while the vessel walls use a similar pathway to generate an equally powerful anti-aggregatory, vasodilator material (prostacyclin; PGI_2). As a corollary of this finding, the belief that thrombosis was merely platelet aggregation in the wrong place gave way to the equally theoretical speculation that thrombosis represented an imbalance between the forces of good (prostacyclin) and evil (TXA_2) so that a shift of this balance would prevent thrombosis [7]. In the real world of thrombotic vascular disease we need to appraise the success in a rebalancing role of old agents used in new ways (aspirin) or of novel agents intended to reduce TXA_2 and to increase prostacyclin synthesis (TXA synthetase inhibitors such as dazoxiben).

11.2.3 CAN WE DISSOLVE OR WEAKEN THE THROMBI?

As well as the pro-coagulatory cascade there is a similar system whereby an inactive precursor, plasminogen, is coverted into a powerful enzyme, plasmin, which digests and solubilizes fibrin [8]. Plasminogen activation can be brought about by intrinsic blood components and by materials released from endothelial cells, kidney cells (urokinase) or haemolytic streptococci (streptokinase). An alternative approach to the management of thrombosis has therefore been to try to lyse the thrombi by activating the fibrinolytic system with urokinase or streptokinase; once again we need to ask whether such thrombolysis has been shown to be of practical value. The final approach has been to try to reduce the amount of fibrinogen in the circulation so that any thrombi formed will be weakly reinforced. The venom of the Malayan pit-viper (arvin or ancrod) has a thrombin-like action but instead of producing tough polymerized fibrin as its end-product, it converts fibrinogen into a weak and readily lysable fibrin monomer, thereby reducing the available plasma fibrinogen [9]. This approach has not yet been applied to the major thrombotic diseases in large clinical trials so the current runners in our race to beat thrombosis are heparin, coumarin anticoagulants, platelet-modifying agents, prostaglandin pathway manipulators and fibrinolytic agents.

Before we study the mode of action and efficacy of each of these in detail we need to remember the limitations of the clinical trial technique. Trials were introduced in diseases with a known cause so they were only trying to answer one question at a time. Thus, the cause of tuberculosis had been known for a century, the bacilli had been grown and studied *in vitro*, so that agents could be developed which killed them on the culture plate. Trials of antituberculous agents such as streptomycin only had to show whether an agent of known *in vitro* efficacy against a known organism could kill the tubercle bacilli in the body without harming the patient. Contrast this with a trial of low-dose aspirin in myocardial infarction which is in effect saying, *if* platelets play a part in the causation of thrombosis and *if* their participation is mediated by an imbalance between TXA_2 and PGI_2 and *if* I can find a dose which reduces the former without depressing the latter, then will such a regime affect outcome? If the trial gives a positive answer, then the whole chain of supposition is validated. If the answer is 'no' or 'maybe', this could be because the underlying assumptions are wrong or because the end-points being used to assess outcome are not directly linked to the process of thrombosis. For example, death after myocardial infarction can indeed be due to reinfarction stemming from further thrombosis but it can also be due to the non-thrombotic consequences of the initial infarction such as ventricular dysrhythmias or pump failure. We must therefore remember that we do not know why thrombi form, so clinical trials in heart attack, stroke and venous thrombo-embolism are testing our theories of causation as well as the properties of the drugs under scrutiny.

11.3 Anticoagulants

11.3.1 DIRECT-ACTING AGENTS: HEPARIN

Heparin is the only widely used member of this group, although hirudin, derived from the leech, and vampire – bat saliva can also interfere with blood clotting. Heparin [10] is not a single chemical entity, nor does it derive from a single biological source; cow lung and pig intestinal mucosa yield a family of straight-chain anionic glycosaminoglycans of variable chain-length and sub-unit structure. The molecular weight of the commercial heparins ranges from 4000 to 30 000 and may vary from 9000 to 16 000 within a single-source batch. The chains consist of alternating sequences of sulphated glycosamines and hexuronic acids but the ratio of these elements and their precise nature depends on the source of the heparin.

(a) Mode of action

After years of debate about the mechanism by which heparin stops blood clotting it is now clear that it acts as an antithrombin in three ways [11]; first, it binds to an α_2 globulin plasma cofactor (antithrombin III) and changes its shape so that it is able to bind and neutralize thrombin avidly; second, it binds to thrombin, bringing it into proximity with the heparin-bound, activated AT III and thereby speeding thrombin inactivation. Third, activated AT III inhibits activated Factor X from the final common pathway and Factors IX, XI and XII from the intrinsic pathway. It is thus an extremely powerful agent because of its many-pronged attack on the amplifying cascade.

(b) Control of dosage

Heparin is digested in the gut so must be given parenterally and the traditional route has been by intermittent intravenous bolus injection, in doses such as 10 000 u. every 6 hours. It seems strange that clinicians who would not contemplate using a biologically – derived and titratable agent such as insulin without measuring the blood sugar are nevertheless prepared to use an agent like heparin without measuring anything and without therefore having any quality control of their therapy.

Heparin is removed from the circulation by the reticulo-endothelial system [10]. The avidity of this mechanism varies widely from person to person, is influenced by disease and is related to the heparin dose. The average half-life is 90 minutes in perfectly normal subjects, but it can range from 30 to 360 minutes; venous thrombosis *per se* does not alter heparin survival in the circulation, but pulmonary embolism does and can shorten it by 50% [12]. Finally, the half-time is dose dependent, being 40 minutes after 3000 u and 69–83 minutes after 10 000 u. It is therefore necessary to make measurements to control heparin treatment, but there is as yet no ideal test; global clotting tests such as the whole-blood clotting time and the activated partial thromboplastin time (APTT) are simple but are relatively insensitive to the effects of heparin, while direct assays of heparin itself, of thrombin, of activated AT III or of Factor Xa inhibition are complex and are of uncertain clinical relevance [11]. At present, all one can say is that it is better to measure something than to measure nothing, and that the APTT, while not ideal, is widely available. The reagents used vary from hospital to hospital so local enquiry is vital, but most reagents give an acceptable level of haemorrhagic complications in patients receiving continuous intravenous heparin when the APTT is kept at 2 to 3 times the control value. Salzman and colleagues, for example, found that major bleeding problems were reduced from 21% to 1% when they moved from uncontrolled bolus doses of heparin to APTT-controlled infusions [13].

(c)   Treatment regimes [14]

To avoid the haemorrhagic complications of conventional intravenous heparin treatment, to obviate the need for laboratory tests and to provide a simple mode of administration which could be delegated to nursing staff, the idea of giving 5000–10 000 u. subcutaneously into the thigh or abdominal wall every 8 or 12 hours has gained wide acceptance. We must note that because heparin is such a powerful and direct anticoagulant, even so-called *'low-dose' regimes* exert a significant effect on clotting. In a major surgical trial of 5000 u. 8 hourly, to which we shall refer later [15], wound haematomas and excessive blood loss during surgery were increased in the heparin group (haematomas occurred in 6% of the control and 8% of the treated patients; bleeding in 6% and 9%) but the differences in blood transfusion requirements and the postoperative fall in haemoglobin did not achieve significance. Even lower dose regimes are now on trial but it is too early to assess their efficacy. The *conventional regime* for using heparin is by continuous intravenous infusion, regulated to an APTT of up to 3 times the initial or control level. The amount needed varies from individual to individual but after an initial bolus of 5000 u. most patients then require between 20 000 and 30 000 u. daily. In pulmonary embolization, heparin may exert a beneficial effect on the secondary consequences of the arrival of fresh thrombotic material in the lungs by reducing the bronchoconstriction and vasoconstriction which the thrombotic plug seems to trigger. In patients whose lives are threatened by major pulmonary emboli a *high-dose regime* of 10 000 u. followed by 60 000 u. for the next 24 hours has therefore been advocated. Because pulmonary embolization shortens heparin half-life, such high-dose schedules do not appear to increase the risk of bleeding.

(d)   Side effects [11, 14]

Bleeding is the only common problem encountered, so in addition to using appropriate regimes and control systems, it is very important to avoid agents which impair coagulation and platelet behaviour such as non-steroidal anti-inflammatory agents or dextran. Heparin may occasionally produce anaphylactic reactions, alopecia or a reduction in platelet count. In long-term use, an alteration of bone matrix leading to osteoporosis and fractures has been observed, but the elevation of free fatty acid levels resulting from activation of lipoprotein lipase by heparin does not seem to be of clinical relevance. If it is necessary to reverse the action of heparin (and this is seldom so because of its rapid natural deactivation) protamine sulphate can be given by slow intravenous injection, 1 mg being able to neutralize 100 u. of heparin given up to 15 minutes before; no more than 50 mg should be used.

(e) The future

The heterogeneity of natural heparin may contribute to the problems outlined above, for the lower the molecular weight the more specific the anti Xa activity, whereas higher-molecular-weight heparins show more diffuse anti-clotting activity [16]. Looking to the future, clarification of the relationship between molecular size and the antithrombotic activity of heparin, together with the development of simple, clinically relevent tests to control its dosage will be invaluable.

11.3.2 INDIRECT AGENTS – THE COUMARINS

Warfarin is widely used, so can serve as the representative of its group. We need, however, to remain aware that other members of the family (phenprocoumon, acenocoumarin and nicoumalone) differ from warfarin in their half-lives, effect on clotting proteins and non-clotting action [5]. As with heparin, the newcomer to a hospital must make himself familiar with the agents and the control systems used locally.

(a) Mode of action

If vitamin K is available, the liver synthesizes a series of proteins with similar amino acid sequences [17], which slot into the clotting cascade as Factors II, VII, IX and X. The contribution of vitamin K is to permit the γ-carboxylation of the glutamic acid residues in these proteins, and during this process the vitamin K shuttles back and forth between its quinol and quinone forms under the influence of an epoxidase enzyme system. The coumarins block this system, so that proteins resembling II, VII, IX, and X but lacking their biological activity [14] are produced (PIVKAs or proteins induced by vitamin K absence/antagonists). The activity which they lack, but which the normal γ-glutamyl groups confer on the active clotting factors, is the ability to bind the calcium and phospholid which is needed for participation in the clotting chain.

If one accepts that thrombosis is related to clotting, then an agent such as warfarin which reduces the activity of the clotting cascade would seem likely to be antithrombotic, but new evidence suggests that the situation is more complex. Circulating blood contains inhibitors of clotting as well as activators; indeed the overall balance is such that the ratio of potential inhibitors to activators is 3:1. We now know that there are three proteins whose amino acid sequence is similar to Factors II, VII, IX and X, but which inhibit clotting by inactivating Factors V and VIII. These clotting antagonists, named proteins C, S and Z are vitamin K dependent [17], so warfarin reduces their activity as well as that of the procoagulant clotting factors. As yet, we do not know whether the dosage, timing or control methods we use for warfarin therapy should be modified to ensure that we do not create the reverse of what we intend by adversely affecting the balance between pro-coagulant and anti coagulant proteins. We do know that low doses of warfarin may depress protein C relatively more than Factor II, which may not be helpful, whereas high-intensity warfarin reduces C and II equally. The final element to our new awareness of vitamin K-dependent proteins is that similar materials exist in bone (osteocalcin) and use their γ-carboxyl residues to bind calcium as part of the natural calcification process [17]. We may therefore need to explore whether warfarin used to prevent venous thrombosis after fractures reduces their healing rate.

(b) Control of dosage

In 1935, Quick found that when a tissue thromboplastin such as brain extract was added to recalcified plasma, clotting occurred in 10–20 s [18]. Link showed that the coumarins which he was then isolating from spoiled sweet-clover hay markedly prolonged this 'Quick one-stage prothrombin (PT) time' when they were fed to cows. So was born the commonest form of oral anticoagulation used throughout the world – namely coumarins, controlled by a simple one-stage PT time [5] to a level just short of that which produces an unacceptable risk of bleeding. Since in many diseases we do not know whether coumarins work at all, still less the precise rebalancing of pro- and anti-clotting factors which they produce, it is foolish to talk of a 'therapeutic range'; as with hypotensive treatment or diabetic control our objective is to lower a measured variable (blood pressure, blood glucose and in this case, clotting factors) as much as we dare without producing hypotension, hypoglycaemia or bleeding. In all these situations we need to strike a compromise between our wishes and the need to avoid overt harm, so I prefer to speak of the 'safe range' for anticoagulant rather than a 'therapeutic range'.

The original simple one-stage test, being a general test of clottability, was not only influenced by those clotting factors from the extrinsic system which were altered by coumarin treatment (Factors II, VII and X) but by other factors which were not (fibrinogen and Factor V). The test was, moreover, insensitive to the alterations in the intrinsic system (Factor IX) produced by coumarins, so the correlation between this early type of one-stage PT test and the risk of bleeding was poor. Improved tests therefore evolved, but unhappily, different countries went along separate paths [19].

In much of Europe, a test which adds back the coumarin-independent factors, and which measures all the coumarin-related ones, is in wide use. The clotting times recorded with this 'Thrombotest' method, which can be done on capillary samples derived by finger-prick, are compared with a standard curve supplied with each pack so that a 'percentage activity' figure is reported to the clinician, whose target for coumarin-treated patients should be 5–10% of normal activity. In Britain and the rest of Europe, a standardized non-commercial agent (the 'Manchester Comparative Reagent' or 'British Comparative Thromboplastin' – BCT) has been widely adopted [19] and reports its results as a clotting time which is compared with a BCT normal clotting value and is then expressed as a simple ratio, the target aimed at being a ratio between patient and control of × 2 to × 4. Finally, in North America, rabbit brain thromboplastins such as Simplastin have remained in wide use. Because they are relatively insensitive to reductions in Factors II, VII and X, they do not fully reflect the effect of coumarins on coagulability; as a result the incidence of haemorrhagic complications is higher. With this method, the ratios to be aimed for between treated and control values should be no higher than ×2 and even with such a conservative goal, parallel testing has shown that had a patient moved to Europe he could have been thought to be overtreated, for his BCT ratio might have been ×8. Conversely a patient moving to America with a BCT ratio of ×2–4 and tested with a rabbit-brain test would be regarded as inadequately treated [19].

It is imperative therefore that any prescriber should ascertain what method is in use in his locality, and familiarize himself with its method of reporting (times in seconds; ratios of times; percentage activity) and the target level to be attained. If he wishes to modify his local system he should join the move towards European and international standardization so that wherever a patient is located a ratio of × 2–4, depending on the clinical condition being dealt with will provide the maximum degree of anticoagulant commensurate with a minimal risk of haemorrhage.

(c) Treatment regime

Warfarin is readily absorbed from the gut and its half-life is about 42 hours. It is avidly bound to plasma albumin so that only 1% may be available for action and any drug which alters albumin-binding will therefore modify the response. In previously fit subjects a loading dose of 30 mg is appropriate, but in the elderly, in patients with liver disease, heart failure, previous bleeding problems or who have received antibiotics, a pre-dosing PT measurement would be wise so that an appropriately judged dose can be given. Because the vitamin K-dependent factors do not fall immediately, the next PT test can be delayed for 48 hours and the subsequent doses adjusted accordingly, towards a daily maintenance dose which can vary from 2 to 21 mg but is usually 6–9 mg. In stable long-term therapy, PT measurements every 4–6 weeks will suffice.

(d) Side effects

Bleeding is, of course, the principal hazard, and any manoeuvre which alters the availability of absorbable vitamin K or which modifies the absorption, transport, protein-binding, liver cell metabolism or excretion of the drug will alter the response to warfarin. The novice should assume that any drug can do so and should consult the lists which have been produced by various bodies [20] or which figure in National Formularies.

As the plasma protein binding of warfarin is high, particular care is needed with non-steroidal anti-inflammatory agents (and especially phenylbutazone), anabolic steroids, sulphinpyrazone, quinidine and amiodarone which compete for the binding site and increase the free warfarin level. Psychotropics and anti-epileptics such as barbiturates can induce liver enzyme activity, leading to an increased warfarin requirement, so when the inducing drug is stopped, warfarin over-dosage can result. Finally, variations in alcohol intake or the degree of heart failure can produce troublesome and erratic deviations.

The action advised [20] in the event of overtreatment is as follows: if the test result is all that is amiss, then stop or reduce the warfarin, repeat the PT and readjust the dose. If an excessive ratio is accompanied by bleeding, or if surgery is required, fat-soluble vitamin K (phytomenadione) 5–15 mg intravenously will reverse the anticoagulation in 3–8 hours, but may render the patient resistant to further treatment for several days. If the bleeding is severe then immediate control can be obtained with fresh-frozen plasma or concentrates containing Factors II, IX and X. Finally, if bleeding occurs with ratios close to the target level look for unrelated and coincidental causes (peptic ulcer, bowel, bladder and lung cancers etc.).

As warfarin crosses the placental barrier it should be avoided wherever possible in the first trimester of pregnancy, because of its teratogenicity and in the last few weeks, because of the risk of fetal intracranial haemorrhage. Although warfarin crosses into breast milk, the concentration is very low so breast feeding poses no problems.

(e) The future

We need to establish how anticoagulants work in those situations in which their antithrombotic potential is not in doubt. New agents which specifically produce this effect can then be developed, and new control methods which are directly relevant to this antithrombotic action can be created, as opposed to our present PT tests, which are assessing safety, and not efficiency. In the meantime we should strive to standardize the ways of performing and reporting PT tests.

11.4 Platelet modifying agents

In the 1960s, when the emphasis began to swing away from thrombosis as a manifestation of disordered clotting, the possible role of platelet misbehaviour as an alternative cause took its place, so the search was on for agents which would modify platelet activity. Three drugs, already widely used for other purposes, were identified [6, 21, 22] and because of the slow natural history of arterial thrombotic disease and the very large numbers of patients needed to confirm or deny clinical efficacy, some 20 years later we still have no clear-cut answers on these agents. Newer platelet-modifying agents can therefore be dealt with more briefly, because we cannot as yet foresee their place in therapeutics.

11.4.1 NEW USES FOR OLD DRUGS

(a) Dipyridamole

My group in Oxford found that adenosine not only modified platelet aggregation *in vitro* but also stopped thrombus formation in injured rabbit arteries. The effect was short-lived because adenosine is rapidly deaminated so when we became aware that the vasodilator drug dipyridamole prevented cells from taking up adenosine and degrading it, we intended to use the agent to prolong the action of adenosine. Before doing so, we tested the drug alone and found that it was a powerful antithrombotic in its own right and was also an inhibitor of platelet activity *in vitro*.

(i) Mode of action [6, 21]
Dipyridamole blocks adenosine uptake, and inhibits cAMP phosphodiesterase, thereby increasing the intracellular cAMP level. As prostacyclin also elevates cAMP by enhancing adenyl cyclase, these effects are additive, but it has been claimed that there may also be a true synergistic action between the two agents or that dipyridamole may modify prostacyclin and thromboxane production. Little evidence exists for these hypotheses so it seems probable that the effect on adenosine uptake and the cAMP enhancement remain the most plausible explanations of dipyridamole's activity. Until its mode of action is clarified it has not been possible to develop successor compounds in a logical way.

(ii) Treatment regime

Dipyridamole is given by mouth in the maximum acceptable dose – usually 200–300 mg daily in divided doses, although some patients can tolerate 400 mg per day.

(iii) Side effects

As with many vasodilators, headache is the major limiting factor but gut symptoms can also occur. There are no adverse interactions with other drugs commonly used in cardiovascular disease.

(b)   Sulphinpyrazone

Fraser Mustard's team in Hamilton were measuring platelet survival in a variety of diseases and having found marked shortening of survival in gouty subjects were surprised to find that some of their patients with gout had normal survival times. They then found that these patients were being treated wih the uricosuric agent, sulphinpyrazone.

(i) Mode of action [6, 21]

Because sulphinpyrazone is related to phenylbutazone, it is a weak cyclo-oxygenase inhibitor, thereby reducing TXA_2 production. Other non-steroidal anti-imflammatory agents with more powerful anti-TXA_2 effects do not, however, prolong survival. The *in vivo* effect of sulphinpyrazone is thus disproportionate to its known *in vitro* properties and has led to speculation that the effect is mediated by an effect on vessel wall or by metabolites such as thio-ethers which take several days to reach peak levels. As with dipyridamole, our inability to identify the mechanism which underlies the drug's ability to normalize shortened survival has prevented the development of successor compounds.

(ii) Treatment regime

Sulphinpyrazone is rapidly absorbed from the gut, is strongly protein bound and has a half-life of 2–3 hours. The usual schedule is 200 mg four times daily.

(iii) Side effects

Gastrointestinal symptoms predominate, but occasional bone-marrow depression has been recorded. The drug enhances the effect of anti-coagulants and oral hypoglycaemic agents.

(c)   Aspirin (acetyl salicylic acid – ASA)

This universally used agent had been suspected for many years of enhancing bleeding when it was used to relieve pain and fever in conditions such as haemophilia. In 1967, Harvey Weiss' team showed that it profoundly modified platelet aggregation and release reactions in response to certain stimuli.

(i) Mode of action [6, 21]

We now know that these effects are due to acetylation of a cyclo-oxygenase enzyme in platelets which produces TXA_2 from arachidonic acid (see Chapter 10). We should note that when other stimuli are provided (collagen, thrombin, or high concentrations of ADP or catecholamines) platelet activity is not suppressed by ASA, so there are prostaglandin/ASA independent pathways; if these are the ones which are involved in thrombosis we cannot expect ASA to be antithrombotic.

(ii) Treatment regime

ASA is rapidly absorbed from the gut, peak plasma levels occurring within 15 minutes, and the half-life being 13–20 minutes. It is rapidly hydrolysed to salicylic acid by esterases present in gut and blood and it has been suggested that the salicylate moiety may interfere with the acetylating action of the rest of the molecule. The dosage schedule depends on the theory being espoused by the prescriber; at the doses of 1g daily or more used in the majority of major trials and which are also appropriate for antipyretic and analgesic purposes, ASA modifies the clotting cascade. If the aim of the prescriber is, however, to rebalance the prostaglandins, then such doses not only acetylate platelet cyclo-oxygenase and cut off the supply of 'bad' TXA_2 but also inhibit vessel wall cyclo-oxygenase, cutting off the supply of the 'good' prostacyclin. Vessel walls can synthesize new non-acetylated proteins whereas platelets cannot, so it was hoped that an ASA dosage schedule could be found which could keep platelet TXA_2 production suppressed while allowing vessel-wall PGI_2 production to remain active. In given individuals, single doses of 40 mg may appear to fulfil this requirement but in some individuals, regular daily dosing produces a cumulative effect so the differential action is lost [22]. Because of this, we may either need to measure the TXA_2/PGI_2 balance and titrate the ASA dose for each individual in future trials, as we do for warfarin by using PT measurements, or use the dose which is likely to produce an acceptable rebalancing in the majority of participants; on present evidence this would be 20–40 mg on alternate days. The problem stems from the naivety of the original concepts; we now know that platelets have two pools of cyclo-oxygenase with different ASA recovery times and different responses to endogenous and exogenous arachidonate, so new questions are being posed all the time in respect of the basic pharmacology of the world's most widely used drug.

330

(iii) Side effects
Upper gut irritation, leading to nausea, pain, vomiting and bleeding have been recorded in 15–20% of the subjects taking part in long-term trials of 1000–1300 mg ASA daily. Low grade gut blood loss and consequent anaemia can occur,, but deafness and tinnitus are rare at these dose levels. Although less troublesome than other non-steroidal anti-inflammatory agents such as phenylbutazone, potentiation of the bleeding hazard from anticoagulants such as heparin and warfarin needs to be remembered.

(iv) The future
There can be no future for these three first-generation platelet modifiers until we know whether they have any antithrombotic activity at all. If they have, we need to clarify the mechanisms involved so that we can develop successor compounds or dosage schedules which will exploit this potential without producing unacceptable side effects. When we characterize their antithrombotic mechanism, we may be forced to ensure that it has been modified optimally in each individual; the apparent attractiveness of simple, side effect-free, platelet modifying regimes which do not require monitoring, in contrast to the hassle required for anticoagulation may be illusory and has not yet been matched by proof of efficacy.

11.4.2 NOVEL AGENTS

(a) Dazoxiben
Because cyclo-oxygenase inhibitors attack both the 'bad' and the 'good' limbs of the TXA_2/PGI_2 system, the search began for agents which would selectively inhibit thromboxane synthetase (TXSIs) [22, 23] thereby allowing the accumulating endoperoxides PGG_2 and PGH_2 to be used to generate 'good' prostacyclin. We need to remember that these cyclic endoperoxides are aggregating agents in their own right so if they accumulate and cannot be transformed to PGI_2 the balance may not have been changed favourably. The use of other agents to re-route the endoperoxides or to potentiate the action of the resulting PGI_2 by enhancing platelet cAMP merits exploration.

(i) Mode of action
In addition to the anticipated effect on platelets which results from the suppression of TXA_2 and the enhancement of PGI_2 we should note that these materials are powerfully vasoactive. Dazoxiben suppresses the forearm vaso-constriction produced by cold stimulation and this effect is abolished by concurrent ASA administration, suggesting that the

331

abolition of constriction is being produced by the rerouting of endoperoxides to PGI_2 [24]. The long-term role of dazoxiben is still being actively explored so we do not know whether this promising material is a 'pharmacological tool or clinical candidate' [23]. If it is the latter, does its future lie in its ability to modify vascular tone (in Raynaud's syndrome, variant angina, migraine etc) rather than in the platelet/thrombosis area, for which it was developed?

(ii) Treatment regime

Dazoxiben is rapidly absorbed from the gut, and a single dose of 100–200 mg produces maximal TXA_2 suppression, with a half-life of 6 hours. Schedules of 100–200 mg three times daily are therefore being studied. Whereas TXA_2 production is predictably suppressed there is considerable variation between individuals in respect of the platelet and vascular-tone effects. This is not due to variable drug kinetics, for the same arbitrary division into 'responders' and 'non-responders' is seen when the drug is added to platelet-rich plasma from these subjects *in vitro*; moreover, responder status can be changed by cAMP-enhancing agents [22]. In clinical trials it may be necessary to ensure that the desired effects are produced in the participants, so blood monitoring may be needed.

(iii) Side effects

These are minimal and there appear to be no interactions with other cardiovascular drugs.

(b) Other candidates

A bewildering array of materials is waiting in the wings and I believe that we do not have the will or the resources to test them adequately in the major thrombotic diseases [22]. Agents to block TXA_2 receptors, materials which stimulate endogenous PGI_2 production, or prevent it being broken down, stable analogues of PGI_2, receptor blockers for the platelet agonists such as ADP and catecholamines, and manipulators of platelet calcium flux are being developed. Existing agents which alter general platelet behaviour such as ticlopidine and suloctidil also offer theoretical antithrombotic potential but I suspect that a follow-up chapter in 20 years time will still not be able to give clear prescribing advice about these newer agents.

11.5 Fibrinolytic agents

If we cannot stop thrombi from forming, can we subsequently dissolve them [25] by activating the lytic system and converting their insoluble fibrin scaffold into soluble degradation products?

11.5.1 STREPTOKINASE

This is produced by beta-haemolytic streptococci and is a single-chain protein with a molecular weight of 48 000. It does not activate plasminogen directly, but complexes with it, and this complex is converted into active plasmin plus streptokinase degradation products. Streptokinase is antigenic so stimulates antibody production; streptococcal infection is common, and pre-existing levels of antibody may block its action. It must be given by intravenous injection and has a half-time of about 90 minutes, although the effects it produces are much longer lasting.

11.5.2 UROKINASE

This is isolated from human urine or kidney tissue cultures, so is not antigenic. It is a beta-globulin consisting of a single polypeptide chain with a molecular weight of 54 000. As with streptokinase it must be given by intravenous injection but unlike streptokinase, urokinase converts plasminogen into plasmin by a direct two-step reaction; more than half the urokinase disappears within 5 minutes but the plasminogen activator it has produced has a half-time of 10–15 minutes.

(a) Treatment regimes

These must be planned in close collaboration with a monitoring laboratory and consist of a priming and a maintenance dose. With streptokinase, an initial dose of 250 000 u is commonly used, followed by a monitored maintenance infusion which can vary from 100 000 to 150 000 u per hour. After 7 days, rising levels of induced antibodies make treatment difficult. With urokinase, 4000 u/kg given over a 30 minute period serves to prime the system and 4000 u/kg hourly thereafter maintains activity. No antibodies develop so this treatment can be continued for prolonged periods.

(b) Control of dosage

Before treatment, it is necessary to exclude abnormalities of haemostasis; with streptokinase it is useful to measure the pre-existing levels of antibodies. During treatment, euglobulin or fibrin plate lysis can be used to monitor efficacy, and the haemostatic tests should be regularly repeated. This is not an area for amateurs so close collaboration with the laboratory is vital.

Antithrombotic agents

(c) Side effects

The most important is bleeding, which can occur in up to 50% of patients treated for more than 12 hours. Contraindications to treatment are therefore recent surgery, trauma or stroke, previous bleeding problems, and pregnancy. If the bleeding fails to respond to cessation of treatment and to local measures, fresh plasma or blood should be given. Fever and allergic reactions are common with streptokinase but are rarely of major clinical significance.

11.6 Do they work?

I propose to examine the three major spontaneous thrombotic diseases – myocardial infarction, stroke and venous thrombo-embolism, plus the problems posed by coronary vein grafts, prosthetic valves and atrial fibrillation. I will do so by drawing on major reviews, which in turn only refer to the few studies which are large enough and sufficiently well conducted to answer the two questions which patients ask – Will I live longer and will I remain free from disability? Where no guidance is given, this indicates that in my view there is no evidence on which clinicians can base a reasoned judgement; in such situations they are on their own and must balance the likelihood of harm against the potential benefit which is claimed.

11.6.1 CORONARY HEART DISEASE

(a) Acute myocardial infarction (AMI)

(i) Anticoagulant therapy [5]
Antithrombotic regimes are unlikely to have a major impact on death or disability after AMI because prognosis is largely determined by the effects of the initial infarct on pumping power and cardiac rhythms, rather than by the risk of further coronary thrombosis and reinfarction. In any event, all the trials performed to date are flawed, and although attempts have been made to turn these sow's ears into silk purses by pooling and recalculating their results, the propriety of this is in doubt. Although there is no clear evidence that anticoagulation modifies mortality after AMI, such patients are also at risk from venous thrombo-embolism and from mural thrombosis which can produce subsequent disability from embolic stroke and limb ischaemia. Table 11.1 shows the rates observed in a well-conducted AMI trial [26] so in my view, until we have the results of new trials, patients with big or complicated AMIs (heart failure, dysrhythmias) should receive prophylactic anticoagulants.

334

(ii) Platelet modifying therapy [21]

No adequate trials have been performed in AMI but a study comparing ASA 324 mg daily with placebo in 1266 men with 'unstable angina' has been reported [27]. Total deaths by 12 weeks were reduced in the ASA group (10 vs 21 on placebo) as was non-fatal MI (21 vs 44). It is difficult to extrapolate to the wider world of AMI from this very selective study (13 666 patients were screened but only 1266 – 18% of the total – were entered) in a condition which not everyone finds easy to define (cardiac pain without evidence of infarction) and which only dealt with men. We should note that this is the first 'low-dose' ASA study to produce positive results.

(iii) Fibrinolytic therapy

The early studies of systemic treatment with intravenous activators made out a suggestive but inconclusive case. For example, a major European collaborative study [28] only enrolled 315 patients out of 2338 suitable patients with AMI into a trial of intravenous streptokinase and all these trial patients were also on coumarins. There was little difference in early outcome (at 21 days, 28 control and 18 streptokinase deaths) but in the next 5 months there were 20 control and only 6 streptokinase deaths, giving a total outcome at 6 months of 48 control and 24 streptokinase deaths. We can only speculate on the way in which an initial 24 hour streptokinase infusion could have influenced late mortality and it seems possible that the haemodynamic effects of fibrinolysis, rather than actual thrombolysis might be responsible (a reduction in cardiac work, systemic and pulmonary pressures by the reduction in fibrinogen and blood viscosity).

Increasing ease of access to occluded coronary arteries led to the infusion of lytic materials directly into them and over the next few years many major trials will be reported. Anderson and colleagues [29] took 50 AMI patients some 2–7 hours after the onset of symptoms and randomly assigned them to receive heparin alone or heparin plus intracoronary streptokinase, the latter being started at 4.0 hours. Reperfusion was

Table 11.1 Thrombo-embolic incidents in MRC AMI trial

	Anticoagulant	Placebo
Systemic arterial occlusion	9	24
Leg vein thrombosis	11	30
Pulmonary embolism	16	40
Thromboembolism rate (%)	4.8	11.0

claimed in 19 of the 24 receiving lytic therapy but no results are given for the control group. The major finding was an improvement in myocardial status judged by enzymes, ECG, isotope images, ejection fraction and echocardiographic wall movement. In sharp contrast to this optimistic view, Khaja and colleagues [30] entered 40 patients into a random comparison of intracoronary streptokinase versus dextrose, the infusions beginning at 5.4 hours. Anticoagulants were not routinely used, although aspirin and dipyridamole were given to all patients from day 2. Reperfusion was established in 12 of 20 streptokinase patients but in only 2 of 20 placebo patients. Despite this, there was no improvement in left ventricular function when measured immediately after the infusion or at 12 days and 5 months. Neither trial was of course big enough to answer the crucial questions about death and disability but in another randomized study [31], where 134 patients with AMI received intracoronary streptokinase while 116 did not, there were 5 deaths by six months in the streptokinase group (3.7%) and 17 deaths in the control group (14.7%). We should note, however, that the mean time from the onset of symptoms to randomization was 276 minutes, and the impracticability of delivering streptokinase into the coronary arteries of everyone with suspected AMI so rapidly after the onset of their symptoms makes it clear that 'even if the current trials show clear evidence of improved survival, it is unlikely for logistic reasons, if for no other, that the technique will make a major impact on the mortality from AMI in the community as a whole' [32].

Another randomized study [33] showed improved survival after thrombolysis with intracoronary streptokinase. Thrombolysis was generally successful (85% patent). There was less ventricular fibrillation, pericarditis or cardiogenic shock, but more bleeding and non-fatal reinfarction on active treatment. The benefit (mortality 9% v 11%) control) was sustained up to 1 year.

The development of fibrinolytics with a greater affinity for fresh fibrin such as tissue-type plasminogen-activator (t-PA) gives a good coronary patency rate (61% v 21% in controls) after a short intravenous infusion [34], suggesting that good clinical results can be obtained without coronary infusion. Even so t-PA is not specific for fibrin and does produce some activation of plasminogen with risk of bleeding [34, 35]. Production by recombinant DNA techniques may be expensive [35] and acylated streptokinase which is also selective for fibrin [35] may be a better approach.

The emphasis is beginning to swing back to systemic fibrinolytic methods that do not demand the full panoply of coronary arteriography; Schröder and colleagues [36] showed that reperfusion could be produced in 11 out of 21 patients by a single 30 minute intravenous streptokinase infusion. Rogers et al. [37] have now compared the effectiveness of 240 000 u of intracoronary streptokinase with 500 000 u and with

1 million units of intravenous streptokinase given 6.5–6.8 hours after onset. Thrombolysis occurred in 76%, 10% and 44% and blood loss requiring transfusions in 4%, 10% and 0% of these groups. If a simple intravenous regime can lyse nearly half the occluding thrombi, whereas an intracoronary regime still seems to fail in about a quarter of all thrombi, then this introduces a new dimension into the acute lytic treatment of MI for 'it could be carried out in any coronary care unit (and could perhaps be initiated even by the family doctor), it avoids the hazards and delays inherent in emergency coronary arteriography, and its use would be immeasurably less demanding of limited resources' [32].

Two final points; once the thrombus has been lysed, the circumstances which produced it still prevail (a thrombotic predisposition and a severely diseased vessel wall). The crucial difference between Anderson *et al.* [29] who claimed to be salvaging myocardium, and Khaja *et al.* [30] who did not, is that the former also used anticoagulants whereas the latter only gave agents which may not have antithrombotic potential. To deal with the abnormal vessel wall which is exposed after successful lysis it is being suggested [38] that percutaneous transluminal balloon angioplasty or coronary artery bypass grafting should also be performed but this moves us back into the cloud-cuckoo land of trying to apply high technology to a condition which kills 160 000 each year in England and Wales alone.

The plan for the future [39] must therefore be to develop effective systemic regimes with a low bleeding risk, which can be given soon after AMI in low-technology areas and follow this through with effective anticoagulation. We should then pick out the small subgroup who require and will benefit from transfer to high-technology units for invasive procedures.

(b)   Long term prevention of recurrent AMI

(i) Anticoagulants
In no area has it been more true that 'the greatest use that anticoagulants may yet have in clinical medicine is their ability to cause controversy' [40]. All we can salvage from the squabbling in the 1950s and 60s is that long-term anticoagulation probably did reduce mortality after infarction by some 20% but the evidence fell tantalizingly short of proof. After a phoney peace, the calm has now been broken by a carefully conducted and reported study from the Netherlands [41], which took a group of 898 elderly patients (mean age 61.6) who had been anticoagulated after an AMI at least 6 months earlier (mean 5.9 years). They were then randomly allocated to continue or to stop their anticoagulation. If one analyses the results on an intention-to-treat basis for total mortality there is no significant difference (Table 11.2) but if one now allows opinions about clinical

Antithrombotic agents

Table 11.2 Dutch over 60's study

Mode of analysis	Placebo (n = 439)	AC (n = 439)	P for difference
(a) distribution of deaths between the groups			
Intention to treat	69	21	0.07
Explicative:			
Protocol adherents	49	28	0.02
Protocol deviants	20	23	—
(b) distribution of recurrent MI (fatal MI)			
Intention to treat	64 (27)	29 (11)	0.0005
Explicative:			
Protocol adherents	58 (24)	20 (4)	0.0001
Protocol deviants	6 (3)	9 (7)	

events (fatal and non-fatal recurrent AMI) to be offered and if one permits separate analysis for the protocol compliers and the protocol deviants, then continued anticoagulation appeared to offer benefit (Table 11.2). All that this trial does is to argue cogently for the whole issue to be re-opened and because it was a trial of stopping treatment in patients who had shown that they could safely weather several years of anticoagulant therapy, it cannot tell us about the benefits or hazards of starting treatment in ordinary patients after their AMI. I hope the matter will be resolved when this chapter is next revised but I doubt it.

(ii) Platelet modifying agents

ASPIRIN. Of the six long-term secondary prevention studies in survivors of myocardial infarction, five showed reductions in total mortality which did not achieve significance within each trial and one showed an equally non-significant increase in mortality [22]. It has been suggested that the results of these trials can be brought together in a way that avoids the statistical traps inherent in simple pooling. If one does so, the probable effect of ASA is to reduce total mortality by 10–15% but the analysis shows that the confidence limits of the pooled 10–15% risk reduction embrace zero, so the 'true' benefit could lie anywhere from zero upwards. One should also remember the problem of ASA dosage set out above: some trials used 1 g daily, others 1.5 g and two used 300 mg. On existing evidence, 'not proven' must be the overall verdict and one can only be sad that so much effort has recently been put into a new trial which does not help us to resolve our dilemma (EPSIM Research Group) [42]. In this study, 652 infarct survivors were randomized to receive oral anticoagulants and 651 to receive ASA, 1.5 g daily. There were 65 deaths in the anticoagulant group and 72 in the ASA group, so the sad, but totally predictable conclusion from the trial was 'that aspirin in the dosage used is probably not different from oral anticoagulants in affecting mortality and morbidity after myocardial infarction. However, this study does not consider the effectiveness of either agent in comparison to no anti-thrombotic therapy – an issue that remains unsettled'.

DIPYRIDAMOLE. The PARIS study [21, 22] compared ASA alone with ASA plus dipyridamole and did not show a beneficial effect in respect of predetermined primary end-points. When secondary data dredging was undertaken, it was suggested that the combination was especially favourable to patients entered soon after their index infarct; to confirm this, a second trial (PARIS II) is now under way, but unhappily ASA plus dipyridamole is being compared with placebo, so whatever the outcome, we will never know whether dipyridamole itself is useful.

SULPHINPYRAZONE. The less that is said about our unhappy experience with this agent the better. The optimistic tone of the reports of the Anturan Reinfarction Trial Research Group was not commensurate with the evidence contained in them. Analysts were able to indentify [43] fundamental flaws in design, conduct, analysis and reporting and to point out that the total intention-to-treat mortality did not differ significantly in the sulphinpyrazone and placebo groups (74 versus 89). The Anturan Reinfarction Italian Study Group [44] recruited too few patients to be able to detect an effect on mortality but total deaths, on an intention-to-treat basis, were 29 on the drug and 27 on placebo. Sulphinpyrazone must therefore share with ASA and dipyridamole the 'not proven' verdict.

11.6.2 STROKE

In cerebrovascular disease we have two different underlying disease processes [2]. About a quarter of strokes are due to intracranial bleeding and the rest to thrombo-embolic infarction. An agent that modified haemostasis and platelet behaviour could have favourable effects on the latter, but devastating effects on the former. Since it is not possible confidently to ascribe stroke to one category or other on simple clinical or investigative grounds, we now know that stroke trials can be carried out only where imaging by computer-assisted tomography or nuclear magnetic resonance is possible. This problem has led investigators to use short-lived neurological deficits (so-called 'transient ischaemic attacks': TIAs) to test drug regimens, but such groups of patients are even less homogenous than those with completed strokes [2].

(a)   Acute stroke

No adequate studies of any of the regimens have been conducted.

(b)   Secondary prevention after an initial stroke or TIA

(i) Anticoagulants

Studies specifically directed to this problem are inadequate but in passing we should note that the Dutch over-sixties post-AMI study found [45] that while there was a modest increase in intracranial haemorrhage in the group continuing on anticoagulants, there was an even more marked reduction in non-haemorrhagic events; the total days of persistent neurological deficit were 1204 in the placebo group as opposed to 120 in the anticoagulant group. As in AMI, we must now re-examine the issue of anticoagulation in stroke prevention.

(ii) Platelet modifying agents

ASPIRIN. Two major TIA trials used 1.2 g daily [46]; in the smaller American study there was no significant effect on stroke-free survival; in the larger Canadian trial a factorial design was used so that some patients received only placebo, some only ASA, some only sulphinpyrazone and some received both. Treating all the ASA takers as homogeneous, the risk of stroke and death was reduced by 31% but this over-all result concealed an apparent disparity between a benefit in men (48% reduction in stroke or death) but no observable benefit in women. A more recent trial [47] compared placebo with ASA 1 g/day, alone and with dipyridamole 225 mg/d, in 604 patients, of whom 16% had presented with TIAs and the rest with completed strokes. In their 3 year follow-up period, the fatal plus non-fatal stroke rate in each group was: placebo – 18%; ASA – 10.5%; ASA + dipyridamole – 10.5%. Unlike the Canadian trial, there was no sex difference in this ASA effect, but as in other ASA trials, the price paid was a significant excess of gastrointestinal symptoms. Unhappily, the trial was too small to tell us what we need to know, which is whether ASA prevents death and disability, so we are now awaiting the results of a large UK trial. This should also help to resolve the question of ASA dosage for it is comparing daily doses of 1g and 300 mg with placebo. Until it reports, I must emphasize that there is no evidence of benefit from low-dose aspirin in cerebrovascular disease.

DIPYRIDAMOLE. No adequate trials have been performed.

SULPHINPYRAZONE. In the Canadian trial [46] there was a 10% reduction in the risk of stroke or death with sulphinpyrazone alone. The lowest stroke-or-death risk was, however, observed in the patients receiving both ASA and sulphinpyrazone, and the trial design did not make it possible to determine whether there was true synergism between these agents. Candelise et al. (1982) [48] have recently reported on 124 patients whom they randomized to ASA (1g) or sulphinpyrazone (800 mg) daily. The opportunity to include a placebo group or a synergistic group was thus not grasped. It was suggested that men benefited from ASA while the women did insignificantly better on sulphinpyrazone but the small numbers do not permit differences in the only end-points that matter to patients (disability and death) to be observed.

11.6.3 VENOUS THROMBO-EMBOLISM

(a) Acute DVT or PE

(i) Anticoagulants

Full anticoagulation [49, 50] should be established at once and it should be remembered that heparin may also reduce other adverse effects of PE by preventing the vasoconstriction and bronchoconstriction which fresh thrombi induce in the lungs.

(ii) Fibrinolytic agents

Systemic streptokinase and urokinase can clear the lung and leg vessels more rapidly than the unaided body but the acid tests of a reduction in total mortality or of long-term disability from the post-phlebitic syndrome or pulmonary hypertension have not yet been satisfied [51].

(b) Prevention of DVT and PE in patients at risk

(i) Anticoagulants

If a risk profile is worked out [52, 54] management becomes very simple; age, severity of insult, obesity and previous DVT/PE are associated with a high risk, whereas youth, minor operation/trauma/illness, normal body build and no previous history of venous problems betoken low risk. For very low-risk patients, cost–benefit analysis suggests that no action is needed; for low-risk patients, compression stockings may suffice or low dose heparin can be used, but as the risk rises, the only regime for which there is hard evidence of an effect on mortality is conventional heparin/ coumarin prophylaxis. Where the insult is a very major one (hip replacement) or has been sustained before prophylactic low-dose heparin can restrain the clotting cascade (hip fracture), conventional anticoagulant regimes have hitherto been thought to be necessary, but Leyvraz et al. [55]

have recently shown that by using the APTT to monitor their low-dose heparin they could produce a DVT rate of only 13% after hip replacement by giving an average of 19 000 u daily, whereas in their fixed low-dose group, receiving 10 500 u daily, the rate was 39%. As previously hinted, the era of regimes which were superficially attractive because they appeared to need no monitoring, may now be giving way to the realization that to maximize benefit and to minimize harm we will still need to make measurements.

The only clinical situation in which additional thought is needed is in pregnancy where the enhanced risk of venous thrombosis has to be weighed against the problems posed by anticoagulation. Warfarin has teratogenic potential in early pregnancy and is thought to present an unacceptable bleeding hazard to mother and baby as term approaches. Heparin is inconvenient and has long-term side effects so the present compromise is to use subcutaneous heparin for the first three months, warfarin until the 37th week, then heparin until the second post-partum day when full warfarin therapy is resumed [56].

(ii) Platelet modifying agents
Having marshalled the confusing and conflicting evidence from 20 trials, Hirsh [21] concludes that none of the drugs has 'been shown to be consistently effective in preventing post-operative venous thrombosis'. A nagging doubt remains, in that in some studies there has been a striking difference in the results obtained in men and women; for example [57] when taking 1.2 g of ASA daily, men undergoing total hip replacement showed a 67% reduction in venographically confirmed thrombosis over those taking placebo, whereas for women the reduction by ASA was only 4%. All the studies so far carried out are however based on small groups of subjects so random variations probably account for these apparent sex differences. For example, in another study [58], which compared placebo with ASA 900 mg plus sulphinpyrazone 800 mg daily, venographically proven DVT after hip replacement was reduced by 75% in women but by only 32% in the men. Future studies should be planned so that the responsiveness of both men and women can be adequately assessed.

(iii) Fibrinolytic agents
Attempts have been made to enhance natural fibrinolysis by oral regimes and the value of anabolic steroids is currently being appraised.

11.6.4 PROSTHETIC HEART VALVES

Here we have a foreign surface (plastic, metal and cloth) which can activate the clotting cascade and the platelets but cannot provide any of the modifying materials found in natural vessel walls (prostacyclin, plasminogen activator, protein C). Embolus rates from aortic and mitral valves have served as the end-point in many trials but, in the majority, oral anticoagulants have also been used. Hirsh [21] concluded that 'the combination of either aspirin or dipyridamole with oral anticoagulants is more effective than anticoagulants alone . . . There is also a suggestion that aspirin alone does not offer adequate protection'.

11.6.5 CORONARY VEIN GRAFTS

The increasing operation rate means that we must take account of the problem of by-pass occlusion [22]. Although the saphenous veins that are used belong to the patient concerned, they are deprived of their normal vasa vasorum and subjected to pressures and mechanical deformations that are greater than in their normal lower-limb site. We therefore should not expect them to behave like normal veins and arteries. In one study, in comparison with a control group, there was no difference in the 6-month graft patency rate in patients given either ASA (975 mg daily) plus dipyridamole (225 mg daily) or tightly controlled warfarin. Another group started dipyridamole (400 mg daily) two days before operation, and continued with dipyridamole (225 mg daily) plus ASA (975 mg daily) immediately after operation. In comparison with a randomly allocated group who received matching placebos, they found that 10 of 351 grafts were occluded within a month in the treated group compared with 38 of 362 in the placebo group. Finally, a third group started sulphinpyrazone (800 mg daily) 24 hours after saphenous vein grafting and found that by 7–14 days, 8 of 212 grafts had become occluded compared with 20 of 219 in patients given matching placebos. The problem is thus not yet resolved.

11.6.6 ATRIAL FIBRILLATION

Atrial fibrillation (AF) occurs in many patients with established heart disease and in up to 5% of the elderly population. It raises the risk of embolic stroke 5-fold in so-called 'lone' AF or 17-fold in AF with valve disease, but to our lasting shame we do not yet know the cost–benefit equation even for such long-used methods as oral anticoagulation [59]. Like many similar treatments, benefit was claimed on the basis of inadequate trials; the regime came into wide use and thus made it impossible or apparently unethical to carry out the proper studies which still need to be done. I believe that controlled coumarin anticoagulation is safer than AF but as in many of the areas we have explored, the clinician must balance the known hazards against the apparent benefits.

Table 11.3 Buyers Guide

		Treatment on offer			
	Anticoagulants	Platelet modifiers			Fibrinolysis
Problem		ASA	Dipyridamole	Sulphinpyrazone	
Myocardial infarction					
Acute	++ (High risk)	+ (Unstable angina)	?	?	+
Prevention	++ (High risk)	+	O	O	?
Stroke					
Acute	?	?	?	?	?
Prevention	?	++ (at 1 g/d or more)	O	?	?
Venous thromboembolism					
Acute	+++	O	O	O	+
Prevention	+++	+	O	O	?
Prosthetic valves	++	+	+	O	?
Coronary grafts	+	+	+	+	?
Atrial fibrillation	++	?	?	?	?

+++ Evidence good – you should do it.
++ Evidence reasonable – I do it.
+ Evidence poor – make up your own mind.
O Evidence suggests no benefit – do not do it.
? Inadequate evidence – wait and see.

11.7 The best buy

Consumer organizations marshall the evidence relating to household goods and then offer the potential purchaser a rating as guidance and I will attempt a similar task for drugs used in thrombotic disease (Table 11.3). It is a dangerous exercise because new products and new evidence about old ones may overturn my rating scales by the time you read them. It is therefore a personal judgment based on the 1984 position.

References

1. Mitchell, J.R.A. (1984) Thrombosis. In *Cardiovascular Disease* (ed. J.R. Hampton), Heinemann, London, pp. 186–97.
2. Mitchell, J.R.A. (1981) Clinical events resulting from thrombosis. In *Haemostasis and Thrombosis* (eds. A.L., Bloom & D.P. Thomas), Churchill Livingstone, Edinburgh, pp. 626–36.
3. Mitchell, J.R.A. (1978) The prevention of thrombosis. In *Advanced Medicine* 14 (ed. D.J. Weatherall) Pitman Medical, Tunbridge Wells, pp. 228–35.
4. Douglas, A.S. (1962) *Anticoagulant Therapy*. Blackwell Scientific, Oxford, pp. 1–7.
5. Mitchell, J.R.A. (1981) Anticoagulants in coronary heart disease – retrospect and prospect. *Lancet*, i, 257–62.
6. Heptinstall, S. and Mitchell, J.R.A. (1984) Platelets and thrombosis. In *Human Blood Coagulation, Haemostasis and Thrombosis* (ed. C.R. Rizza), Blackwell Scientific, Oxford, pp. 380–414.
7. Mitchell, J.R.A. (1981) Prostaglandins in vascular disease; a seminal approach *Br. Med. J.*, **282**, 590–4.
8. Gaffney, P.J. (1981) The fibrinolytic system. In *Haemostasis and Thrombosis* (eds. A.L. Bloom & D.P. Thomas), Churchill Livingstone, Edinburgh, pp. 198–224.
9. Reid, H.A. and Chan, K.E. (1968) The paradox in therapeutic defibrination. *Lancet*, i, 485–6.
10. Wessler, S. and Gitel, S.N. (1979) Heparin: new concepts relevant to clinical use. *Blood*, **53**, 525–44.
11. Barrowcliffe, T.W. and Thomas, D.P. (1981) Anti-thrombin III and heparin. In *Haemostasis and Thrombosis* (ed. A.L. Bloom & D.P. Thomas), Churchill Livingstone, Edinburgh, pp. 712–24.
12. Hirsh, J. van Aken, W.G., Gallus, A.S., Dollery, C.T., Cade, J.F. and Yung, W.L. (1976) Heparin kinetics in venous thrombosis and pulmonary embolism. *Circulation*, **53**, 691–5.
13. Salzman, E.W., Deykin, D., Shapiro, R.M. and Rosenberg, R. (1975) Management of heparin therapy. Controlled prospective trial. *N. Engl. J. Med.*, **292**, 1046–50.
14. Prentice, C.R.M. (1983) Anticoagulant therapy. In *The Thromboembolic Disorders* (eds J. Van de Loo, C.R.M. Prentice & F.K. Beller), Schattauer, Stuttgart, pp. 159–81.
15. International Multicentre Trial Group (1975) Prevention of fatal post-operative

pulmonary embolism by low doses of heparin. *Lancet*, ii, 45–51.

16. Kakkar, V.V., Djazaeri, B., Fok J., Fletcher, M., Scully, M.F. and Westwick, J. (1982) Low-molecular-weight heparin and prevention of postoperative deep vein thrombosis. *Br. Med. J.*, **284**, 375–9.

17. Gallop, P.M., Lian, J.B. and Hauschka, P.V. (1980) Carboxylated calcium-binding proteins and vitamin K. *N. Engl. J. Med.*, **302**, 1460–6.

18. Loeliger, E.A. (1979) The optimal therapeutic range in oral anticoagulation: history and proposal. *Thromb. Haem.*, (Stuttgart), **42**, 1141–52.

19. Poller, L. (1982) Oral anticoagulants reassessed. *Br. Med. J.*, **284**, 1425–6.

20. Sharp, A.A. (1982) Problems with anticoagulants. *Br. Med. J.*, **285**, 242–3.

21. Hirsh, J. (1982) Antiplatelet agents; their mode of action, rationale and clinical effectiveness. *Prog. Pharmacol.*, **4**, 21–50.

22. Mitchell, J.R.A. (1983) Clinical aspects of the arachidonic acid – thromboxane pathway. *Br. Med. Bull.*, **39**, 289–95.

23. Tyler, H.M. (1983) Dazoxiben: a pharmacological tool or clinical candidate? *Br. J. Clin. Pharmacol.*, **15**, 13 S–16 S.

24. Cowley, A.J., Jones, E.W. and Hanley, S.P. (1983) Effects of Dazoxiben, an inhibitor of thromboxane synthetase, on forearm vasoconstriction in response to cold stimulation and on human blood vessel prostacyclin production. *Br. J. Clin. Pharmacol.*, **15**, 107S–112S.

25. Genton, E. (1983) Fibrinolytic therapy. In *The Thromboembolic Disorders* (eds. J. Van de Loo, C.R.M. Prentice & F.K. Beller), Schattauer, Stuttgart, pp. 183–97.

26. Report of Working Party on Anticoagulant Therapy in Coronary Thrombosis to the Medical Research Council (1969) Assessment of short-term anticoagulant administration after cardiac infarction. *Br. Med. J.*, **1**, 335–42.

27. Lewis, H.D., Davies, J.W., Archibald, D.G., *et al.* (1983) Protective effects of aspirin against acute myocardial infarction and death in men with unstable angina. *N. Engl. J. Med.*, **309**, 396–403.

28. Mitchell, J.R.A. (1979) Fibrinolytic therapy in myocardial infarction. *Br. Med. J.*, **3**, 1017–8.

29. Anderson, J.L., Marshall, H.W., Bray, B.E. *et al.* (1983) A randomized trial of intracoronary streptokinase in the treatment of acute myocardial infarction. *N. Engl. J. Med.*, **308**, 1312–8.

30. Khaja, F., Walton, J.A., Brymer, J.F. *et al.* (1983) Intracoronary fibrinolytic therapy in acute myocardial infarction. Report of a prospective randomized trial. *N. Engl. J. Med.*, **308**, 1305–11.

31. Kennedy, J.W., Ritchie, J.L., Davis, K.B. and Fritz, J.K. (1983) Western Washington randomized trial of intra-coronary streptokinase in acute myocardial infarction. *N. Engl. J. Med.*, **309**, 1477–82.

32. Brooks, N. (1983) Intracoronary thrombolysis in acute myocardial infarction. *Br. Heart J.*, **50**, 397–400.

33. Simoons, M.L. *et al.* (1985) Improved survival after early thrombolysis in acute myocardial infarction. *Lancet*, **ii**, 578–82.

34. Vestraete, M. *et al.* (1985) Double-blind randomized trial of intravenous tissue-type plasminogen activator versus placebo in acute myocardial infarction. *Lancet*, **ii**, 965–69.

35. Sherry, S. (1985) Tissue plasminogen activator (t-PA): will it fulfill its promise? *N. Engl. J. Med.*, **313**, 1014–17.

36. Schröder, R., Biamino, G., von Leitner, E.R., Linderer, T., Brüggemann, T., Heitz, J., Vöhringer H.F., & Wegscheider, K. (1983) Intravenous short-term infusion of streptokinase in acute myocardial infarction. *Circulation*, **67** 536–48.

37. Rogers, W.J., Mantle, J.A., Hood, W.P., Baxley, W.A., Whitlow, P.L., Reeves, R.C. and Soto, B. (1983) Prospective randomized trial of intravenous and intracoronary streptokinase in acute myocardial infarction. *Circulation*, **68**, 1051–61.

38. Swan, H.J.C. (1982) Thrombolysis in acute myocardial infarction: treatment of the underlying coronary artery disease. *Circulation*, **66**, 914–6.

39. Collen, D. and Verstraete, M. (1983) Systemic thrombolytic therapy of acute myocardial infarction? *Circulation*, **68**, 462–5.

40. Breckenridge, A. (1976) Oral anticoagulants – the totem and the taboo. *Br. Med. J.*, **1**, 419–23.

41. Report of the Sixty-plus Reinfarction Study Research Group (1980) A double-blind trial to assess long-term oral anticoagulant therapy in elderly patients after myocardial infarction. *Lancet*, **ii**, 989–94.

42. The EPSIM Research Group (1982) A controlled comparison of aspirin and oral anticoagulants in prevention of death after myocardial infarction. *N. Engl. J. Med.*, **307**, 701–8.

43. Mitchell, J.R.A. (1980) Secondary prevention of myocardial infarction – the present state of the art. *Br. Med. J.*, **280**, 1128–32.

44. Report from the Anturan Reinfarction Italian Study (1982) Sulphinpyrazone in post-myocardial infarction. *Lancet*, **i**, 237–42.

45. Second Report of the Sixty-plus Reinforcement Study Research Group (1982) Risks of long-term oral anticoagulant therapy in elderly patients after myocardial infarction. *Lancet*, **i**, 64–8.

46. Mitchell, J.R.A. (1981) Anticoagulants, aspirin and anturan in transient cerebral ischaemic attacks. In *Advanced Medicine* (ed. W.M.G. Tunbridge), Pitman Medical, London, pp. 276–86.

47. Bousser, M.G. Eschwege, E., Haguenau, M., Lefauconnier, J.M., Thibult, N., Touboul, D., and Touboul, P.J. (1983) 'AICLA' controlled trial of aspirin and dipyridamole in the secondary prevention of atherothrombotic cerebral ischaemia. *Stroke*, **14**, 5–14.

48. Candelise, L., Landi, G., Perrone, P., Bracchi, M. and Brambilla, G. (1982) A randomized trial of aspirin and sulfinpyrazone in patients with TIA. *Stroke*, **13**, 175–9.

49. Anonymous (1981) Pulmonary embolism – therapeutic dilemma? *Lancet*, **ii**, 1396.

50. Ruckley, C.V. (1982) Management of pulmonary embolism. *Br. Med. J.*, **285**, 831–3.

51. Anonymous (1981) Streptokinase and deep venous thrombosis. *Lancet*, **i**, 1035–6.

52. Davies, G.C. and Salzman, E.W. (1981) Cost effectiveness of prophylaxis of venous thromboembolism. *J. Roy. Soc. Med.*, **74**, 177–80.

53. Hull, R.D., Hirsh, J., Sackett, D.L. and Stoddart, G.L. (1982) Cost-effectiveness of primary and secondary prevention of fatal pulmonary embolism in high-risk surgical patients. *Can. Med. Assoc. J.*, **127**, 990–5.

Antithrombotic agents

54. Salzman, E.W. (1983) Progress in preventing venous thromboembolism. *N. Engl. J. Med*, **309** 980–2.
55. Leyvraz, P.F., Richard, J., Bachmann, F., *et al.*, (1983) Adjusted versus fixed-dose subcutaneous heparin in the prevention of deep-vein thrombosis after total hip replacement. *N. Engl. J. Med.*, **309,** 954–8.
56. Anonymous (1975) Venous thromboembolism and anti-coagulants in pregnancy. *Br. Med. J.*, **2,** 421–2.
57. Harris, W.H., Salzman, E.W., Athanasoulis, C.A., Waltman, A.C. and DeSanctis, R.W. (1977) Aspirin prophylaxis of venous thromboembolism after total hip replacement. *N. Engl. J. Med.*, **297,** 1246–9.
58. Sautter, R.D., Koch, E.L., Myers, W.O. *et al.*, (1983) Aspirin-sulfinpyrazone in prophylaxis of deep venous thrombosis in total hip replacement. *J. Am. Med. Assoc.*, **250,** 2649–54.
59. Milliken, J.A. (1983) Atrial fibrillation and embolisation. *Can. Med. Assoc. J.*, **128,** 1370–2.

12   The management of the hyperlipidaemias

N.I. JOWETT and D.J. GALTON

12.1   Introduction

The hyperlipidaemias are a common and heterogeneous group of metabolic disorders which affect more than 10% of the population of Western industrialized countries [1–3]. Although hypertension and diabetes mellitus are well established as predisposing factors for the development of atherosclerotic disease [4, 5] the role of dietary fat and altered lipoprotein metabolism is not so well understood [6–8]. Epidemiological studies have demonstrated that increased levels of plasma cholesterol may be associated with premature coronary heart disease [2, 3] and the United States Lipid Research Clinics trial [9] has given clear evidence that reducing high cholesterol levels in men will lower the incidence of coronary heart disease (CHD), and additionally will significantly reduce deaths, myocardial infarcts, angina and the need for coronary artery bypass surgery. These results confirm previous similar reports [10–12].

The role of hypertriglyceridaemia in the aetiology of coronary heart disease is a little harder to interpret. In 1972, Carlson [13] reported that in his 9 year study of over 3000 men, elevation of both plasma cholesterol and triglyceride were independently and linearly associated with the incidence of CHD, and at 14 years it was the plasma triglyceride level which was a strongly associated risk factor [14]. However, some epidemiologists remain sceptical over the independent role of plasma triglycerides in coronary heart disease and Hulley [15] believes that the association is not due to hypertriglyceridaemia *per se*; but because of its association with hypercholesterolaemia. Nevertheless, hypertriglyceridaemia can cause acute pancreatitis or may draw attention to other cardiovascular risk factors such as diabetes.

It is also difficult to assess the value of therapeutic intervention because whilst atheroma is generally progressive, it may regress spontaneously [16, 17]. The results of a study on femoral atheroma [18] suggest that effective hypolipidaemic treatment favourably influences the natural

349

The management of the hyperlipidaemias

history of symptomatic peripheral atherosclerosis in patients with hyperlipidaemia. Unfortunately we do not know whether the rest of the arterial system will also respond in the same way to this or to other forms of risk factor reduction.

12.2 Lipids, lipoproteins and the hyperlipidaemias

The major lipids found in man are triglycerides, phospholipids and cholesterol. The former are found predominantly in adipose tissue and the others are cell membrane components. All three are insoluble in water and for transport in blood they are converted into water-soluble complexes called lipoproteins by binding to specific proteins (apoproteins). These lipoproteins are distinguished by the types of carrier apoprotein present and the proportion of the various lipids carried. The main lipoproteins are:

(1) Chylomicrons. Chylomicrons are the largest lipoproteins and consist mainly of exogenous (dietary) triglyceride which has been absorbed from the small intestine. They are cleared rapidly from the plasma, and are not usually found after a 12–14 hour fast.

(2) Very low density lipoproteins (VLDL). These are small triglyceride-rich (50%) lipoproteins bearing endogenous lipids synthesized mainly by the liver.

(3) Low density lipoproteins (LDL). LDL is the main transport vehicle for both endogenous and exogenous cholesterol. Cellular uptake is governed by specific surface LDL receptors.

(4) High density lipoproteins (HDL). These are the smallest lipoproteins and are made up of two subfractions – HDL2 and HDL3. They are phospholipid rich but contain some cholesterol which may be transported away from cells to the liver. High levels of HDL, particularly HDL2, are negatively correlated with atheromatous disease, and raised levels are often found in premenopausal women, joggers and moderate, regular drinkers of alcohol. The role of lipoproteins in enzyme regulation has recently been reviewed by Galton et al. [19].

12.3 Classification of the hyperlipidaemias

The hyperlipidaemias may be subdivided into either primary (idiopathic) or the more common secondary forms. The former are often familial and should only be diagnosed by exclusion of known underlying causes, the commonest of which are diabetes, thyroid disease, renal disease,

Table 12.1 Classification of hyperlipidaemias

Type	Other names	Incidence in UK	Lipoprotein increased	Plasma Chol.	Plasma Trigs.	Plasma appearance (4 C/12 h)
I	Exogenous hypertrigly-ceridaemia	0.1%	Chylomicrons	+	+++	Milky with clear infranatant
IIa	Monogenic and polygenic hypercholes-terolaemia	20–25%	LDL	+++	N	Clear
IIb	Familial combined hyperlipidaemia	20–25%	LDL VLDL	++	+	Turbid
III	Floating or broad beta disease	2–5%	Abnormal LDL	++	++	Turbid
IV	Essential or carbohydrate induced hypertrigly-ceridaemia	35–50%	VLDL	N/+	++/+++	Turbid
V	Exogenous and endogenous hyperlipidaemia	2–3%	VLDL Chylomicrons	N/+	++/+++	Milky with turbid infranatant

Key to plasma lipid levels: N = Normal levels, + = Slight elevation, ++ = Elevated, +++ = Marked elevation

The management of the hyperlipidaemias

cholestasis, alcohol and drugs (q.v.). The hyperlipidaemias have been classified into six types by the World Health Organization [20]. This classification is shown in Table 12.1

12.4 Management of the hyperlipidaemias

12.4.1 PATIENT SCREENING

There are certain groups of patients who should always be screened for plasma lipid or lipoprotein abnormalities. These include patients with diabetes mellitus, renal disease, pancreatitis and those with premature cardiovascular disease. Physical findings suggesting vascular disorders, such as absence of peripheral pulses, arterial bruits or the finding of cutaneous xanthomata should lead to measurement of serum lipids. This screening procedure is especially important where there is a family history of hyperlipidaemia, diabetes or early onset of cardiovascular disease.

The most commonly employed screening test is the measurement of total cholesterol and triglyceride levels in a sample of venous blood taken, preferably without stasis, after an overnight (12 hour) fast. It should be noted that acute illness such as infection, trauma (including surgery) or myocardial infarction may alter serum lipoprotein concentrations. For example, for about three months after acute myocardial infarction, plasma triglycerides may be higher and total cholesterol lower than in the pre-infarction state. The upper limits of normality will vary between laboratories, and take into account both differing analytical methodology, and the population that is being assessed. Commonly, values above the 95th percentile for the age-adjusted population are termed abnormal. There is little sex difference in total cholesterol levels, but this is not so for triglyceride levels which are lower in females.

Plasma lipids also vary with age. Low levels are found in babies and levels rise sharply in childhood. Levels continue to rise until the age of 70–80 years [21] after which levels start to fall again. These changes should perhaps not be viewed as normal, but may reflect the increased incidence of obesity, and lack of exercise. Usually, normal ranges do not allow for these small differences which in a London population only varied by about 8% [22]. The values defining normal ranges employed at St Bartholomew's Hospital, London are shown in Table 12.2.

If abnormal values are discovered, our practice is to re-measure fasting samples on three occasions at weekly intervals, before a diagnosis of hyperlipidaemia is established.

If the total cholesterol is elevated, the HDL level should be obtained, because it is the HDL/LDL cholesterol ratio and not the total concentra-

Table 12.2

Lipid	
Total cholesterol	< 6.5 mmol/l
HDL cholesterol	> 1.0 mmol/l
LDL cholesterol	< 5.0 mmol/l
Triglycerides (men)	< 2.0 mmol/l
(women)	< 1.7 mmol/l

tions that are important. Low HDL levels and high LDL levels are associated with atherosclerotic disease [23], and the ratio of these two lipoprotein subfractions appears to be an important predictor of coronary heart disease [24].

12.4.2 FAMILY SCREENING

Many of the primary hyperlipidaemias are familial and lipoprotein abnormalities may be found in first degree relatives. Measurement of serum lipids should therefore always be offered to first degree relatives, particularly the younger males where early therapy will be of most value. This is especially important in monogenic familial hypercholesterolaemia, a dominantly inherited disorder which carriers a high risk of very early coronary death. Early diagnosis and therapy is the only hope of improving the prognosis.

12.4.3 EXERCISE

The advantages of regular exercise for the cardiovascular system are difficult to demonstrate but most physicians advise it. Exercise increases HDL levels and HDL/LDL ratios [25] and may decrease the incidence of atherosclerotic heart disease [26]. However, its role in the post-coronary patient is unknown, and certainly should not be embarked upon unless cardiac evaluation has been carried out.

12.4.4 DIET

Dietary modification must be the first line of treatment for all types of hyperlipidaemia, although the response will depend both on the underlying lipoprotein abnormality and its severity. Fat intake should be reduced to about one-third of total energy requirements, and the proportion of these ingested as polyunsaturated (as opposed to saturated) fats should be increased from the typical 25% found in Western diets to about

353

The management of the hyperlipidaemias

75% of the total fat intake. This action alone will reduce cholesterol levels and increase the HDL/LDL ratio, as well as making the fat-depleted diet more tolerable.

The calorific deficit can be replaced by unrefined, high-fibre carbohydrates, although replacement should not be complete in the overweight. This applies particularly to those patients with predominantly raised VLDL levels, as attainment of correct body weight will often be the only therapy required. Alcohol excess may produce hypertriglyceridaemia, but unfortunately 'excess' will vary from patient to patient, and abstention may sometimes be the only way of reducing VLDL triglyceride.

12.5   Drug therapy for hyperlipidaemia

Although the value of drug therapy in every type of hyperlipidaemia has not been assessed, evidence from the many trials carried out over the last few years suggests that it is reasonable to reduce raised plasma lipid levels, particularly cholesterol, by any measure which is effective and not obviously harmful. Assessing the benefits and risks must be made for each patient and constantly re-evaluated throughout the course of therapy. Trials off medication may be as important as the use of new drugs, particularly following weight loss or when other medication has been changed or discontinued.

Three classes of drug are commonly used:

(1) Drugs inhibiting lipid or lipoprotein synthesis (antilipogenic agents).

(2) Drugs inhibiting breakdown of stored lipid (antilipolytic agents).

(3) Bile acid sequestrants.

12.5.1   ANTILIPOGENIC AGENTS

These drugs may inhibit metabolic pathways involved in the hepatic synthesis of lipoproteins.

(a)   Clofibrate

Clofibrate (Atromid-S) and a number of recently introduced analogues such as bezafibrate (Bezalip) and fenofibrate are derivatives of *P*-chlorophenoxyisobutyric acid (CPIB) and all have qualitatively similar modes of action [27]. One of their actions is to stimulate hepatic and lipoprotein lipase. These enzymes are located on capillary endothelium and are responsible for initiating VLDL triglyceride hydrolysis resulting in the production of LDL. Hence, the CPIB derivatives are effective in hypertriglyceridaemic patients who will commonly show a 30% reduction in plasma triglyceride when treated with these agents. Unfortunately this may often be accompained by a rise in LDL, although if plasma triglyceride levels are normal, LDL levels often fall. This suggests that in addition to promoting LDL synthesis, these fibric acid derivatives may also accelerate LDL catabolism, possibly by activation of the high affinity LDL receptor pathway. The CPIB derivatives usually have no effect on plasma HDL.

Until the late 1970s, clofibrate was widely (and probably inappropriately) dispensed, until two large-scale trials seemed to indicate that clofibrate not only had little therapeutic benefit, but actually increased overall morbidity and mortality [28, 29]. The interpretation of these findings has probably been over emphasized and when appropriately used – as part of an integrated approach to hyperlipidaemia – there appear to be few problems. Clofibrate is mainly used in hypertriglyceridaemia, and is also of value for resolving cutaneous xanthomas and prevention of relapsing pancreatitis [30]. It is of particular use in Type III hyperlipidaemia, an uncommon primary lipaemia characterized by widespread xanthomata and early onset of coronary heart disease. After dietary intervention, clofibrate is very effective at lowering plasma lipids and clearing cutaneous lipid deposits.

The fibric acid derivatives are usually very well tolerated but gastrointestinal problems may occur. Anticoagulants may be displaced from albumin-binding sites increasing the prothrombin time. The biochemical response to the fibric acid derivatives is variable and it is not always possible to predict which patient will respond to therapy. The drug should not be continued in those who do not show a significant fall in plasma lipids. As yet there is no evidence that bezafibrate has any advantage over clofibrate, which is cheaper. Fenofibrate is at present undergoing trials in this country.

(b) Probucol

The chemical structure of this recently introduced agent is entirely different from other hypolipidaemic agents, and so presumably is its mode of action. It is thought to lower cholesterol both by inhibiting its synthesis and by blocking its absorption. Only about 10% is absorbed orally, although this may be aided by simultaneous ingestion of fat. Probucol lowers plasma cholesterol by about 20% without affecting triglyceride levels [31] and so is mainly used as an adjunct to bile acid sequestrants (q.v.) in hypercholesterolaemia. However, both LDL and HDL fall during treatment and the effect on the latter appears to be greater. Whilst the significance of this in relation to ischaemic heart disease is not clear, it may be disadvantageous. Animal studies have shown that disturbances of cardiac rhythm (including ventricular tachycardia and fibrillation), associated with QT prolongation in the electrocardiogram, may occur with prubucol, but QT changes are slight in man at the usual doses, and there is no record of any problem.

12.5.2 ANTILIPOLYTIC AGENTS

These drugs reduce the release of free fatty acids from adipose tissue and consequently reduce substrate for hepatic synthesis of trigylceride. Occasionally there may be additional actions leading to a fall in plasma lipids which cannot be explained by their antilipolytic effect alone.

(a) Nicotinic acid

Nicotinic acid reduces plasma levels of both trigylceride and cholesterol. Its primary action is on the flux of free fatty acids to the liver, generated by triglyceride hydrolysis of adipose tissue. Nicotinic acid suppresses the responsible enzyme – hormone sensitive lipase – and reduces the plasma levels of free fatty acids below that requred for hepatic VLDL synthesis and secretion. Hence triglyceride levels fall, often sharply, and in proportion to the height of pretreatment levels. In severe hypertriglyceridaemia this may be as much as 90%, although about a 40% reduction is more often seen. There is a secondary reduction in LDL synthesis (VLDL being its precursor) and plasma cholesterol falls by about 15%. Since HDL and VLDL have common structural components (such as apoproteins and phospholipids), their concentrations in the plasma are often reciprocal. Hence as VLDL levels fall there is often a beneficial rise in HDL concentrations, particularly the HDL2 subfraction [32]. However, use of nicotinic acid in men with coronary heart disease in the Coronary Drug Project [28] did not reduce the overall mortality rate. The decrease in the number of non-fatal myocardial infarctions was offset by an increase in fatal cardiac arrhythmias, suggesting caution when prescribing for patients with a history of rhythm disturbance. Nicotinic acid is particularly useful as a second line agent to lower cholesterol in patients who do not respond to bile acid sequestrants alone [33] and this combination is often used in patients with familial hypercholesterolaemia. The drug has a vasodilator action and may thus exaggerate the effect of other peripheral vasodilators. A fall in blood pressure may accentuate myocardial ischaemia and could account for the provocation of arrhythmias suggested above. The most common side effects are cutaneous flushing and pruritis, although both usually decline in intensity after the first few weeks of therapy. If there are still problems, then a slow release form (Bradilan) may be tried, although this drug sometimes affects liver function. Gastrointestinal problems can occur and glucose intolerance or hyperuricaemia may be precipitated occasionally, resulting in clinical diabetes and gout.

(b) Acipimox

This is a new lipid-lowering agent whose structure is similar to nicotinic acid but seems to be better tolerated. It inhibits lipolysis and additionally stimulates lipoprotein lipase leading primarily to a reduction in plasma triglyceride. It is at present undergoing clinical trials in this country.

(c) Insulin

In addition to its hypoglycaemic action insulin will lower circulating plasma free fatty acids by its direct antilipolytic action upon adipose tissue and stimulation of fatty acid re-esterification. The net effect is a fall in free fatty acids with a consequent reduction in hepatic VLDL triglyceride synthesis. Additionally, insulin may also lower triglyceride levels by inducing lipoprotein lipase. This enzyme is situated in the capillary bed of many tissues (heart, skeletal muscle, adipose tissue) and is responsible for the initial breakdown of VLDL triglyceride to fatty acids. Many patients with severe hypertriglyceridaemia also have mild glucose intolerance and in these subjects insulin may be required to treat both sugar and lipid disturbances which can occasionally be resistant to other forms of therapy.

12.5.3 BILE ACID SEQUESTRANTS

Bile acid sequestrants (anion-exchange resins), such as cholestyramine (Questran) and colestipol (Colestid) act by binding to bile acids in the gut lumen and interrupting their enterohepatic circulation. This alters the activity of several key hepatic enzymes whose function is normally regulated by these bile acids returning to the liver in the portal blood. The rate-limiting enzyme in bile acid synthesis is activated and initiates the conversion of cholesterol into bile acids, thus increasing the efflux from the hepatic cholesterol pool. Two compensatory mechanisms counteract this decline. First, endogenous cholesterol synthesis in the liver increases and secondly, LDL cholesterol assimilation by the liver is promoted via the high affinity LDL receptor pathway on hepatocyte membranes. Bile acids also affect the rate-limiting step in trigylceride synthesis and interruption of the enterohepatic circulation of bile acids stimulates hepatic VLDL-triglyceride synthesis and secretion [34]. As a result levels of LDL fall by about 25%, and VLDL levels rise often dramatically in patients with pre-existing hypertriglyceridaemia [35–37]. There is no change in total plasma HDL concentrations, although the HDL2 subfraction increases, probably as result of increased HDL protein synthesis by the gut.

The management of the hyperlipidaemias

Bile acid sequestrants are thus very effective in type II hyperlipidaemia, but are of little value in hypertriglyceridaemia. Initially, small doses (one sachet) of the powder are taken before meals mixed with water. These instructions are important because ingestion of dry resin may cause intestinal obstruction, and absorption of cholesterol is decreased only if taken before the meal. The daily dose is gradually increased up to a maximum of 9 sachets in divided doses as required. Constipation is frequent and other gastrointestinal side effects such as nausea, vomiting or unpleasant tastes may occur. As a result of bile acid sequestration, there may be malabsorption of many substances which depend upon bile acids for absorption, particularly lipophilic agents. These include fat-soluble vitamins, folate and iron, so that dietary supplements may be required. The absorption of many drugs, including digoxin, thiazide diuretics and thyroxine may be similarly affected. It is therefore advisable to take these medications at least one hour before the resins.

12.5.4 A SUMMARY OF THERAPY IN RELATION TO LIPID TYPES

Dietary modification is the first line of therapy for all patients. Then:

(1) Patients with Type IIa/IIb hyperlipidaemia (primarily hyper-cholesterolaemia). Therapy should be started with bile sequestrant resins. Response is variable and total cholesterol levels may fall by up to 20%. If after several months levels are still elevated, nicotinic acid may be added and will produce an additive effect as well as raising plasma HDL-LDL ratios. If control is still not obtained, compliance to diet, exercise and drugs should be checked. A third-line drug (e.g. Probucol) may then be considered or possible surgical intervention (q.v.).

(2) Patients with types III, IV and V hyperlipidaemia (primarily hyper-triglyceridaemia). Clofibrate or other fibric acid derivatives are the first choice in hypertriglyceridaemia. Nicotinic acid may be added after a few months if an adequate response is not obtained.

Once long-term control has been achieved using either of the above approaches, therapy may be reduced or simplified, by withdrawing the last-added drug first. Constant follow-up is always needed to check compliance, and to reassess therapeutic requirements.

12.6 Non-drug therapy

12.6.1 ILEAL BY-PASS

Surgical by-pass of the distal third of the small intestine attempts to reduce the intestinal surface available for resorption of bile acids and provides an interruption in the enterohepatic circulation [38]. Its metabolic effects are similar to those seen during cholestyramine therapy and plasma cholesterol falls by about 35%. The main complication of this procedure is watery and often severe diarrhoea caused by increased amounts of bile salts reaching the colon [39]. The concurrent use of bile acid sequestrants may reduce the concentration of free bile acids and relieve this problem. Vitamin B12 supplements are always required and it is also advisable to give small doses of calcium and vitamin D.

12.6.2 PLASMAPHERESIS

This has been used to reduce very high serum cholesterol levels in type II hyperlipidaemia [40]. Blood is withdrawn into a continuous blood flow separator, where the cells are separated from the cholesterol-rich plasma. This is then replaced with plasma protein fraction which is combined with the cells and returned to the patient as lipid-depleted whole blood. Cholesterol levels have been controlled in some type II patients by plasmapheresis sessions at three-weekly intervals, without the need for any other therapy [41].

12.7 Other drugs which affect lipoprotein levels

There are many drugs which influence lipid metabolism. Some of the commoner ones are as follows.

12.7.1 BETA-ADRENERGIC BLOCKING AGENTS

In general beta-blockers increase plasma triglycerides and reduce HDL cholesterol [42]. Both of these effects are probably due to impaired catabolism of trigylceride-rich lipoproteins. Patients with pre-existing hypertriglyceridaemia are most at risk and acute pancreatitis may be provoked. The appearance of cutaneous xanthomata, or episodic abdominal pain after starting beta-blocker therapy should lead to examination of serum for turbidity, particularly in diabetics, where secondary hypertriglyceridaemia is common.

12.7.2 OTHER ANTIHYPERTENSIVE AGENTS

Methyldopa (Aldomet) has been reported to lower HDL levels without affecting either LDL cholesterol or trigylceride levels. Prazosin (Hypovase) lowers serum triglycerides and LDL cholesterol, whilst having no effect (or producing a small increase) in HDL levels [42].

12.7.3 DIURETIC THERAPY

Thiazide diuretics increase serum triglycerides and LDL without affecting HDL levels [43]. These effects are occasionally worsened (if not caused) by the associated deterioration in glucose tolerance. Similar problems have been reported in association with the loop diuretics (e.g. frusemide), but not with spironolactone.

12.7.4 STEROIDS

Glucocorticoids increase both plasma LDL and triglycerides, and again this may be partly due to their diabetogenic action. Although oestrogens alone may increase both triglycerides and HDL cholesterol, their effect in oral contraceptives, in which they are generally formulated with a progestogen, is more variable. Progestogens tend to lower HDL levels and so will counteract the oestrogen rise depending on the particular agents involved. Hence care must be taken when prescribing for hyperlipidaemic patients, particularly those with co-existing glucose intolerance.

12.8 Conclusions

Hyperlipidaemia is a major risk factor for cardiovascular disease, and if raised blood lipids are found, the hyperlipidaemia must first be confirmed by serial assays, and then fully evaluated. A secondary hyperlipidaemia must always be considered so that underlying disorders, such as diabetes, obesity, hypothyroidism and alcohol excesses may be detected and treated. Patients with primary hyperlipidaemia should initially be treated with dietary modification and exercise, probably for a trial period of 3 months [44]. Patients whose lipids are still significantly elevated at this time should receive additional (drug) therapy. It must be emphasized that this is additional and not alternative therapy, and that the success of any treatment programme is dependent on continued adherence to proper diet and weight control. Of great importance is the simultaneous correction of other known atheromatous risk factors, particularly smoking, hypertension and glucose intolerance. The resort to hypolipidaemic therapy in non-compliant patients is futile, expensive and potentially dangerous. Since no currently available hypolipidaemic agent will correct the underlying metabolic abnormality, long-term therapy is necessary and consideration of drug efficacy, patient compliance, long-term safety and drug cost is essential.

References

1. Carlson, L.A. and Linstedt, S. (1969) The Stockholm Prospective Study. The initial values for plasma lipids. *Acta Med. Scand.*, Suppl., 493.
2. Kannel, W.B., Castelli, W.P., Gordon, T. *et al.* (1971) Serum cholesterol, lipoproteins and the risk of coronary heart disease. *Ann. Intern. Med.*, **74**, 1.
3. Fuller, J.H., Pinney, S., Jarrett, R.J. *et al.* (1978) Plasma lipids in a London population and their relation to other risk factors for coronary heart disease. *Br. Heart J.*, **40**, 170.
4. Marks, H.H., Krall, L.P. and White, P. (1971) Epidemiology and detection of diabetes mellitus. In *Joslin's Diabetes Mellitus* (ed. Marble, White, Bradley and Krall), Lea and Febiger, Philadelphia.
5. Walker, W.J. (1976) Success story: the Program against major cardiovascular risk factors. *Geriatrics*, **31**, 97.
6. Walker, A.R.P. (1978) Diet and coronary heart disease. *S. Afr. Med. J.*, **53**, 587.
7. Mann, G.V. *et al.* (1978) Diet-heart era: premature obituary? *N. Engl. J. Med.*, **298**, 106–8.
8. Ahrens, E.H. (1979) Dietary fats and coronary heart disease: unfinished business. *Lancet*, **ii**, 1345.
9. The Lipid Research Clinics coronary primary prevention trial results (1984) *J. Am. Med. Assoc.*, **251**, 351.
10. Dayton, S., Pearce, M.L., Hashimoto, S. *et al.* (1969) A controlled trial of a diet high in unsaturated fat in preventing complications of atherosclerosis. *Circulation*, **40**, (Suppl. 2), 1.
11. Hjermann, I., Byre, K.V., Holme, I. *et al.* (1981) Effect of diet and smoking intervention on the incidence of coronary heart disease. Report from the Oslo study group of a randomised trial in healthy men. *Lancet*, **ii**, 1303.
12. WHO Clofibrate Trial Committee of Principal Investigators (1978) A cooperative trial in the primary prevention of ischaemic heart disease using clofibrate. *Br. Heart J.*, **40**, 1069.
13. Carlson, L.A. and Bottiger, L.E. (1972) Ischaemic heart disease in relation to fasting values of plasma triglycerides and cholesterol: Stockholm Prospective Study. *Lancet*, **i**, 865.
14. Carlson, L.A., Bottiger, L.E. and Ahfeldt, P.E. (1979) Risk factors for myocardial infarction in the Stockholm Prospective Study: A 14 year follow-up focussing on the role of plasma triglycerides and cholesterol. *Acta Med. Scand.*, **206**, 351.
15. Hulley, S.B., Rosenman, R.H., Bawol, R.D. *et al.* (1980) Epidemiology as a guide to clinical decisions: The association between triglyceride and coronary heart disease. *N. Engl. J. Med.*, **382**, 1383.
16. Chivers, A.G., Lea Thomas, M. and Browse, N.L. (1974) The Progression of arteriosclerosis. A radiological study. *Circulation*, **50**, 402.
17. Gensini, G.G., Esente, P. and Kelly, A. (1974) Natural history of coronary disease in patients with and without coronary bypass graft surgery. *Circulation*, **50**, 98.
18. Duffield, R.G.M., Lewis, B., Miller, N.E. *et al.* (1983) Treatment of hyperlipidaemia retards progression of symptomatic femoral atherosclerosis. *Lancet*, **ii**, 639.

19. Galton, D.J., Stocks, J. and Dodson, P.M. (1982) Lipoproteins – their role in enzyme regulation. In *Clinical Biochemistry Review*, Vol. 3. (ed. D.M. Golberg) Wiley, New York.
20. Beaumont, J.L., Carlson, L.A., Coooper, G.R. *et al.* (1970) Classification of hyperlipidaemias and hyperlipoproteinaemias. *Bull. Wld. Hlth, Org.*, **43**, 891.
21. Fredrickson, D.S., Goldstein, J.L. and Brown, M.S. (1983) in *The Metabolic Basis of Inherited Disease*, 5th edn, (eds J.B. Stanbury, J.B. Wyngaarden, & D.S. Fredrickson). McGraw-Hill, New York.
22. Lewis, B., Chait, A., Wootton, I.D.P. *et al.* (1974) Frequency of risk factors in a healthy British population. *Lancet*, i, 141.
23. Tall, A.R. and Small, D.M. (1978) Current concepts. Plasma high density lipoproteins. *N. Engl. J. Med.*, **299**, 1232.
24. Gordon, T. (1980) HDL and coronary heart disease (letter). *Lancet*, ii, 1139.
25. Durstine, J.L., Miller, W., Farrell, W.M. and Ivy, J.L. (1983) Increases in HDL-cholesterol and the HDL/LDL cholesterol ratio during prolonged endurance exercise. *Metabolism*, **32**, 10.
26. Morris, J.N., Everitt, M.G. and Pollard, R. (1980) Vigorous exercise in leisure-time: Protection against coronary heart disease. *Lancet*, ii, 1207.
27. Schlierf, G., Chwat, M., Feverborn, *et al.* (1980) Bezafibrate and clofibrate in hyperlipidaemia. *Atherosclerosis*, **36**, 323.
28. Coronary Project Group (1975) Clofibrate and niacin in coronary heart disease. *J. Am. Med. Assoc.*, **231**, 360.
29. Committee of Principal Investigators (1980) WHO cooperative trial on the prevention of ischaemic heart disease using clofibrate to lower serum cholesterol. Mortality follow-up. *Lancet*, **11**, 379.
30. Keen, H., Lewis, B., Miller, N.E. *et al.* (1980) Clofibrate and hyperlipidaemia. *Lancet*, ii, 1241.
31. Lelorier, J., Dubrenil-Quidoz, S., Lussier-Cacan, S. *et al.* (1977) Diet and probucol in lowering cholesterol concentrations. *Arch. Intern. Med.*, **137**, 1429.
32. Shepherd, J., Packard, C.J., Patsch, J.R. *et al.* (1979) Effects of nicotinic acid therapy on plasma high density lipoprotein subfraction distribution and composition and apoprotein A metabolism. *J. Clin. Invest.*, **63**, 858.
33. Kane, J.P., Malloy, M.J., Tun, P. *et al.* (1981) Normalization of low-density-lipoprotein levels in heterozygous familial hypercholesterolaemia with a combined drug regimen. *N. Engl. J. Med.*, **304**, 251.
34. Witztum, J.L., Schonfield, D. and Weldman, S.W. (1976) The effect of colestipol on the metabolism of very low density lipoproteins in man. *J. Lab. Clin. Med.*, **88**, 108.
35. Hashim, S.A. and Van Italie, T.B. (1965) Cholestyramine resin therapy for hypercholesterolaemia. *J. Am. Med. Assoc.*, **192**, 289.
36. Levy, R.L., Fredrickson, D.S., Kwiterovich, P.O. *et al.* (1969) Normalisation of lipids in familial hypercholesterolaemia. *Circulation*, **40**, (Suppl.3), 15.
37. Glueck, C.J., Ford, S. Scheel, D, *et al.* (1972) Colestipol and cholestyramine resin. *J. Am. Med. Assoc.*, **222**, 676.
38. Buchwald, H., Moore, R.B. and Varco, R.L. (1981) in *Atherosclerosis V* (eds A.M. Gotto *et al.*), Springer-Verlag, Berlin, pp. 462–5.
39. Chalstrey, L.J., Winder, A.F. and Galton, D.J. (1982) Partial ileal bypass in the treatment of familial hypercholesterolaemia. *J. Roy. Soc Med.*, **75**, 851–6.
40. Thompson, G.R., Lowenthal, R. and Myant, N.B. (1975) Plasma exchange in

the management of homozygous familial hypercholesterolaemia. *Lancet*, **i,** 1208.

41. Brook, G., Winterstein, G. and Aviram, M. (1983) Platelet function and lipoprotein levels after plasma-exchange in patients with familial hyper-cholesterolaemia. *Clin. Sci.*, **64,** 637.

42. Lerne, P., Foss, P.O., Helgeland, A. *et al.* (1980) Effect of propranolol and Prazosin on blood lipids. The Oslo Study. *Lancet*, **ii,** 4.

43. Grimm, R.H., Leon, A.S., Hunninghake, D.B. *et al.* (1965) Effects of thiazide diuretics on plasma lipids and lipoproteins in mildly hypertensive patients. A double-blind controlled trial. *Ann. Intern. Med.*, **94,** 7.

44. Samuel, P. (1980) Drug treatment of hyperlipidaemia. *Am. Heart J.*, **100,** 573.

13 Techniques for the blood level measurement of cardiac drugs and their application

A. JOHNSTON

13.1 Introduction

It is indisputable that the ability to measure accurately the concentrations of cardiac drugs in biological fluids has greatly improved their use in clinical practice. The need for drug level measurements in research is obvious. Measurement of drug bioavailability, drug pharmacokinetics, effects of disease, patient age, drug interactions etc. have to be investigated to define dosage regimes of new drugs. However it does not follow that the measurement of cardiac drug levels in individuals will enhance patient treatment.

The majority of drugs are first prescribed to a patient at an 'average' dose. If this dose does not produce the desired therapeutic action or results in adverse side effects then the regimen is adjusted. In certain diseases, e.g. hypertension, the clinician has a well-defined goal and can measure the effectiveness of the drug treatment easily and adjust drug dosage accordingly. In these diseases a patient's drug regimen can be tailored to the individual's need by the physician's clinical measurement, and any drug level measurement is a waste of resources and may confuse or conflict with an otherwise straightforward clinical judgement.

If there is a direct relationship between the serum concentration and the therapeutic or toxic action of a drug then there are several indications for the estimation of blood levels of cardiac drugs in routine clinical practice:

(1) To check patient compliance. The incidence of patients failing to take a prescribed course of treatment is high. The reasons for this non-compliance are many, e.g. occurrence of side effects, fear of addiction, complicated dosage regimen, or conflicting medical direction, and patients are often unwilling to admit they are not taking their medication.

(2) To ensure serum drug levels are sufficently high to prevent an event for which the drug is being given prophylactically. There can be

great difficulty in the clinical assessment of the efficacy of preventive treatment and the first indication of a treatment's failure, e.g. the occurrence of ventricular fibrillation, may result in the patient's demise.

(3) To distinguish situations where similar clinical symptoms are caused by the patient's disease or drug toxicity. The toxic effects of overdosage with some drugs may be subtle and their development can mimic underlying disease, e.g. high levels of cardiac glycosides will cause progressive heart failure due to their depressant action on the myocardium and this can be wrongly attributed to the patient's heart disease worsening.

(4)To optimize drug dosage in those patients with known alterations in pharmacokinetics. Many cardiac patients have gross alterations in haemodynamics and the resulting changes in hepatic blood flow and renal function can cause unpredictable changes in drug handling, e.g. the elimination half-life of lignocaine in a group of cardiac patients has been shown to vary between < 2 and > 24 hours [1].

The abnormalities and variabilities in the pharmacokinetics of cardiac drugs in the very young and the very old makes correct drug dosage in these patients difficult to achieve. Neonates for example have been shown to require disproportionatley higher doses of the antiarrhythmic drugs disopyramide and mexiletine than do adults [2] and the variability in the half-life of lignocaine is up to 4 times greater in the elderly compared to young adults [1].

In patients whose changing pathology causes unpredicable variations in drug levels, e.g. renal failure which alters the elimination of disopyramide [3], measurements of serum drug concentrations will aid correct dose prescribing.

(5) To investigate idiosyncratic patient responses. Occasionally patients may have adverse reactions or an exaggerated therapeutic response to a low dose of drug. This may be due to a drug interaction, e.g. cimetidine increases the serum levels of propranolol [4], or the patient may have a genetically slow metabolism as can occur with poor metabolisers of debrisoquine (only about 8% of the population) or with slow acetylators. Where a drug showing such polymorphism must be used and there is no reliable clinical measure of effectiveness then there is little choice but to monitor serum drug levels [5].

Conversely patients may fail to respond or respond poorly to seemingly high doses of drug. If non-compliance can be ruled out then another reason may be increased drug elimination due to enzyme induction. This can be caused by long-term treatment with other drugs, e.g. anticonvulsants, or may be the result of a short course of antibiotics, e.g. rifampacin [6].

13.2 Measurement of cardiac drugs

The techniques used to measure cardiac drug concentrations can be arbitrarily divided into physical and immunological methods. Research laboratories tend to place a heavy emphasis on physical methods as it is unusual for immunological methods to be set up at an early stage of drug development. Laboratories which deal with a large number of routine clinical measurements of cardiac drugs will rely on immunological methods. The physical techniques of drug analysis are flexible but very capital and labour intensive and depend very much on the skill of the operator to achieve best results. Immunological techniques require only modest operator skills and can process large numbers of samples in a short time but are inflexible and can have very high reagent costs.

It is impossible in a chapter of this size to give detailed descriptions of every available method of drug analysis and a critique of strengths and weaknesses of each. Instead this section contains a brief outline of the methods in common usage to give the reader a feel for the subject.

13.3 Physical methods

13.3.1 THE INITIAL SEPARATION STEP

The separation step is often the most crucial part of any drug assay. It is of little use having an analytical method which is sensitive to minute amounts of pure drug but which cannot measure the drug against a background of other compounds. The separation step fulfils two important purposes; removal of drug from the potentially interfering matrix and, usually, concentration of the drug.

The commonly used separation methods used are outlined below.

(a)   Direct use of sample

If the assay method used is not affected by other compounds present then the sample can be used directly without any cleanup.

(b)   Protein precipitation

This is the most straightforward way of separating the drug from extraneous material. The serum sample is treated with some agent which denatures the protein, for example trichloroacetic acid, centrifuged and the supernatant used directly. This method has the advantage of speed and minimal sample manipulation, but does not remove low-molecular-weight compounds or concentrate the drug.

(c) Filtration

Interfering compounds of high molecular weight (usually > 1000) can be removed by ultrafiltration of the sample through a semipermeable membrane. The same effect can be achieved by dialysis. However, it should be noted that protein-bound drug will not pass across the membrane.

(d) Solvent extraction

Here the physicochemical properties of the drug of interest are exploited to remove the drug from the biological matrix. The pH of the serum is altered so that the drug becomes unionized, for basic drugs the pH is increased, for acidic drugs decreased. A suitable organic solvent is then added and the mixture shaken to hasten equilibrium. The unionized drug partitions preferentially into the solvent phase, leaving the interfering compounds in the aqueous phase. The drug can then be concentrated by evaporating the organic layer to small volume or dryness.

Unfortunately not all the biological material is left in the discarded aqueous phase since some, in particular the lipids, will also partition into the solvent layer. If this is a problem the drug can be back-extracted and further purified. This involves removal of the drug from the organic solvent by extracting it back into fresh aqueous phase at a pH opposite to that of the first extraction, e.g. basic pH for acidic drugs. The lipid contaminants are left in the organic phase and the aqueous phase can then be used directly or can be re-extracted with solvent after once again reversing the pH.

(e) Column extraction

The sample material containing the drug is poured through a small column of adsorbent material, the drug of interest is retained on the column and the interfering compounds are lost in the eluant. The drug can then be removed by washing the column with solvent. This eluant can then either be used directly or evaporated to small volume. Selectivity can be obtained by altering either the absorbent material and/or the eluting solvents.

13.3.2 SPECTROPHOMETRIC METHODS

(a) Spectrophotometry

The amount of light absorbed by a solution containing the drug can be measured using a spectrophotometer. Drugs absorb ultra violet, visible and infra red light but in practice it is the UV and visible end of the spectrum that is used to quantitate cardiac drugs in biological fluids. This is because the solvents used to dissolve the drugs absorb infra red light very strongly and mask the weaker absorbance of the drugs. Many cardiac drugs contain chromophores, parts of their chemical structure that absorb light, and can be measured by spectrophotometry. However the majority of other drugs and biochemicals also contain chromophores (e.g. Clarke [7, 8] lists over 150 drug substances which have absorbance maxima in the range 250–260 nm). Spectrophometry is therefore very non-specific and requires an efficient separation step or chemical derivatization to achieve satisfactory results.

The chemical reaction of the drug to form a coloured derivative which can then be measured, colorimetry, not only increases the specificity of spectrophotometric methods but usually results in a large increase in sensitivity. Practolol, for example, has a relatively weak absorbance but following derivatization can be quantitated at the levels found in biological fluids [9].

(b) Spectrofluorimetry

Some compounds having absorbed light of one wavelength then emit light of another wavelength, i.e. they fluoresce. The wavelength of the incident light is known as the excitation wavelength, and that of the emitted light the emission wavelength. The former wavelength is always greater than the latter since energy is lost during the process.

The specificity of spectrofluorimetry is much greater than spectrophotometry, as only a small proportion (about 2%) of molecules fluoresce naturally, and a drug can be characterized by both excitation and emission wavelengths. Moreover the sensitivity of fluorescence methods is usually greater, e.g. propranolol can be measured down to 10 μg/l in serum after solvent extraction and back-extraction into hydrochloric acid [10]. Compounds which do not show native fluorescence may be chemically modified to produce fluorescent species. This is usually achieved by reacting the drug with a fluorophore, e.g. the beta-adrenoreceptor antagonist pindolol can be measured in serum following reaction with *o*-phthaldaldehyde [11].

Although, in general, fluorimetric assays are more specific than spectrophotometric assays, it should be realized that as with spectrophotometry, metabolites which are present in the assay solutions are likely to contribute to the results of both methods.

13.3.3 CHROMATOGRAPHY

Following the initial separation step spectrophotometry and spectrofluorimetry are rarely sensitive or specific enough to measure cardiac drugs directly. It is therefore necessary to use these techniques in conjunction with other methods which will perform a more rigorous separation of the drug or drugs of interest and will concentrate them to enhance sensitivity. This further separation is usually brought about using chromatography.

Chromatography was first used at the beginning of the twentieth century by the Russian chemist, Tswett, who described the separation of coloured pigments in a chalk column. The general principle of all chromatographic methods is similar. The compounds of interest are separated from each other by differential partitioning between a mobile phase and a stationary phase. The degree of separation can be altered by changing either the mobile phase composition or the nature of the stationary phase.

(a) Thin-layer chromatography (TLC)

An absorbant material, usually silica gel, is evenly coated onto an inert backing plate as a thin layer. This is the stationary phase. The mobile phase is a solvent which is allowed to rise up the plate by means of capillary action. The drug-containing solution is applied near the bottom of the plate and is drawn upwards with the mobile phase. The components of the mixture move at different speeds up the plate and are separated as discrete spots or bands. These can then be visualized by examining the plate under UV light, spraying with a reagent which reacts with the compounds to produce colours or by scanning the plate for radioactivity if labelled drug was used.

Although TLC can be used to measure cardiac drugs quantitatively in plasma, e.g. measurement of disopyramide [12], its main use is in qualitative drug analysis. It is particularly useful in the early stages of drug development for the separation of radio labelled metabolites for further analysis.

(b) High performance liquid chromatography (HPLC)

Early liquid chromatography was used to purify bulk material and required wide, long columns, kilograms of stationary phase and gram quantities of sample. High performance (or pressure) liquid chromatography developed from this, but because of the very small particle size ($< 10\mu m$) of the stationary phase used, the columns could perform very efficient separations on small samples. However very high pressures, between 30 and 400 bar, are needed to pump the mobile phase through the columns. As with TLC, the stationary phase is usually silica or modified silica and the mobile phase aqueous or non-aqueous solvent.

The sample or extract containing the drug is introduced into the solvent flow and thence onto the analytical column by means of a loop injector valve, which ensures uninterrupted solvent flow. The effluent from the column is passed through a suitable detector, for cardiac drugs the most commonly used are spectrophotometric or spectrofluorimetric detectors, and quantitated.

HPLC is without doubt the most versatile method of drug analysis available today,and methods exist for the measurement of the majority of cardiac drugs in plasma, with the exception of the cardiac glycosides.

(c) Gas–liquid chromatography

In gas–liquid chromatography (GLC or GC) the mobile phase is gaseous and referred to as carrier gas, the stationary phase is wax or gum coated onto a powder of inert support material. At the temperatures used for GLC, 100–350°C, the stationary phase can be considered as a liquid, hence gas–liquid chromatography. The separation of drugs occurs in the vapour phase. The drugs are introduced into the stream of carrier gas flowing through a column packed with support coated with the stationary phase, and the column effluent is fed to a detector. In recent years the use of capillary columns for GLC has been increasing. These are very long (> 10m) small-bore columns (< 0.5mm) with the stationary phase coated directly onto the inside of the tubing and they offer a spectacular degree of specificity.

In the most commonly encountered detector, flame ionization (FID), the effluent is mixed with hydrogen and air and burnt. The combustion products of drugs present in the flame cause measurable changes in potential between the flame jet and an electrode. The specificity of this form of detector can be increased by addition of halide salts to the flame. This selectivity enhances the detector sensitivity to nitrogen and phosphorus (referred to variously as: NPD, nitrogen phosphorus detector; AFID, alkali flame ionization detector; TSD, thermionic selective detector). Drugs which contain groups with a high affinity for electrons can be detected using an electron capture detector (ECD); here the effluent is passed through a stream of beta particles and again drugs passing through the beam cause measurable changes in potential. Drugs which do not contain electron capturing groups can be chemically derivatized to add or enhance their electron affinity.

GLC is as specific and as sensitive as HPLC for measuring cardiovascular drugs in plasma, but the range of compounds that can be measured is limited to those which are volatile, or can be made volatile, are not heat labile and, since retention time is to a large extent proportional to molecular weight, have a molecular weight lower than about 500 daltons.

(d) Mass spectrometry

In a mass spectrometer molecules are broken into fragments by fast-moving electrons. The positively charged fragments are then accelerated through a magnetic field towards a negatively charged target and their separation can be very accurately related to their mass and charge. The specificity of mass spectrometry is unrivalled since the fragmentation pattern produced is unique to the each compound. The spectrometer can be selectively tuned for specific mass fragments by adjusting the electrode voltage and the strength of the magnetic field. Mass spectrometry is not in itself a chromatographic technique but is usually used as a sophisticated detection system in conjunction with gas chromatography (GCMS) and more recently HPLC. Mass spectrometers alone and in combination with other techniques have been much used for the identification of drug metabolites as the fragmentation pattern or mass spectrum produced can be used to elucidate the structural changes from the parent compounds.

Used in conjunction with stable isotopes, commonly carbon-13 or deuterium, mass spectrometry allows a variety of sophisticated measurements of labelled cardiac drugs without the inherent toxicity of radiopharmaceuticals. For example oral drug bioavailability can be measured in one experiment by giving isotopically labelled drug by intravenous administration and the unlabelled drug by mouth, because the blood levels of each form can be followed independently.

A mass spectrometer is very expensive to buy, maintain and run and requires a specialist operating staff, consequently mass spectrometers tend to be in centralized, shared facilities and mainly devoted to research. However modified mass spectrometers called selective ion detectors are now marketed specifically for use with gas chromatographs. This has reduced their cost and complexity and although these detectors are not able to scan the whole spectrum they can selectively measure about six masses at any one time which is sufficient for drug measurements.

13.3.4 RADIOACTIVE ISOTOPES

Drugs can be synthesized incorporating radioactive forms of their constituent atoms; this usually is done by substituting carbon-14 or tritium for 'cold' carbon or hydrogen. If these radiolabelled drugs are administered their concentration can be easily measured in biological fluids by quantifying the amount of radioactivity present using scintillation counting. This is straightforward and can be measured directly, provided there is no metabolism of the compound concerned. If metabolism has occurred then the measured radioactivity may be a mixture of the parent drug and metabolites and a separation step, e.g. TLC, will have to be incorporated.

Radiolabelled drugs are used at an early stage in drug development because of the ease with which radioactive compounds can be detected and quantitated. This method of drug analysis is used both in animal and human studies, in conjunction with other methods, to work out the metabolic fate of new compounds.

13.4 Immunoassays

Since the first edition of this book in 1979 there has been a large increase in the number and type of immunoassays available for cardiac drugs. Most immunoassays rely on the competitive binding to antibody of the drug and a suitably labelled form of the drug. The antibodies are usually raised against the drug by conjugating the compound with protein and injecting the conjugate into an animal, which then responds by producing antibodies specific to the drug moiety. When the drug-containing solution is mixed with antibody and labelled drug then both the drug and the labelled species compete for binding sites on the antibody. The degree of binding of each is dependent on the other. Therefore if the concentration of labelled drug remains constant then its binding can be related to the concentration of unlabelled drug, i.e. as unlabelled drug concentration rises the proportion of labelled drug bound falls. If the free and bound drug can be separated and/or the amount of bound labelled drug quantitated, then the concentration of drug in solution can be calculated. It is the various strategies employed to separate and measure the bound and free drug that distinguish the various methods of immunoassay.

There are three major disadvantages with immunoassay techniques; specificity, precision and cost. The specificity of the assay is dependent on the specificity of the antibody for the drug. Often the antibody will bind not only the drug but also structurally similar compounds or metabolites and this can produce misleading results. Occasionally antibodies are too specific and bind only one isomeric form of a drug and since most drugs are administered as racemic mixtures this will produce biased results. The precision of immunoassays is governed by the antibody dilution used. In most cases the calibration is optimized to produce good precision over a selected range, e.g. the therapeutic window of a drug, and concentrations outside this range will be measured with less precision. The cost of developing a new immunoassay for a drug is very high, consequently assays are often developed by firms specializing in the production of diagnostic reagents and the immunoassay is sold in kit form. This tends to make analysis by immunoassay expensive. However the high cost per sample should be balanced against the staff savings that can be made due to the high capacity of this type of assay.

13.4.1 RADIO-IMMUNOASSAY (RIA)

In radio-immunoassay the sample containing drug is incubated with radiolabelled drug and drug antibodies. After a period of equilibration the free and bound drug are separated, e.g. by adsorption of the free drug onto charcoal, and the amount of labelled drug bound is then estimated by scintillation or gamma counting. The amount of labelled drug bound is inversely proportional to the concentration of drug in the sample.

The separation step in RIA is often the most difficult to perform and tends to be error prone. The classical separations involve either adsorption of the free drug onto charcoal or precipitation of the bound drug using polyethyleneglycol (PEG) followed by centrifugation to sediment the solid material before decanting the liquid phase. More recent methods have utilized a second antibody to bind the first. The second antibody can be precoated onto tubes, plastic beads or magnetic particles which hold the bound drug while the free drug is decanted. Because of the separation step ratio-immunoassay is referred to as a heterogeneous assay.

RIA using ^{125}I has until recently been the method of choice for the measurement of cardiac glycosides. However the inherent drawbacks of radioactive labels, short shelf-life, designated laboratories and areas for handling radioactive material, decontamination and waste disposal, staff health monitoring etc., has resulted in a shift towards newer, non-radioactive, methods of immunoassay.

13.4.2 HETEROGENEOUS ENZYME-IMMUNOASSAY

In this assay system, antigen from the sample, i.e. drug, is incubated with drug tagged with an enzyme, often peroxidase, and antibody to the drug. Again the amount of labelled drug bound is related to the amount of drug in the sample. Following separation of bound and free, substrate is added to estimate the activity of bound enzyme and this can be used to calculate the amount of drug which was present in the sample.

To aid separation of the bound and free, the antibody is linked to the surface of the tube as in the case of ELISA (Enzyme Linked Immuno-Sorbant Assay). The bound can be separated directly from the free by simply decanting the tubes. Enzyme substrate is then added to the tubes and the activity measured. This is the basis of a commercially available digoxin assay (Enzyme-Test^R, Boehringer Corporation Ltd, Bell Lane, Lewes, BN7 1LG, UK).

13.4.3 HOMOGENEOUS ENZYME-IMMUNOASSAY EMIT

This assay system was the first real alternative to RIA for the measurement of cardiac drugs. It is commercially available for a wide range of compounds and is referred to by the acronym EMIT (Enzyme Mediated Immunoassay Technique, Syva UK, Maidenhead, Berkshire, SL6 1RD, UK).

The drug-containing sample is mixed with antibody and drug-labelled enzyme. Once again equilibrium is reached between the drug and the drug-labelled enzyme; on addition of enzyme substrate and cofactors there is a change in optical density of the mixture which can be measured spectrophotometrically. The enzyme, bacterial glucose 6-phosphate dehydrogenase, has had the drug of interest covalently coupled to it in such a way that when antibody is bound to the drug the active site is blocked and therefore no substrate can be broken down. Enzyme activity will therefore increase in proportion to the amount of drug present in the sample and there is no requirement to separate the bound from the free, hence a homogeneous assay.

13.4.4 SLIFA

Substrate Labelled Fluorescence ImmunoAssay differs from EMIT in that the competing antigen, the labelled drug, is attached to the substrate rather than the enzyme. A fluorogenic enzyme substrate, beta-galactosylumbelliferone, is covalently coupled to the drug to be assayed. The labelled drug does not fluoresce until it reacts with the enzyme beta-D-galactosidase to release the fluorescent product. When the labelled drug is bound to antibody the enzyme is sterically hindered and cannot use it as a substrate. Competition by drug from the sample for the antibody will produce an increase in the fluorescent signal and thus the drug can be quantitated. This assay system is available as the Ames TDA (Miles Laboratories Ltd, Stoke Court, Stoke Poges, Buckinghamshire, SL2 4LY, UK).

13.4.5 FLUORESCENCE QUENCHING IMMUNOASSAY

This assay exploits the quenching of fluorescence caused by the binding of a quencher-labelled antibody to a fluorophore-tagged antigen. Sample containing the analyte is mixed with fluorescence-labelled analyte and quencher-labelled antibody. The competition of the unlabelled drug for the antibody causes a measurable rise in the fluorescence signal which is proportional to concentration. This reaction is the basis of the Advance fluorescence immunoassay (Syva UK Ltd).

Fluorescent polarization immunoassy

If polarized light is used to excite a low-molecular-weight fluorophore in aqueous solution the resulting emitted light is depolarized because during the small time lag between excitation and emission the orientation of the molecule has altered. However if the molecular weight of the fluorophore is large, or if it is associated with another molecule of high molecular weight than the extent of depolarization of the light will be reduced, since the rotation of large molecules is much slower. This fact is exploited in fluorescence polarization assays where the degree of polarization produced by a solution is governed by the equilibrium set up between the drug in the sample, fluorophore-labelled drug and the high-molecular-weight antibody. The Abbott TDX assay system functions on this principle (Abbott, The Business Centre, Molly Millars Lane, Wokingham, Berkshire, RG11 2QZ, UK).

13.4.6 NEPHELOMETRIC INHIBITION

The principle of this assay differs from the other immunoassays described as the labelled species is a high-molecular-weight conjugate with four drug molecules attached to it so that four antibody molecules can combine with it. When this occurs the complexes formed precipitate from solution and the solution becomes turbid. When unconjugated antigen (cardiac drug) is added to the turbid solution, antibodies are displaced from the antibody/antigen–conjugate complex and the solubility of the complex increases, decreasing the tubidity of the solution. The reduced turbidity of the solution can be measured, using a nephelometer, as a decrease in light scattered by the solution. The decrease in the amount of light scattered is proportionally related to the concentration of cardiac drug (Beckman Instruments Ltd, Progress Road, Sands Industrial Estate, High Wycombe, Buckinghamshire, HP12 4JL, UK).

13.4.7 DRY REAGENT STRIPS

This assay uses dry reagent strips which are similar in appearance to urine dip sticks. The reagent pad of the stick contains a monoclonal antibody to the drug, drug labelled with enzyme cofactor, enzyme and substrate. No reaction occurs until the strip is wetted. A measured amount of diluted plasma containing drug is placed on the reagent pad, the drug competes with the drug-labelled cofactor for the antibody and the enzyme reaction proceeds at a rate proportional to the amount of unbound cofactor to produce a blue colour. The intensity of the colour is quantitated in a specially designed spectrophotometer which measures the reflectance from the strip and incorporates a temperature controlled strip holder (Ames Seralyzer, Miles Laboratories). The Seralyzer, which is smaller than most text books of general medicine, is designed for single sample stat use and takes approximately two minutes to produce a result, and is at present only available for the measurement of theophylline.

References

1. Nation, R.L., Triggs, E.J. and Selig, M. (1977) Lignocaine kinetics in cardiac patients. *Br. J. Clin. Pharmacol.*, **4**, 439–48.
2. Holt, D.W., Walsh, A.C., Curry, P.V. and Tynan, M. (1979) Paediatric use of mexiletine and disopyramide. *Br. Med. J.*, **2**, 1476–7.
3. Johnston, A., Henry, J.A., Warrington, S.J. and Hamer, N.A.J. (1980) Pharmacokinetics of oral disopyramide phosphate in patients with renal failure. *Br. J. Clin. Pharmacol.*, **10**, 245–8.
4. Heagerty, A.M., Donovan, M.A., Castleden, C.M. Pohl, J.F., Patel, L. and Hedges, A. (1981) Influence of cimetidine on the pharmacokinetics of propranolol. *Br. Med. J.*, **282**, 1917–18.
5. Lancet (1984) Polymorphic drug oxidation – much ado about nothing? *Lancet*, **ii**, 1337.
6. Aitio, M.-L., Mansury, L., Tala, E., Haataja, M. and Aitio, A. (1981) The effect of enzyme induction on the metabolism of disopyramide in man. *Br. J. Clin Pharmacol.*, **11**, 279–85.
7. Clarke, E.G.C. (1969) *Isolation and Identification of Drugs.* Vol.1, Pharmaceutical Press, London.
8. Clarke, E.G.C. (1975) *Isolation and Identification of Drugs.* Vol. 2, Pharmaceutical Press, London.
9. Fitzgerald, J.D. and Scales, B. (1968) Effect of a new adrenergic beta-blocking agent (ICI-50 172) on heart rate in relation to its blood levels. *Int. J. Clin. Pharmacol.*, **1**, 467–74.
10. Shand, D.G., Nuckolls, E.M. and Dates, J.A. (1970) Plasma propranolol levels in adults with obervations in four children. *Clin. Pharm. Ther.*, **11**, 112–20.
11. Pacha, W.L. (1969) A method for the fluorimetric determination of 4-(2-hydroxy-3-isopropylaminopropoxy)-indole (LB46), a beta-blocking agent, in plasma and urine. *Experientia*, **25**, 802–3.
12. Gupta, R.N., Eng. F., Lewis, D. and Kumana, C. (1979) Fluorescence photometric determination of disopyramide and mono-N-dealkylated disopyramide in plasma after separation by thin layer chromatography. *Anal. Chem.*, **51**, 455–8.

Index

Index

Index

Index

Index

Gastrectomy, partial, digoxin
  absorption 179
Glomerular filtrate, absorption,
  Henle's loop 212
Glucocorticoids, lipoprotein level
  effects 360
Gluconeogenesis, beta-blocker
  effects 66
Glucose metabolism, beta-blocker
  effects 65–7
Glucose tolerance
  beta-blocker effects 65
  impaired, diuretic-induced 230, 239
Glyceryl trinitrate, nifedipine
  comparison, coronary artery
  disease 88
cGMP see Cyclic GMP
Gout
  diuretic-induced 229, 239
  polyvalent diuretics 229
Great arteries, transposition,
  prostaglandin E 307
Guanabenz 254
Guancydine, vasodilatation 260
Guandrel sulphate, hypertension 244
Guanethidine
  hypertension 243–4
  tolerance 244
Guanfacine 254
Guyton concept 275

Haemostasis 317–18
Hallucinations, beta-blocker-
  associated 41–2
Heart failure
  cardiovascular haemodynamics,
    digitalis action 157–73
  digitalis long-term activity 163–9
  loop diuretics 215–16
  nifedipine/digoxin co-
    administration 168
  positive inotropic drugs 195–206
  volume-overloaded, digitalis 161–2
  see also Congestive heart failure
Heart valves, prosthetic,
  antithrombotic agent trials 342–3,
  344
Henle's loop
  glomerular filtrate absorption 212
  thick ascending limb 212–13
Heparin
  action mode 321

direct anticoagulant activity 321–24
discovery (1916) 319
dosage control 322–3
half-life 322
side effect 323–4
treatment regimes 323
Heterogeneous enzyme-
  immunoassays, cardiac drugs 374
High density lipoproteins (HDL) 350
  LDL ratio, beta-blocker effects 35–6
  plasma levels, beta-blocker
    effects 35–6
Hirudin 321
His bundle ablation, high energy
  endocardial shocks 6
His-Purkinje fibres, digitalis
  effects 173–4, 175
Homogeneneous enzyme-
  immunoassays (EMIT), cardiac
  drugs 374–5
Hydralazine
  aortic incompetence 288
  congestive heart failure 281
  digoxin renal tubular secretion 180
  hepatic acetylation 258
  hypertension 257–8
  mitral regurgitation 288
  postitive inotropic effects 281
  primary pulmonary
    hypertension 287
  side effects 258
  tachyphylaxis 281
  tolerance 289
Hydrofluazides, TAL action site 217
Hyperaldosteronism
  primary, spironolactone 241
  secondary potassium loss 239
Hypercalcaemia
  digitalis toxicty 182
  primary hyperparathyroidism,
    diuretic effects 239
Hypercholesterolaemia
  coronary heart disease 349
  familial, nicotinic acid/bile acid
    sequestrant combination 356
  probucol/bile acid sequestrant
    combination 355–6
Hyperkalaemia
  antikaliuretics 222
  triamterene-induced 241
Hyperlipidaemias
  classification 360–2

386

Index

Index

Index